THE LAW–MEDICINE RELATION:

A PHILOSOPHICAL EXPLORATION

PHILOSOPHY AND MEDICINE

VOLUME 9

THE LAW–MEDICINE RELATION: A PHILOSOPHICAL EXPLORATION

PROCEEDINGS OF THE EIGHTH TRANS-DISCIPLINARY SYMPOSIUM ON PHILOSOPHY AND MEDICINE HELD AT FARMINGTON, CONNECTICUT, NOVEMBER 9–11, 1978

Edited by

STUART F. SPICKER

University of Connecticut Health Center, Farmington, Conn., U.S.A.

JOSEPH M. HEALEY, JR.

University of Connecticut Health Center, Farmington, Conn., U.S.A.

H. TRISTRAM ENGELHARDT, JR.

Kennedy Institute of Ethics, Georgetown University, Washington, D.C., U.S.A.

SPRINGER-SCIENCE+BUSINESS MEDIA, B.V.

Library of Congress Cataloging in Publication Data

CIP

Trans-disciplinary Symposium on Philosophy and Medicine (8th: 1978: Farmington, Conn.). The law–medicine relation.

(Philosophy and medicine; v. 9)
Includes bibliographies and index.
1. Medical laws and legislation—Congresses. 2. Medical laws and legislation—United States—Congresses. 3. Medical ethics—Congresses. I. Spicker, Stuart F., 1937– . II. Healey, Joseph M. (Joseph Michael), 1947– . III. Engelhardt, H. Tristram (Hugo Tristram), 1941– . IV. Title. V. Series. [DNLM: 1. Forensic medicine—Congresses. 2. Forensic psychiatry—Congresses. 3. Philosophy, Medical—Congresses. W 3 PH609 v. 9 1978 / W 700 T772 1978L]
K3601.A55T7 1978 344'.041 81–757
AACR2

DOI 10.1007/978-94-009-8407-3

Originally published by D. Reidel Publishing Company, Dordrecht, Holland in 1981
MyCopy version of the original edition 1981

EDITORIAL PREFACE

This volume is a contribution to the continuing interaction between law and medicine. Problems arising from this interaction have been addressed, in part, by previous volumes in this series. In fact, one such problem constitutes the central focus of Volume 5, *Mental Illness: Law and Public Policy* [1]. The present volume joins other volumes in this series in offering an exploration and critical analysis of concepts and values underlying health care. In this volume, however, we look as well at some of the general questions occasioned by the law's relation with medicine. We do so out of a conviction that medicine and the law must be understood as the human creations they are, reflecting important, wide-ranging, but often unaddressed aspects of the nature of the human condition. It is only by such philosophical analysis of the nature of the conceptual foundations of the health care professions and of the legal profession that we will be able to judge whether these professions do indeed serve our best interests. Such philosophical explorations are required for the public policy decisions that will be pressed upon us through the increasing complexity of health care and of the law's response to new and changing circumstances. As a consequence, this volume attends as much to issues in public policy as in the law. The law is, after all, the creature of human decisions concerning prudent public policy and basic human rights and goods. And medicine is indeed the means to realize a large proportion of what we hold to be human well-being.

This volume developed from a symposium directed to this theme: 'The Law–Medicine Relation: A Philosophical Critique'. This, the Eighth Symposium on Philosophy and Medicine, was held at the University of Connecticut Health Center in Farmington, on November 9, 10, and 11, 1978. During this period of gestation, much has been altered and some additions have been made. Its final shape emerged from discussions between the participants and the authors of papers and commentaries. We acknowledge our appreciation to the many individuals who attended this symposium and who, through their comments and discussions with the authors, enabled them to revise and frame their essays as they now appear in this volume. We wish, as well, to thank all of those who have aided us in developing this volume from the proceedings of the symposium. From among the many to whom we are in debt, we would especially like to mention Susan G. Engelhardt, Series Editorial Assistant, and Mrs. Gail Fitzgerald, who inherited the post-symposium manuscripts. We are grateful to her for her careful preparation of the final manuscript.

We want to express our thanks to all who helped to make possible the symposium from which this volume grew. We are grateful to the Division of Humanistic Studies in Medicine of the Department of Community Medicine and Health Care in the School of Medicine, University of Connecticut, who sponsored the symposium. The project was supported by a grant from the Connecticut Humanities Council, the State Committee of the National Endowment for the Humanities; however, the viewpoints or recommendations expressed in the volume are not necessarily those of the Council or the Endowment. The editors wish to express their gratitude to the Council and its Executive Director, Ronald A. Wells, for their support of the symposium. In addition, the University of Connecticut Research Foundation through its material support enabled the symposium directors to execute their original program without revision. We stand in special debt to the School of Medicine of the University of Connecticut for the many ways its administration encouraged and made possible this meeting of clinicians, lawyers, philosophers and other scholars. Many individuals labored unselfishly in the preparation and conduct of this symposium in the philosophy of medicine. We are deeply grateful to them all, but wish to recognize our special indebtedness to Robert U. Massey, Dean of the School of Medicine, and James E. C. Walker, Head, Department of Community Medicine and Health Care. Through them, a symposium came into being that allowed sustained cross-disciplinary discussion concerning the interrelations of the major secular learned professions, law and medicine.

After the eighteen months of development from the proceedings of this symposium to this volume, a set of sustained analyses has been forged. As a series of interwoven discussions in print, it ranges in focus from public policy to the basic ethical underpinnings of the relation of law and medicine with special attention being given to epistemological concerns. It makes no claim to encompass all of the issues, or even all of the central issues at stake. However, it is offered as an introduction to some of the central philosophical roots of the law-medicine relation.

September 19, 1980

H. TRISTRAM ENGELHARDT, JR.
JOSEPH M. HEALEY, JR.
STUART F. SPICKER

BIBLIOGRAPHY

[1] Brody, B. A. and Engelhardt, H. T., Jr. (eds.): 1980, *Mental Illness: Law and Public Policy*, D. Reidel, Dordrecht, Holland / Boston, U.S.A. / London, England.

TABLE OF CONTENTS

SECTION III / THE PSYCHIATRIST'S DILEMMA: DUTY TO PATIENT OR DUTY TO SOCIETY?

SECTION IV / DECISION MAKING AT THE BEGINNING OF LIFE: MEDICINE, ETHICS AND THE LAW

SECTION V / ROUND TABLE DISCUSSION – LEGAL RIGHTS AND MORAL RESPONSIBILITIES IN THE HEALTH CARE PROCESS

INTRODUCTION

> Making therefore due allowance for one or two shining exceptions, experience may teach us to foretell that a lawyer thus educated to the bar [i.e., without benefit of a liberal education], in subservience to attorneys and solicitors, will find he has begun at the wrong end. If practice be the whole he is taught, practice must also be the whole he will ever know: if he be uninstructed in the elements and first principles upon which the rule of practice is founded, the least variation from established precedents will totally distract and bewilder him: *ita lex scripta est* is the utmost his knowledge will arrive at; he must never aspire to form, and seldom expect to comprehend, any arguments drawn *a priori*, from the spirit of the laws and the natural foundations of justice.
>
> WILLIAM BLACKSTONE,
> *On the Study of the Law* [5]

In this volume, we take as our touchstone these reflections of William Blackstone, that the law well practiced requires an insight into its basic principles and concepts. This need becomes more acute as one brings the law to bear in new areas and in the framing of new public policy. In such circumstances especially it is necessary, as Blackstone suggests, to be clear concerning the spirit of the law, and its relationship to the natural foundations of justice. It is unquestionably out of these needs that a great deal of the philosophical reflections on law and medicine has sprung, for it is often unclear how the law should function, when it is brought to bear in new areas of medicine. But it is not simply in these special areas where new public policy is being framed that such reflections can be useful. As Blackstone intimates, the everyday practice of the law requires an insight into the law's fundamental ideals and purposes. Many of the disputes concerning the proper function of law in medicine, even in more commonplace areas, suggest that some of these understandings may be imperfect, misapplied, or mistaken.

Contemporary controversies concerning medicine have elicited ever more

S. F. Spicker, J. M. Healey, and H. T. Engelhardt (eds.), The Law–Medicine Relation: A Philosophical Exploration, xiii–xxvii.

attention from the law. Where medical law, in the past, may have more narrowly concerned itself with forensic issues, such as the determination of the cause and circumstances of death, with issues involving the medical 'police power' regarding the control and prevention of contagious diseases, and with issues of malpractice, the concerns are now much more broadly cast. This, in part, reflects increased interest in human research and experimentation, as well as, in part, reflecting the view that medicine is now better able to predict and prevent untoward consequences of pathological processes. Among the latter, one must include the reflections in this volume focused on the proposed right of children to sue for having been born under circumstances that fail to meet some minimal standards. Here, as well, one would place discussion of claims of paternalistic rights to enforce the best interests of patients, or to violate confidentiality in protecting third parties in the context of psychiatric medicine. In addition, the very interest in such reflections brings to public debate policies previously accepted silently and without discussion. One might think here of the fact that Western countries in some cases properly allow de facto, if not de jure, passive infanticide. For example, it is generally not the policy to attempt to do anything to insure the survival of anencephalic children. The question, however, at once arises as to what the policy should be with regard to infants with less disastrous defects. Indications for intervention, or for refraining from treatment, will reflect judgments concerning not only possible qualities of life for the person the infant may become, but also likely costs of intervention. By employing such indications one will have decided when established duties to beneficence will be overridden by a combination of financial and other burdens, and unlikelihood of sufficient success.

These basic ethical issues that undergird law and public policy in health care presuppose, as well, issues often placed within the philosophy of science. Law and public policy must deal with notions of causal relations that establish lines of responsibility and accountability. Here, as the passage from Blackstone suggests, reflections in the law are indistinguishable from reflections in philosophy. The borders between jurisprudence and philosophy are often vague at best. One must think, for example, of H. L. A. Hart and A. M. Honoré's classic study, *Causation in the Law* [18]. These epistemological questions assume practical importance at the interface of law and medicine, where it often appears that law and medicine are making appeals to quite different notions of causality or causation. The issues addressed by medical law and reflections upon it are therefore wide-ranging.

In this volume, 'medical law' is used in an expansive sense and includes not only analyses of the cases arising out of health care but the jurisprudential reflections that they occasion. This use of the term 'medical law' services to signal contemporary departure from a long-standing Anglo-American legal tradition. This recent development calls for the participation of attorneys in various legal specialties: family law, hospital law, health insurance law, and others. The recent addition of medical law courses in colleges of medicine and law represents an acknowledgement of this sub-specialty now viewed by the layman and the professional community as deserving serious attention.

With the establishment of medical law in the health care context, there is a tendency to conflate legal and ethical analyses and to fail to distinguish legal questions from moral or ethical questions. Clearly, law and ethics share many common concerns. However, laws can fail to receive ethical sanction, and ethical points of view are not always reflected in legislation or court decisions. More problematic still is the fact that judges and legislators may avoid examining the moral principles presupposed in requirements established by law. Whatever confusions occur here at the law/ethics interface, one thing is certain: a legal analysis of particular problems is and should be open to philosophical exploration and critique. In our time, increasing attention is being paid to issues germane to the patient's rights and duties, as well as the duties and rights of health care providers. The dramatic rise of biomedical technology has given extensive power to the health professional, a power which is not always with legitimate authority, and which is open to possible abuse. This power leads some to demand that medicine and the health professions be formally regulated through the legal process. The ever-increasing demand for regulation through law raises the question of the physician's mandate from society – clearly not a single, unchanging expression of the public's will.

In the search for a health policy, medicine and law will of necessity have to share a common normative base. Although there is some historical precedent for this relation, the recent call for the legal regulation of medicine and the health professions could, if not pursued carefully, perpetuate an adversarial relation between medicine and law. This would be unfortunate, for the patient is the one who would suffer most. As is perhaps obvious, the relationship between medicine and the law has not always been characterized by harmony and mutual respect. An unhealthy antagonism between these professions can only lead to the isolation of each from the other, which, at the least, discourages a multidisciplinary approach to problems of mutual concern to the professional, and, at worst, threatens the welfare of the patient. In the end, then, the efforts of the contributors to this volume, as well as others writing on similar and related issues, are directed to serve those who suffer most from our rejection of inter-professional cooperation and the subsequent retreat into professional isolation – the patient whom we are all committed to serve.

Because of this isolation, the conceptual roots that law and medicine share in common are often unrecognized. Though these two secular, learned professions focus on preserving and restoring human goods, in often overlapping ways, their communality is as often obscured by their conflicts as professions competing for esteem, prestige, and the prerogative to pursue, without hindrance, their goals. As a consequence, the relationship between medicine and the law is often perceived to be adversarial. This perception, one must recognize, is well entrenched, for bitter complaints concerning the law's intrusions into medicine, as in malpractice suits, extend back, for example, to the early 19th century in America. Consequently, it has become commonplace to perceive the law as interfering in the conduct of health care, rather than as helping the patient or the common weal.

Criticisms of this sort come from both ends of the political spectrum and have become commonplace. Dr. Franz Ingelfinger, the late editor of the *New England Journal of Medicine*, protested what he described as 'legal hegemony' in medicine:

> Examples of the lawyer's pervasiveness in medical decision-making abound. Who needs to be reminded of his role in the current malpractice mania? If medical care is costly, the doctor defensive, and the patients suspicious, the referee must share part of the blame. By the means of actual or threatened court action, lawyers determine not only the particulars of treatment, but also who will get blood transfusions, and whether or not treatment will be meted out in a given case. Courts decide on who will get medical education. Even when doctors try to clean their own house, courts may order reinstatement of a suspended staff member. Courts may also decide on the overall administrative practices of medicine, on who may or may not practice, on the payment of the physician, on the conversation permitted and required between the doctor and patient, and on the kinds of records kept ([20], pp. 825–826).

Professor Elliot Krause has criticized the law's complicity in allowing patterns of professional dominance:

> We found that credentialing processes are being used at present at least as much to protect the interest of the occupational group as to protect the interests of the public. That programs to control the growth and efficiency of health care settings have been given to the hospital interests; that regulation of food, drugs, technology, and supplies, where it exists at all is very carefully limited by corporate interests in their influence on the executive branch, and that every indirect attempt to regulate costs has failed, because

the politics of the formation of the law gives a place for the spenders in the regulation of their spending ([21], p. 293).

Chancellor W. Allen Wallis of the University of Rochester admonished the School of Medicine and Dental Medicine graduates in 1974 with the following:

You may find lawyers defining the range of treatments that you are allowed to use in specified circumstances. Lawyers may prescribe the criteria by which you are to choose among the allowable treatments. Lawyers may specify the priorities you must assign to different patients. Lawyers may require you to keep detailed record to establish at all times that you are in full compliance. Lawyers may punish you unless you can refute beyond a reasonable doubt their presumption that your failures result from not following all of their regulations and requirements.

The lawyers have you outnumbered, but on the average they are no match for you in intelligence or dedication. Just don't let them ambush you while you are absorbed in caring for the sick [30].

As these quotations suggest, there is a great deal of dissatisfaction with the current law-medicine relation [10, 20]. Many physicians are convinced that the law is playing an excessive role in regulating medical care. Their concerns are part of a general belief in our society that we are experiencing a period of excessive reliance on the legal system and excessive imposition of public regulatory mechanisms.

The evidence clearly suggests that medicine has been the center of a great deal of regulatory attention. In his classic work of 1869, *The Jurisprudence of Medicine* [25], Ordronoux describes statutory enactments relating to the practice of medicine. For example, an individual engaged in the practice of medicine or surgery in the Connecticut of the 1860's encountered little regulation: there was no licensure system, only minimal reporting requirements (births, deaths, pestilential diseases), though some guidelines for the performance of post-mortem examination and dissection were required. In contrast, a contemporary practitioner is faced with an imposing array of regulations. The current index of *Connecticut General Laws* (the collected state statutes) reveals more than 275 references and cross-references to statutes regulating the practice of medicine and surgery. This number does not include the additional references to other health care providers or to health care facilities. This ever-increasing volume of regulations is enormous and its impact upon the health care process remains uncertain.

Law and medicine are respected professions whose histories are virtually coterminous with the rise of Western civilization [6, 9, 12, 13]. Each is characterized by a long-standing heritage of independence and authority. It is not unexpected that they should participate in a relationship that even in the best of times is tainted with suspicion, detachment, and even hostility. In the worst of times, the hostility and antagonism can reach such a degree as to limit the effectiveness of each. It is a recurring frustration that these two respected professions are so frequently in conflicting rather than cooperative roles.

Understanding the long and often bittersweet relationship between law and medicine is complicated by the fact that at least two distinct areas of the relationship have histories of more than three thousand years. The first area is concerned with the use of scientific/medical evidence in the legal process and includes a range of issues from evidence supporting claims of personal injury to determination of cause of death as established by post-mortem examination [14, 23]. The second area is concerned with legal regulation of medical practice and includes a range of issues from the imposition of licensure requirements to patient's rights to recover damages if injured by health care providers [1, 2, 11, 19]. From the Code of Hammurabi and the Code of the Hittites to contemporary legislative enactments and judicial decisions, each of these areas of concern has been the focus of medicolegal interest. Deeply rooted in specific societal contexts and influenced by a variety of social, political and economic forces, these areas of concern have developed throughout history. Exploration of this development remains a major task for medical historians. A parallel task is the central focus of this volume: exploration by lawyers, physicians and philosophers of what the relation can be and should be.

The possibility of excessive regulation is present in a wide variety of settings in our society. Increasing reliance upon the formal mechanisms of our legal system, to replace informal mechanisms of conflict resolution, demonstrates the insufficiency of those informal mechanisms. However, such a reliance on formal mechanisms can distort the role of the law and lead to confusion about legitimate justification for legal involvement in regulating the particular activity under scrutiny. Medical care is just such an example.

In the United States, legal regulation of the health care process has its roots in the police power, the power "to enact and enforce laws to protect and promote the health, safety, morals, order, peace, comfort and general welfare of the people" ([17], p. 5). This power is often held to be an inherent power of a sovereign government, derived from its very nature as a government. In point of fact, the police power is the source of such health care regulation as medical licensure and vaccinations. Since the federal government is a government of delegated powers, it does not possess police power in its broadest sense.

A second source of legal authority to regulate the health care process may be found in the law's role in adjudicating conflicts involving the rights and duties of individual citizens. By applying principles of the law to interpersonal relationships in general, and to the physician-patient relationship in particular, the law has played a major role in the resolution of disputes within society. While some might disagree with the outcome of specific conflicts, even those disturbed by the increased role of the law in regulating medicine must admit the importance of the law's involvement in this process and the need for a just resolution of these issues.

The concern remains, however, that health care providers frustrated with the present volume of legal regulation will proclaim that health care is, or should be, beyond the scope of legal regulations. Those who argue to this conclusion fail to appreciate the legitimate goals for legal regulation of the health care process. It is the understanding of these goals that is a primary task for those who would examine the law-medicine relation. It is for this reason that this volume has been created. We hope, through this volume, better to display the concepts and goals that frame the proper role of law in medicine. These examinations fall naturally within a series in philosophy and medicine.

Philosophy can establish standpoints from which one can explore critically, and where possible clarify, conceptual confusions that have resulted in a failure to identify the commitments that bring law and medicine together. These confusions have often sprung from a mismanaged use of concepts or of language. The last point is poignantly captured by Ludwig Wittgenstein's remark that "philosophy is a battle against the bewitchment of our intelligence by means of language".[1] This maxim, of course, cuts two ways (which is quite different from saying that it is ambiguous): for it means, on the one hand, that the 'refined' use of language is the only way of overcoming the bewitchment caused by language; on the other hand, the maxim suggests that the use of language has produced the very bewitchment that we wish to overcome. Indeed, it is often because we are trapped in our own languages or jargons that we fail to appreciate the standpoints and arguments of those in sibling professions.

This interdisciplinary volume has, in part, been directed across those barriers in order to disclose the often unnoticed interdependencies of the professions, the nature of the concepts to which they appeal, and the fact that they often share common puzzles and goals in coming to terms with the human condition. It has not, however, endeavored to encompass all issues of pressing contemporary concern. The contemporary discussions of the law-medicine relation of interest to physicians, lawyers, and philosophers are wide-ranging; they include abortion [7, 8, 9, 24, 27], care for the incompetent adult [3, 4, 28, 29], and compulsory public health measures [17, 33]. However, in this volume we have directed attention to none of those three, and to only some of the many issues that merit attention. Though the topical focus is often narrow, the discussions reach deeply into the presuppositions of the contemporary concerns regarding the law-medicine relationship. We have hoped to touch some central leitmotifs in the discussions of the interplay of law and medicine.

Thus, the first section, which examines the mandates physicians and researchers receive from their society to engage in their activities, addresses issues of physician responsibility, patients' rights, the regulation of research involving humans, and the social responsibility of medicine and physicians. Siegler and Goldblatt initiate discussion of the physician's mandate by identifying the difficulties in the physician-patient relationship concerning respective rights and duties. They acknowledge the contemporary antagonism between law and medicine as a source of confusion for both physicians and patients, and as a barrier to a clearer understanding of how physicians are expected to satisfy their duties to their patients. Using the example of critically ill patients who have easily treatable diseases, yet who refuse life-saving therapy, and the example of ambulatory patients with self-defined senses of disease or illness who demand specific services, Siegler and Goldblatt recommend a decision-making process they call 'clinical intuition' as one method of clarifying the rights and duties of both patients and physicians. They suggest that within the emerging framework of a physician-patient relationship, in which the patient is the major decision-maker, there needs to be an acknowledgement of the physician's ethical obligations as a physician and as a moral agent. However, it is clear that much must be done to specify the force of clinical intuitions, as another volume in this series attests [15]. In any event, one frequently fails to clarify the duties of the patient and the rights of the physician in speaking of the mandate of physicians. It is towards such clarification that Siegler and Goldblatt direct their energies.

In contrast with this rather individualistic understanding of the physician-patient relationship, John Ladd focuses upon the social responsibilities of physicians. A major source of the confusion about the physician's mandate is, as Ladd shows, the dramatic evolution of 19th century medicine and the 19th century role of physicians into the contemporary doctor-patient relationship, which is inextricably embedded in a societal matrix. In the process, the model of the medical professional has changed, altering traditional notions of professional independence, autonomy, and self-regulation. Physicians have become a powerful élite in society, who, due to their position and power, affect numerous social goods that are, at least in part, open to competent lay assessment. In short, these developments establish the basis for the entry of the law into regulation of the medical profession.

William J. Curran and Robert M. Veatch examine these issues of power and responsibility in detail. Curran examines the use of populations in developing countries in the establishment of the clinical effectiveness of new drugs and treatments. Often, such investigation can be pursued with less regulation and with less cost than in the more developed nations. The use of such populations, however, raises the question of whether it is appropriate to ask individuals from less developed countries to subject themselves to risks to which members of more advanced countries would not be exposed, even if individuals from such less developed countries receive more in medical services and other benefits than would be otherwise available to them. Does one respect their right to make such exchanges freely, or does one paternalistically preclude them? Further, will the absence of adequate regulation of research in less developed countries, in contrast to more developed countries, lead not only to members of less developed countries agreeing freely to engage in more risky experiments, but to those populations being coerced, deceived and actually abused?

Robert Veatch addresses such questions more generally by focusing on society's right to regulate the medical decisions of its members, as well as to regulate the professional conduct of its physicians. While recognizing that intrusions of regulation will have both social and individual costs, he warns that

> If, however, there is a good reason to believe that the professional group will base its decisions on a different set of values or beliefs than those held by the broader society and the differences in behavior will not be trivial, then it is foolish for a society to fail to exercise its right to regulate. [32]

To resolve such questions, one will need, as Veatch indicates, to decide when it is prudent not to regulate, even when it may be legitimate to regulate the decisions of citizens or of medical professionals. In these explorations, Veatch provides a survey of issues ranging from experimentation to medical licensure, indicating their place in the law-medicine relationship.

In the second section, Kenneth Schaffner, H. Tristram Engelhardt, Jr., and Thomas Halper explore the roles of causal explanations in law, medicine, biomedicine and science. The essays indicate some of the relationships among the practices of making predictions, forwarding explanations for events, and assigning responsibility and accountability for the outcomes of various processes and activities. In the first essay, Schaffner analyzes contemporary reflections on the notion of causality that have been offered by philosophers such as Carl Hempel, J. L. Mackie, Wesley Salmon, and Michael Scriven. He argues that both science and medicine share a sense of causality, which is shared as well with at least some areas of the law, and which relies upon 'gappy' probabilistic generalizations. Such incomplete generalizations are tacitly compared in the generation of a causal account. As Engelhardt indicates, the choice among rival causal explanations will be guided in medicine and the law by practical considerations as to where and under what circumstances it will be most useful to identify some factors rather than others as *the* causes. In the law this takes place, as H. L. A. Hart and A. M. Honoré indicate, by distinguishing between causes and conditions, where conditions are those causal factors that are taken to be normal, expected, and defining of social roles, that is, not useful in assigning responsibility or accountability for harms [18]. As Engelhardt suggests, a similar phenomenon occurs in medicine in selecting some among the various causal variables to be addressed by treatment. Finally, Thomas Halper stresses these practical considerations in the development of such practices as strict liability in the law. As he indicates, causal language and the assignment of responsibility in the law grow out of everyday concerns with explanation and the fixing of responsibility. These essays, though at times technical in their treatment of the nature of causality, provide important links among the concerns of philosophers of science, physicians, and lawyers.

The limits of paternalism and of duties to confidentiality are explored in the third section with a special focus upon the problems of the psychotherapist. William Winslade, in his essay, addresses the re-examination of the practice of strict confidentiality in the patient-psychotherapist relationship that was occasioned by the tragic events surrounding the death of Tatiana Tarasoff. These events raised the question whether a psychiatrist or psychologist should warn a third party who may be endangered by a patient under that therapist's care. Winslade approaches this question through an exploration of two important cases, *People v. Poddar* (1974) [26] and *Tarasoff v. Regents of University of California* (1976) [31], occasioned by Tarasoff's death. These cases have served as foci for reassessing the responsibility of psychotherapists in settings where a duty of confidentiality owed to a patient may conflict with the duty to warn a possible victim of danger to him or her. Winslade argues that the two decisions serve as evidence that the law may have only limited effectiveness in intervening in the context of human conduct generally, and in psychotherapy particularly.

In the second essay in this section, Charles Culver and Bernard Gert evaluate the ethical issues involved in the involuntary hospitalization of the mentally ill. They forward an argument for limited paternalistic interventions. Michael Peszke concludes the section, analyzing the dilemmas engendered by concerns about paternalism and confidentiality. As he shows, a psychotherapist is recurringly torn by conflicting duties to the patient and to society. The practice of maintaining confidentiality in order to secure a good psychotherapist/patient relationship may be jeopardized by the fear that material may eventually have to be disclosed through legal pressures. On the other hand, a desire to protect the freedoms of individuals may prevent one from committing for treatment individuals who are, in fact, incompetent.

Judgments concerning the quality of life of defective infants and of fetuses are analyzed in Section IV. Stuart Spicker and John Raye indicate the complexity of the issues involved in the prognoses employed in making decisions whether to treat or not to treat defective newborns. One is never simply making a prediction when making a prognosis, as Spicker and Raye show. One is, in addition, weighing the consequences of having acted upon incorrect predictions. Such consequences are incorporated in criteria for treatment choices that reflect prognoses. This involves assigning different values to different possible outcomes. For example, the controversy that has been engendered by such individuals as John Freeman [16] and John Lorber [22] turns, in part, on different views of the consequences of over- or under-treating defective children. If one overtreats, that is, decides to treat a defective newborn who will not survive, or not survive at a level worthwhile for that infant (or for its parents), one will have needlessly committed expenditures not only of time and medical resources, but of parental agony. However, if one undertreats, that is, does not give full treatment in expectation that the child will die, and it fails to die, but survives with greater handicaps due to the delay in treatment, one may have allowed irreparable damages. If one is not willing to treat all infants maximally, no matter how severely deformed and how unlikely their chances of survival, one will have to develop criteria for prognoses authorizing treatment that reflect the various risks of being wrong, and therefore of over- or under-treating. Spicker and Raye develop these issues with special focus on the public policy implications of different decision procedures for the treatment of children born with myelomeningocele manifesta, a congenital anomaly. These discussions are then closed by

John Robertson's legal analysis of the criteria that should properly be employed in selecting infants for non-treatment.

The final brace of papers in the fourth section addresses the quality of life issue in terms of the putative right of fetuses not to be born into circumstances worse than non-existence. Angela Holder reviews the cases at law in which individuals have attempted to recover for having been born under circumstances of deprivation, where the only alternative would have been not to have been born at all. As she indicates, such cases raise the notion of the right to have a healthy baby and perhaps a duty to support abortions in order to prevent a tort for wrongful life. Peter Williams suggests in his commentary that such cases have fared poorly in the courts because of their challenges to well-entrenched views of the integrity of the family (e.g., one would not want to have children suing parents for being born into less than optimal circumstances) and of the integrity of the court system, which would need to calculate damages that would often be somewhat speculative. However, though such cases may not become generally successful at law, they offer us a set of important tests of our intuitions concerning the liability of physicians, parents, and others for their children being born with defects that could have been prevented only by abortion. As more such defects can be diagnosed prenatally, these issues will undoubtedly become more pressing for both law and public policy.

The closing section, which addresses legal rights and moral responsibilities, draws upon the expertise of a historian of medicine, a pediatrician, two lawyers, and two philosophers. It provides a view of the historical origins of the regulation of health care, as well as the moral and legal roots of patient, health-care provider, and societal rights and responsibilities. The reflections by William Bartholome, for example, raise the issue of the moral and legal integrity of the family. Should the family, for example, have the *prima facie* right to decide with regard to the treatment or non-treatment of its infant members? That is, should taking the family seriously as a social unit place the burden upon others who would intrude into its decisions, rather than placing the burden upon the family to justify its decisions with regard to its infant members? Bartholome deals critically with such parental prerogatives. Such criticisms, however, remind us of the importance of deciding the proper boundaries between families and society at large, and the extent to which taking the family seriously as a social entity will commit us to tolerating choices that many in society might find to be ill-advised.

The essays in this volume thus address basic conceptual and moral questions that underlie controversies engendered by the interrelations of law and medicine. As these essays show, it is only by becoming clearer about these questions, and the fundamental conceptual geography to which they point, that the interrelation of law and medicine will be better understood. Blackstone's remarks, cited at the beginning of this introduction, are usefully recalled here. If one simply reviews, one by one, the cases and controversies engendered by the relation of law and medicine, one will not be able to understand well the relations between these, the two major secular learned professions. These professions, after all, arise out of a social context structured by views of the nature of man, of morals, and of what is proper to the human condition. As Blackstone's remarks can be taken to suggest, such basic issues of the liberal arts, indeed, of philosophy, are keys to an in-depth understanding of the law's relation with medicine. It is towards the better appreciation of these issues that this volume was developed.

As a consequence, the discussion of issues in malpractice and litigation bearing on medicine does not have central place here. What we have attempted instead is to provide an understanding of some of the conceptual controversies that underlie disputes concerning the proper relation of law and medicine. These explorations do, though, provide information concerning current controversies in medical litigation. However, by looking deeper to the roots of such controversies, we hope to suggest the ways in which these two major learned professions can act in better consort for the good of patients, citizens and the common weal. We will have to explore with greater care our concerns for patients' rights, the capacity of physicians to act upon their better judgment, our interests in being free and self-determining, our concerns to protect ourselves and others from ill-advised choices, our views concerning the lines between human biological and human personal life, and our interests in assigning responsibility and accountability for harms. In short, these basic philosophical and ethical issues undergird concerns with regulation, paternalism, parental consent for the treatment of children, and all such central issues in the debates occasioned by the relation of law and medicine. It is for this reason that this volume is offered as the ninth in this series on philosophy and medicine.

July, 1980

H. TRISTRAM ENGELHARDT, JR.
JOSEPH M. HEALEY, JR.
STUART F. SPICKER

NOTES

[1] The original text of Wittgenstein's remark reads: "Die Philosophie ist ein Kampf gegen die Verhexung unseres Verstandes durch die Mittel unserer Sprache" ([34], par. 109).

BIBLIOGRAPHY

1. Annas, G.: 1972, 'Medical Remedies and Human Rights: Why Civil Rights Lawyers Must Become Involved in Medical Decision-Making', *Human Rights* **2**, 151–167.
2. Annas, G.: 1978, *The Rights of Hospital Patients*, Avon Press, New York.
3. Baron, C.: 1978, 'Assuring "Detached but Passionate Investigation and Decision": The Role of Guardians Ad Litem on Saikewicz-Type Cases', *American Journal of Law and Medicine* **4**, 111–130.
4. Baron, C.: 1978, 'Medical Paternalism and the Rule of Law: A Reply to Dr. Realman', *American Journal of Law and Medicine* **4**, 337–365.
5. Blackstone, W.: 1803, *Blackstone's Commentaries*, 5 vols., W. Y. Birch and A. Small, Philadelphia, Book 1, Part 1, p. 32.
6. Burns, C. (ed.): 1977, *Legacies in Law and Medicine*, Science History Publications, New York.
7. Callahan, D.: 1970, *Abortion: Law, Choice and Morality*, The Macmillan Company, New York.
8. Callahan, D.: 1980, 'Contemporary Biomedical Ethics', *New England Journal of Medicine* **302**, 1228–1233.
9. Camps, F. (ed.): 1968, *Gradiwohl's Legal Medicine* (3rd ed.), Wright and Sons Ltd Publication, Chicago.
10. Chayet, N.: 1976, 'Hegemony in Medicine Revisited', *New England Journal of Medicine* **294**, 547–548.
11. Curran, W. and Shapiro,: 1970, *Law, Medicine and Forensic Science* (2nd edition), Little Brown and Company, Boston.
12. Curran, W., McGarry, A. and Petty, C.: 1980, *Modern Legal Medicine, Psychiatry and Forensic Science*, F. S. Dorris Company, Philadelphia.
13. Curran, W.: 1976, 'The Proper and Improper Concerns of Medical Law and Ethics', *New England Journal of Medicine* **295**, 1057–1058.
14. Curran, W.: 1975, 'Titles in the Medicolegal Field: A Proposal for Reform', *American Journal of Law and Medicine* **1**, 1–11.
15. Engelhardt, H. T., Jr., Spicker, S. F., and Towers, B. (eds.): 1979, *Clinical Judgment: A Critical Appraisal*, D. Reidel, Dordrecht, Holland/Boston, Mass.
16. Freeman, J. M.: 1973, 'To Treat or not to Treat', in R. H. Wilkins (ed.), *Clinical Neurosurgery: Proceedings of the Congress of Neurological Surgeons, Denver, Colorado, 1972*, Williams and Wilkins, Baltimore, Maryland, pp. 134–146.
17. Grad, F.: 1975, *Public Health Law Manual*, American Public Health Association, Washington, D.C.
18. Hart, H. L. A. and Honoré, A. M.: 1959, *Causation in the Law*, Clarendon Press, Oxford.
19. Healey, J.: 1979, 'Medical Law and the Health Care Process', *Connecticut Medicine* **43**, 181.

20. Ingelfinger, F.: 1975, 'Legal Hegemony in Medicine', *New England Journal of Medicine* 293, 825–826.
21. Krause, E.: 1977, *Power and Illness*, Elsevier North Holland, New York.
22. Lorber, J.: 1974, 'Selective Treatment of Myelomeningocele: To Treat or Not to Treat?', *Pediatrics* 53, 307–308.
23. Luke, J.: 1976, 'Forensic Pathology', *New England Journal of Medicine* 295, 32–33.
24. Noonan, J.: 1979, *A Private Choice: Abortion in America in the Seventies*, Free Press, New York.
25. Ordronoux, J.: 1973, *The Jurisprudence of Medicine*, Arno Press, (A New York Times Company), New York. Originally published in 1869 under *The Jurisprudence of Medicine in Its Relations to The Law of Contracts, Torts, and Evidence*, T. & J. W. Johnson & Company, Philadelphia.
26. *People v. Prosenjit Poddar*: 1974, 16C.3d 750, 111 Cal. Rptr. 910, 518 P. 2d 342.
27. Ramsey, P.: 1978, *Ethics at the Edges of Life*, Yale University Press, New Haven.
28. Relman, A.: 1978, 'The Saikewicz Decision: A Medical Viewpoint', *American Journal of Law and Medicine* 4, 233–242/
29. Relman, A.: 1978, 'The Saikewicz Decision: Judges as Physicians', *New England Journal of Medicine* 298, 508–509.
30. Schwartz, H.: 1975, 'Will Medicine Be Strangled in the Law?', *The New York Times*, February 26, p. 58.
31. Tarasoff v. Regents of Univ. of Calif.: 1976, 17 Cal. 3d 425, 131 Cal. Rprt. 14, 551 P. 2d 334.
32 Veatch, R. M.: 1981, 'Federal Regulation of Medicine and Biomedical Research: Power, Authority and Legitimacy', in this volume, pp. 75–91.
33. Wing, K.: 1976, *Law and the Public's Health*, C. V. Mosby and Company, St. Louis.
34. Wittgenstein, L.: 1953, *Philosophical Investigations*, G. E. M. Anscombe, R. Rhees, and G. H. von Wright (eds.), transl. by G. E. M. Anscombe, Macmillan, New York, Part I.

ROBERT U. MASSEY

PROLOGUE TO THE SYMPOSIUM

It is my honor to welcome you to the Eighth Symposium on Philosophy and Medicine. I am pleased and proud that this program with its distinguished faculty is being held at the University of Connecticut Health Center, School of Medicine, under the auspices of our Division of Humanistic Studies in Medicine. These symposia, which were inaugurated in May, 1974, have served to bring together scholars and practitioners from many disciplines to consider how their special insights may contribute to the practice of medicine. Philosophy, history, literature, art, biology, physics, chemistry, sociology, technology, and law are elements which are combined by a kind of alchemy determined by our human nature in the science and practical art which we call medicine.

If it is useful to recognize two cultures, as Lord Snow maintained – and this is not the time or the place to reconsider that debate, should we suppose we had the wit to do so – these two cultures, in his sense, are compelled to unite at some points by the very nature of the matter of medicine. It is not possible to consider a human being, whether well or sick, apart from his body, his religion or his ultimate concern, his society, his history, or his laws. But this audience does not require any instruction from me about the place of these disciplines in medicine, nor admonition that both the sciences and the humanities are incomplete and in intellectual trouble without each other.

Law and medicine have a long and ancient liaison. The earliest cultures that we know about had laws governing medical practice, malpractice, and fees. Medical licensure laws first appeared in formal fashion in the late Middle Ages and have continued to change, especially in the most technologically advanced nations of the West.

As law has surrounded the practice of medicine, so medicine has been woven into the substance of law, and all the serious questions asked by either physicians or lawyers are ethical questions. Since that is so, our two professions stand open on the one hand to all of natural science, and on the other to all of custom, art, literature, philosophy, and religion.

In his *Idea of a University*, John Henry Newman quotes Edward Copleston to support his own views on the importance of the liberal arts to the professions:

S. F. Spicker, J. M. Healey, and H. T. Engelhardt (eds.), The Law–Medicine Relation: A Philosophical Exploration, xxix–xxx.

"There can be no doubt that every art is improved by confining the professor of it to that single study. But, *although the art itself is advanced by this concentration of mind in its service, the individual who is confined to it goes back*. The advantage of the community is nearly in an inverse ratio with his own.

"Society itself requires some other contribution from each individual, besides the particular duties of his profession. And, if no such liberal intercourse be established, it is the common failing of human nature, to be engrossed with petty views and interests, to underrate the importance of all in which we are not concerned, and to carry our partial notions into cases where they are inapplicable, to act, in short, as so many unconnected units, displacing and repelling one another".

This will be an important Symposium and, I am certain, a successful one. The School of Medicine is honored to be part of it.

University of Connecticut, School of Medicine
Farmington, Connecticut

SECTION I

THE PHYSICIANS AND RESEARCHER'S MANDATE FROM SOCIETY: BIOMEDICAL, LEGAL, AND ETHICAL CONSIDERATIONS

PATRICIA KING

INTRODUCTORY COMMENTS

I have been asked to introduce the opening section of essays concerning the physician's and the researcher's mandate from society and particularly the legal aspects of that mandate. I should like to offer a few brief comments concerning the legal obligations of the physician in contemporary society, particularly in light of the ever-evolving nature of the physician-patient relationship.

Traditionally, the physician has been vested with an authority rarely found in professional relationships. The patient by virtue of his illness was viewed as abdicating responsibility for himself and transferring it to the physician. It was the role of the patient with respect to the treatment of his disease to accept and follow the advice of the physician who possessed superior skills and information.

To be sure the behavior and conduct of physicians and researchers with respect to their patients and subjects were constrained by ethical principles, professional standards, codes of ethics, peer review and hospital authority. These constraints were, however, determined, evaluated and interpreted by the profession.

Traditionally, the law has served as the only formal external constraint on the medical profession. While it was possible for a patient to recover damages in assault and battery for an unconsented touching and in negligence for care falling below prevailing medical practice, as a practical matter the law re-enforced the physician's autonomy and authority in relation to his patient.

A combination of legal rules made it highly unlikely that an injured patient or subject would recover for negligent treatment. For example, in the usual case, testimony of experts was required to establish the standard of care and the fact that the standard had been breached. Since patients were usually unable to obtain expert testimony because of a notable reluctance on the part of physicians to testify against one another, patients were discouraged from resorting to the legal system; were they brave or presumptuous enough to file suit anyway, their cases usually failed for lack of proof. In effect, then, the medical profession, because testimony of physicians was needed in malpractice suits, 'controlled' even this external constraint.

As John Ladd correctly observes, however, modern medicine has changed.

S. F. Spicker, J. M. Healey, and H. T. Engelhardt (eds.), The Law–Medicine Relation: A Philosophical Exploration, 3–4.

There has been a perceptible movement toward regarding the physician as merely a provider of skills, a provider of information or the key to obtaining access to technical services. The physician has lost much of his autonomy and authority with respect to his patients. This change is the result of many factors too detailed to discuss here. Suffice it to say, these changes in the physician-patient relationship have occasioned a re-examination of the adequacy of the traditional constraints which controlled physician conduct.

As might have been expected, the nature and kinds of legal constraints are also changing. Plaintiffs now find it easier to recover against physicians in negligence. There is a renewed emphasis on patient autonomy. The doctrine of informed consent, for example, is just one aspect of this phenomenon. Numerous appeals for legislation which would permit competent adults to control the manner in which they will die is another aspect. In short, the changing character of legal constraints raises critical questions for the law. How should we characterize current legal constraints on physician conduct? Are these constraints reflective of the changing character of the physician-patient relationship? For example, does the recent emphasis on patient autonomy adequately take into account the fact that the patient is still the disadvantaged or weaker party in the relationship? Furthermore, do the present legal constraints unduly favor those patients who are often reluctant to exercise their autonomy? Finally, should the external constraints on physician conduct continue to be primarily legal ones? These and other equally important questions are raised by the essays which open this volume. The contributors surely initiate an exploration sorely needed in our time.

Georgetown University
Washington, D. C.

MARK SIEGLER AND ANN DUDLEY GOLDBLATT

CLINICAL INTUITION: A PROCEDURE FOR BALANCING THE RIGHTS OF PATIENTS AND THE RESPONSIBILITIES OF PHYSICIANS

I. INTRODUCTION

The assumption underlying the subtitle of this paper is that medicine in the 1970's has become an adversarial practice, requiring a procedure for adjudicating between the rights of patients and the responsibilities of physicians. It is ironic that the relationship between doctor and patient – traditionally a vital element in the healing process – should deteriorate at precisely the time when medicine has become more effective. Although the doctor-patient relationship appears to be evolving in a libertarian direction, emphasizing individual autonomy, self-determination, and rights, an ambivalence remains; witness the unclarity of attitude of the courts and legislatures. Precisely because this uncertainty exists, it is not surprising that at times the practice of medicine seems to juxtapose the interests of patients and those of physicians. This essay will consider these questions by examining two very different issues in modern medicine:

(1) the rights of patients and the responsibilities of physicians in situations in which acutely, critically ill patients who have easily treatable diseases refuse life-saving therapy, and

(2) the rights of patients and the responsibilities of physicians in situations in which ambulatory patients with self-defined senses of dis-ease or illness demand specific services from physicians.

We will attempt to show by reference to these limiting cases that the libertarian model has serious weaknesses and limitations. An attempt will be made to articulate a decision-making process which we refer to as 'clinical intuition', which takes account of both patients' rights and physicians' responsibilities. We will strive to justify our conclusion with reference to legal and philosophical principles. First, we will consider the situation of the patient refusing treatment; we will subsequently examine problems posed by the demanding patient.

The central concern of this essay – balancing the general rights of patients to self-determination with the responsibility of physicians, occasionally, to override patient decisions – has been examined frequently in recent years. One aspect of this examination has been a consideration of the change in the

S. F. Spicker, J. M. Healey, and H. T. Engelhardt (eds.), The Law–Medicine Relation: A Philosophical Exploration, 5–31.

doctor-patient relationship [DPR], a change from a paternalistic model to one that emphasizes the patient's autonomy and right of self-determination. The contributions of humanists and social scientists have been instrumental in the reassessment of the DPR. Their commentaries have structured the issues and, in general, have resolved them in accord with libertarian principles of self-determination.

Unfortunately, practicing physicians have contributed little to the analysis of this issue, although it has a direct effect on the practice of medicine and the care of patients.[1] This essay will analyze the issue of patients' rights and physicians' responsibilities from the perspective of professionals actively involved in clinical situations, rather than by conjuring hypothetical circumstances. It is not that the judgment of medical professionals is always correct merely because they are professionals or because they possess technical expertise. However, their viewpoint merits careful consideration in the resolution of these complex issues.

The role of the professional is unique. The professional's relationship to a client or patient is premised on specific technical training and on competency. This specialized knowledge and proficiency is used to assist patients in curing or ameliorating their illness and disease, and to assist them in overcoming the fear, pain and suffering that are often associated with ill health. Once sought out by the client, a professional (in this case, a medical doctor) becomes involved in the client's concerns. He is never a mere observer. He cannot rely on the counterfeit courage of the non-combatant. The physician is accountable to the patient if he fails to perform his task adequately because of lack of skill, because of negligence, or because he fails to act in the client's behalf. This special quality of the professional enterprise was described eloquently by the Roman General Lucius Aemilius Paulus in 168 B.C.

> Commanders should be counselled, chiefly, by persons of known talent; by those who have made the art of war their particular study, and whose knowledge is derived from experience; from those who are present at the scene of action, who see the country, who see the enemy; who see the advantages that occasions offer, and who, like people embarked in the same ship, are sharers of the danger. If, therefore, any one thinks himself qualified to give advice respecting the war which I am to conduct, which may prove advantageous to the public, let him not refuse his assistance to the state, but let him come with me into Macedonia. He shall be furnished with a ship, a horse, a tent; even his travelling charges shall be defrayed. But if he thinks this too much trouble, and prefers the repose of a city life to the toils of war, let him not on land assume the office of a pilot. The city, in itself, furnishes abundance of topics for conversation ([13], pp. 326–327).

Although we do not endorse Paulus's concept that only professionals are capable of criticizing their professional enterprise, we do endorse the principle that professionals should contribute to the analysis and criticism of their own endeavors. This essay offers and defends a position on proper actions of physicians towards acutely, critically ill patients. It is intended to complement those commentaries on this issue proffered by non-physicians.

II. THE CHANGING DOCTOR-PATIENT RELATIONSHIP [DPR]

The DPR has changed dramatically within the last sixty years. The traditional paternal model, premised on trust in the physician and characterized by the patient's dependency and the physician's control, has been replaced by a more bilateral relationship where patients are increasingly involved in decision-making which concerns their own care. In a companion essay in this volume, Professor John Ladd discusses this change and concludes that the earlier medical model has crumbled: "The ultimate authority in medical matters has shifted away from the physician. . . . The patient or administrator can now tell the doctor what he needs and what he must do . . . ". [12].

Professor Alan Donagan has arrived at a similar conclusion. He suggests that the expressed legal and moral requirements of the informed consent doctrine represent a formal recognition of today's changes in the DRP. He notes that there has been a gradual but unmistakable change from a 'physician decides' to a 'physician proposes, patient decides' model of medicine ([3], p. 313; [19]). This dramatic change in the DRP has three major causes: the successes of scientific medicine, the increase in medical research, and the public perception of health care as a 'right'.

Paradoxically, the successes of medicine have contributed to a decreased trust in physicians and a decline in the paternalistic approach to health care. The continuity of the relationship between a patient and his personal physician has been interrupted by an increased use of medical specialists and by institutional and team care.

Increased medical research has led to distrust of medical practitioners as the public has come to see physicians as applied biologists rather than as healers. Frank mistrust of physician-scientists has been augmented by documentation of various abuses in research involving human subjects. Finally, broad social changes, including a general decline in trust in public institutions and experts and the rise of the consumer movement, has encouraged the recent claim that medical care is a 'right'. This assertion has led to another: that the physician is a mere provider of a product or service – medical care – and that this product can be purchased and consumed at the will of the consumer. All these changes have occurred in a political environment that emphasizes individual rights and liberties. There is no doubt, then, that our society's understanding of medicine is unclear and the paternalistic approach to the patient is under attack.

III. SIDGWICK AND THE PUBLIC UNDERSTANDING OF INSTITUTIONAL AND SOCIETAL PROMISES

Moral dilemmas arise in any period of social uncertainty and change. The old paternalistic model of the DPR was widely embraced and rarely questioned. The proper end and limits of medicine were accepted, and the determination of these ends was assumed to be the province of the medical practitioner. Now a new model of medicine is evolving; many new questions are being asked. Eventually, the public and the medical profession will accept and articulate a new vision of the end and limits of medicine. Until this new definition of medicine emerges, however, concepts about the proper ends of medicine will differ. The public and the profession will be unsure which model of medicine – the paternal or the libertarian – is prevailing.

In the *Methods of Ethics*, published in 1874, Henry Sidgwick discussed institutional and societal promises [17]. His discussion was particularly perceptive and remains helpful in considering the problems presently faced by physicians and patients. Sidgwick noted that social promises must change when values and expectations change. But until such a change in societal values is recognized and institutionalized, different people will have conflicting understandings of the expressed and implicit promises on which certain public activities (in the present context the practice of medicine) are based. Sidgwick stated:

> We have now to observe that in the cases of promises made to the community, as a condition of obtaining some office or emolument, a certain unalterable form of words has to be used if a promise is to be made at all .... It may be said, indeed, *that the promise ought to be interpreted in the sense in which its terms are understood by the community*; and, no doubt, if their usage is quite uniform and unambiguous, this role of interpretation is sufficiently obvious and simple ....
>
> The question then arises, how far this process of gradual ... relaxation ... can modify the moral obligation of the promise for a thoroughly conscientious person. It seems clear that when the process is complete, we are right in adopting the new understanding as far as good faith is concerned ... although it is always desirable in such cases that the form of the promise should be changed to correspond with the changed substance. *But when, as is ordinarily the case, the process is incomplete, since a portion of the community understands the engagement in the original strict sense, the obligation*

becomes difficult to determine, and the judgment of conscientious persons respecting it becomes divergent and perplexed ([17], pp. 308–310, emphasis added).

In this period of increased 'rights consciousness' and reduced medical authority, we appear to be in a phase of incomplete redefinition of a social promise, the promise of the medical profession. Sidgwick provides a method to analyze the community's perception of the DPR. He maintains that "the promise ought to be interpreted in the sense in which its terms are understood by the community". To use this method, we must inquire how the medical relationship is understood by the public and the profession. Our answer is that we have indeed reached the stage described by Sidgwick as one in which judgments of conscientious persons have become divergent and perplexed, and in which there is no societal consensus.

IV. ACUTE CRITICAL ILLNESS: A LIMITING CASE

What is the judgment of conscientious persons on the question of how one reconciles the rights of patients and the responsibilities of physicians within a gradually evolving model of medicine? Are there limits to a patient's rights within the medical relationship? Conversely, and starkly stated, should a physician ever override the expressed wishes of a patient who has not been found legally incompetent?

We are concerned that the movement towards patients' rights and the libertarian model of medicine has gone too far. The proper end of medicine may require a shared obligation between patient and physician. The recent tendency to move toward a patient-dominated model of medicine, led by medical ethicists and philosophers, and more recently by lawyers, is probably unworkable. We suspect that the implications of this movement are unacceptable to many patients. There is little doubt that in the case of medicine when "a portion of the community understands the engagement in the original strict sense, the obligation becomes difficult to determine, and the judgements of conscientious persons regarding it become divergent and perplexed".

We think there are medical situations in which the judgment of technically competent physicians ought to dominate regardless of the patient's statements. It must be acknowledged that situations in which it is legitimate, perhaps even mandatory, to ignore the refusal of consent to treatment by a patient who has not previously been found legally incompetent are exceptional. But if these exceptional cases are shown to warrant a limited exercise of medical paternalism, it may be possible to isolate the details of such cases and to develop guidelines for an adjudication of conflicts between the patient and the physician. For conceptual clarity we prefer to examine cases in which third party interests – the family, the community, the state – are not used to justify overriding the wishes of an individual. We wish to examine the narrower issue of whether a physician is ever justified in usurping the will of a patient in the *patient's own interest*. The two limiting cases we propose to examine are (1) the right of an acutely, critically ill patient to refuse simple, life-saving treatment, and (2) the right of a patient to demand specific services from physicians. We will return to the issue of the demanding patient in a later section of this essay. We turn now to the question of whether an acutely, critically ill, but treatable, patient has an absolute right to refuse treatment.

For our purposes, we define 'acute, critical, treatable illness' as an unanticipated, immediately life-threatening condition which begins acutely and is caused by factors beyond the patient's control. The conditions we are considering are those for which treatment is relatively easy, standardized and conventional. Further, if treatment were withheld then the prognosis would be very poor in terms of high mortality, and severe long-term disability would result if spontaneous recovery occurred. Prognosis with treatment, however, is excellent in terms of both survival and survival without long-term disability. Indeed, we will assume that with adequate treatment these patients can be restored to the level of health and functioning they enjoyed prior to the onset of the acute critical illness.

Several of the terms in this definition require additional clarification. 'Acute critical illness' must be contrasted with 'chronic illness'. 'Unanticipated illness' distinguishes these conditions from expected and predictable life-threatening crises that inevitably occur in the course of chronic diseases or terminal illness. Thus, we are not thinking of an episode of acute respiratory failure that may occur once or several times during the progression of an underlying illness such as chronic obstructive or restrictive pulmonary disease.

The term 'immediately life-threatening condition' describes a disease process in which events unfold in minutes or hours rather than in days or weeks. 'Cause beyond an individual's control' is used to exclude patients who directly try to end their own lives or to injure themselves. Infectious illnesses, traumatic injuries and myocardial infarctions are considered diseases 'beyond an individual's control', even if certain life choices may in a statistical sense predispose some individuals to these diseases.

The notion of treatment which is 'relatively easy, standardized and conventional' is meant to imply short-term, 'one shot' therapy such as an operation or a short course of medication. This must be distinguished from high risk, experimental treatment, or long-term painful treatment such as cancer chemotherapy. The concept of 'prognosis' is of course based on probabilities, but in this context is used to refer to the outcome of diseases for which the data is relatively unambiguous, such as pneumococcal meningitis, acute respiratory failure, or exsanguinating hemorrhage, diseases in which immediate treatment has a very great probability of preventing death and disability.

Our model cases are not examples of terminal illness, chronic disease, suicidal patients, or even patients who assert a so-called 'right to die'. We wish to examine the responsibility of physicians to acutely, critically ill patients who somehow come to the attention of a physician, either by presenting voluntarily or by being admitted to hospital, and who then refuse life-saving treatment. Consider the following cases:

Case 1. The patient presents at an emergency room with high fever, headache and stiff neck. Consent is given for a spinal fluid examination to rule out meningitis. The lumbar puncture confirms non-epidemic bacterial (pneumococcal) meningitis. Pneumococcal meningitis can be treated by administering a course of antibiotics. This treatment usually will provide a total cure. If untreated, this form of meningitis is fatal in approximately 75% of its instances. Those who survive without treatment usually have severe, permanent, physical and mental impairment. The patient refuses treatment upon learning of the confirmed diagnosis.

Case 2. The patient has completed initial treatment for second and third degree burns extending over 50% of the patient's body. Therapy has entered a stage of debridement which is extremely painful, although the pain is partially palliated by analgesic and sedative medication and occasionally by anesthesia during debridement procedures. If the therapy is completed, the patient will regain nearly normal function. If treatment is terminated prior to its completion, a fatal bacteremia will probably result. The patient refuses to continue treatment.

Case 3. A patient is brought unconscious to a hospital emergency room. Initial examination reveals serious injuries including a punctured lung, a ruptured spleen and a probable concussion. While the patient is unconscious, plans are made to proceed with emergency abdominal surgery. The patient regains consciousness, refuses to consent to surgery, and demands to leave the hospital. The patient offers no specific reason for this decision.

Case 4. A patient presents to an emergency room with severe crushing chest pain. An electrocardiogram reveals an acute myocardial infarction and greater than 20 multifocal, premature ventricular contractions per minute. The patient refuses to be admitted to hospital but requests analgesic medicine for use as an outpatient.

Case 5. A consenting, hospitalized patient is started on cancer chemotherapy with high dose methotrexate. Twelve hours later the patient refuses to accept oral leucovoran 'rescue' which is necessary to prevent severe and probably fatal bone marrow depression. The patient gives no reason for the refusal.

V. CLINICAL INTUITION

It is tempting to search for simple rules or principles which will enable one to resolve all cases of critically ill patients who refuse to consent to life-saving treatment. Several years ago, one of us (M.S.) published a case in which an acutely, critically ill patient's choices were respected and he died of his illness [18]. In that paper the physician adopted a basically libertarian stance and imposed a stringent burden on those who would wish to disregard a competent patient's refusal. The major issue was whether the patient understood the consequences of his refusal or whether his critical illness so impaired his thought processes that the soundness of his mentation was in question. Because of the difficulty of distinguishing competent, rational, and authentic decisions from incompetent, irrational and inauthentic judgments, there was a temptation to choose an existential position in which any decision was acceptable.

Eric Cassell, M.D., has explored the same problem and has argued the contrary position in an essay entitled "The Function of Medicine" [1]. He argued that most acutely, critically ill patients should be presumed to be devoid of autonomy. He relied on Gerald Dworkin's definition of autonomy as 'authenticity plus independence' [4]. Cassell suggested that the function of medicine was to *restore* autonomy by treating the patient, even if this meant disregarding the patient's competent, 'rational' refusal.

Cassell's justification for overriding a patient's wishes, on the grounds that illness renders individuals inauthentic, seemed excessively broad. It raised the possibility that acute, critical illness might provide grounds for a paternalistic intervention. One might consider that all critically ill patients lacked the knowledge and emotional capacity to make decisions about life and death. They would thus be like children for whom paternalistic intrusions might be permissible. One could consider acutely, critically ill patients to be ignorant of the potential dangers involved in refusing the therapy (i.e., the probability of imminent death) and therefore temporarily restrain them, just as one might restrain a blind individual who wished to cross a bridge and did not realize the bridge had been washed away.

A colleague of ours, Martin Cook, pointed out that both we and Dr. Cassell were trying to stay off the slippery slope of determining what was a competent, rational, and authentic decision, although we did so with different results. Cassell argued that each patient should be presumed to be deprived of autonomy simply by virtue of his illness. We argued that almost any choice should be acceptable. All of us were looking for a conceptually neat solution. H. L. Mencken once remarked: "For every complex problem there is a solution that is simple, neat and wrong". We now believe that some patients with acute illness are, and some are not, able to make authentic choices; it is necessary, then, to formulate criteria for assessing individual judgments.

Unable to discover a single principle or a number of general rules to delimit coercive medical intervention, we have developed an approach we call 'clinical intuition'. Clinical intuition is based on a determination and a balancing of those clinical indications which should be considered by a physician when faced with an acutely, critically ill patient who declines life-saving treatment. We have constructed a list of *prima facie* considerations which should be used, and have attempted to rank them in order of importance.[2] Although this list is not exhaustive, the factors noted should always be taken into account by conscientious physicians before deciding whether to usurp the expressed will of critically ill patients who have not been found to be legally incompetent.

(1) The most important consideration is the patient's ability to choose: to understand the nature of his problem, to be able to express the medical alternatives and to understand the prognosis with and without treatment. If this ability is absent, as it is in unconscious or profoundly irrational patients, the physician's legal and moral duty to treat and to preserve life prevails. Even if the acutely, critically ill patient is able to express a choice and articulate the consequences of his choice, the physician should attempt to determine two additional things: first, whether the patient retains sufficient intellect and rationality to make this irreversible choice, and second, whether his choice reflects a 'true will' or is merely a reaction to the pain, fear, and uncertainty of his critical condition.

(2) In addition to assessing the rationality of the patient's particular choice, the physician should also ask another question: is this choice authentic? Is

it consistent with the 'kind of person' this patient is? Is the choice consistent with the patient's enduring values, with his previous choices, with the convictions he has previously asserted and defended?

Authenticity may be established in several ways. It may be established by antecedent actions. The writing of a living will, the pre-existing appointment of an agent/surrogate, membership in a religious group which has a particular stance with respect to certain kinds of therapy, all support authenticity of particular choices which otherwise might be incomprehensible. The arguments of the Jehovah's Witness who refuses potentially life-saving blood transfusions are not only convincing because the courts have upheld them as expressing a free exercise of religion, but also because these convictions have been held and defended by individual Witnesses over a period of time; they have been temporally authenticated.

Authenticity, however, does not necessarily require antecedent statements or action. All people, even acutely, critically ill persons, have the right to change their minds. Thus, the quality and character of the refusal is also relevant. This is a kind of psychodynamic demonstration. It is achieved most easily when a long-standing DPR exists, but it can be accomplished when the patient is being seen for the first time. It depends upon the physician's understanding and acceptance that the patient is committed irrevocably to his determination not to be treated.

There is always a temptation to regard any choice which is not immediately comprehensible to physicians as an irrational or incompetent choice. Authentic choices are usually, but not always, understandable to others. Choosing death rather than intractable pain or financial ruin are comprehensible choices. An observer might not make the same choice, but he could perceive the factors that had been considered relevant and that had been weighed by the agent before reaching a decision. When authentic choices are based on private, secret, personal factors not easily comprehended by an observer (for example, a private religious belief against antibiotics), it is more difficult for the patient, particularly the acutely, critically ill patient being seen for the first time, to demonstrate the authenticity of his refusal.

It is true that the determination both of rationality and of authenticity is made by the physician. Many critics of medicine would prefer that the patient's condition – i.e., his rationality or competence or authenticity – rather than the physician's judgment of his condition, actually control whether the physician overrides a patient's wishes. This notion is unworkable. Rationality, competence and authenticity are not absolute standards such as 'Middle C.' Rather, they are states of mental responses that must be construed. While one would hope for a rule of action that would eliminate subjectivity and avoid wrong decisions, we have seen why conceptually neat alternatives – either libertarianism or an all encompassing medical paternalism – are even more unacceptable.

(3) A third factor is the nature of the disease. Our discussion involves acute, critical illness in the hospital setting. Patients with chronic disease or even acutely, critically ill patients who present to a physician's office can more easily reject treatment. But in cases of acute, critical illness, one important fact is its prognosis if untreated and the probability of improvement if treatment is administered. Where diagnostic uncertainty is minimal, a simple treatment is curative, and the probability of death without treatment is high, the physician will be more likely to disregard the hospitalized patient's refusal. Examples would include conditions such as life-threatening but treatable, infectious illnesses (Case 1), severe hemorrhage after an injury (Case 3), or acute myocardial infarction with a life-threatening arrhythmia (Case 4).

Our decision in the three cases noted is based upon the acute, critical illness of the patient and the extremely favorable prognosis of those illnesses if treated quickly and appropriately. In contrast, if these illnesses were left untreated, the patient would almost certainly die or become permanently disabled. Our decision is also based on the uncertainty of the patient's rationality. The patient's choices appear inauthentic; no sound reasons are advanced for them. They are incomprehensible to the neutral observer. The physical pain present in each of these circumstances raises additional questions about the patient's true wishes. The probability of metabolic brain derangement from either the infectious meningitis or the impaired cardiac output associated with shock and cardiac arrhythmias would further encourage us to intervene even when these patients had not been declared legally incompetent. In these three cases, and in cases similar to them, we would tend to override the patient's expressed wishes.

(4) Several clinical variables can modify this determination, even in cases of acute, critical illness. If the patient has an underlying terminal disease or a severely disabling chronic condition, this should weigh in favor of respecting his refusal of treatment for the acute, critical condition. The same is true if an acute condition would result in permanent physical or mental disability even if treated promptly. To the contrary, if there is considerable uncertainty concerning diagnosis and prognosis, this may weigh in favor of disregarding a patient's refusal. However, if such an undiagnosed disease is unresponsive to therapy, and if the probability for successful intervention decreases, the balance can shift again.

(5) Another consideration is the patient's age. Unquestionably, age influences clinical decisions involving the patient's refusals. The older the patient, the more likely his choice will be accepted.

These are considerations physicians should weigh whenever an acutely, critically ill patient refuses treatment. No formula or simple rule will resolve all clinical dilemmas, but physicians who use clinical intuition to help determine their actual decisions in individual cases have a potentially coherent procedure which can be applied, explained and subjected to public scrutiny.

VI. FURTHER THOUGHTS ON CLINICAL INTUITION

Alvan Feinstein, M.D., published his book *Clinical Judgment* in 1967 [5]. He urged clinicians to utilize the methods of scientific reasoning to improve their ability to make *therapeutic* decisions, one type of clinical decision. In contrast to therapeutic decisions, Feinstein noted that there was another type of clinical decision which he called 'environmental' and which he believed was not susceptible to scientific analysis. Feinstein writes:

> . . . the multiple human personal attributes considered in the environmental decisions are often too complex to be catalogued, analyzed, and rationally dissected by any conventional contemporary logic. The clinician's approach to evaluating the patient exclusively as a person is still an artful aspect of care that depends on human perception and understanding. These components of clinical care are properties of heart and spirit, of instinct and psyche, and cannot be easily identified, assessed, or quantified by ordinary methods of reasoning.

He continues:

> . . . the personal environmental management of a patient is a challenge to the clinician's judgment as a humanistic healer. The treatment of the patient is a challenge to the clinican's judgment as an experimental scientist. It is this latter aspect of clinical judgment – the performance and appraisal of therapeutic decisions – with which these essays are primarily concerned ([5], pp. 28–30).

Feinstein concludes that environmental decisions, unlike therapeutic decisions, are not easily resolvable by the application of the traditional methods of experimental science. Earlier in this essay, we concluded that certain environmental decisions, such as how to manage the acutely, critically ill patient who refuses life-saving treatment, are not easily resolvable by the application of rigid ethical principles or moral rules. Some guidelines are desirable, however, particularly when environmental decisions must be made.

Guidelines for decision-making are necessary for several reasons. The clinician must decide. He is forced to act (even inaction is an act); he must 'sin bravely'. In emergency situations there is limited time to gather information about the patient's values; the physician often must apply ethical principles to a particular clinical case without knowing his patient's true wishes. Guidelines would be desirable and helpful. If the guidelines for such decision-making were articulated, this would allow educators to teach these principles to medical students and physicians-in-training. This would also encourage intra-professional examination and criticism of the guidelines. Enunciated, published guidelines for action, as opposed to unspoken, personal clinical maxims, would permit public scrutiny of such guidelines. If some were unacceptable they could be restructured through intra-professional decisions or legislation. The point here is that it is useful to have articulated action-guiding principles which are subject to criticism.

Clinical intuition is a preliminary excursion into this domain. Clinical intuition includes both conventional scientific clinical judgment and the informed, moral intuition of physician-clinicians. These guidelines for decision-making in acute, critical illness are premised upon the traditional professional ethic of medicine. At the same time, they are, as they must be, sensitive to the changing moral understanding of patients and society. The principles of clinical intuition presented here are not absolute; it is certainly appropriate to criticize, refine, modify or abandon them if they prove inadequate or unworkable.

The process of clinical intuition is analogous to that proposed by W. D. Ross ([16], pp. 16–29) and consists of two components. First, it may be possible for physicians to elaborate a series of technical-moral guidelines which can serve as *conditional considerations* similar to Ross's *prima facie* duties. Such a conditional duty would always be a straightforward actual duty except that in certain circumstances there are other moral considerations which must also be weighed. The enumeration of a list of conditional duties for physicians – that is, principles of action which would always be binding in the absence of countervailing duties – is not an arbitrary exercise. It is based upon personal moral values, and upon those special moral guidelines which pertain to the profession of medicine. Homiletic injunctions such as: 'help and do no harm', or 'preserve life', or 'do unto others as you would have others do unto you', are all traditional moral guidelines for physicians. These general maxims probably include Ross's more clearly stated *prima facie* duties of fidelity, reparation, gratitude, justice, beneficence, non-maleficence and self-improvement. It is entirely appropriate, indeed it is essential, that society and its institutions, particularly legislatures and courts, be involved in the construction of this list of conditional considerations and in the attempt to rank and give weight to such considerations. This, then, is the first step in the process of clinical intuition.

The second stage, again analogous to Ross's, is to try to determine what our actual duty is in situations when conflicts exist among *prima facie* duties. In this process we are balancing the various *prima facie* duties in order to decide what specific action is appropriate, i.e., offers the greatest balance of positive considerations over negative ones. In this paper we have examined appropriate responses to acutely, critically ill patients who refuse therapy. Such cases seem to involve several conditional considerations which include (1) fidelity – what is the promise of the medical profession to critically ill individuals?, (2) beneficence; and (3) non-maleficence. But even if we agree that non-maleficence is the highest good, we are still left with the dilemma of whether to usurp the acutely ill patient's conscious wishes (in the context of being uncertain as to his competency) or to let him die. Which is the greater evil?

It is in situations like this, after a rational ordering of all conditional considerations, that physicians must exercise clinical intuition to decide what their actual duty is. We do not claim that physicians can rely solely upon intuition to *know* with certainty what their actual duties are. Rather, we argue that the physician must utilize clinical intuition, an inductive form of reasoning, to appreciate what clinical action is suitable to the situation. Clinical intuition is fallible, but it is preferable to any existing system for making such determinations. It can be criticized and corrected. In this sense, it is similar to Rawls's concept of reflective equilibrium, a "mutual adjustment of principles and considered judgments . . . " ([15], p. 20).

We are sensitive to many of the criticisms of intuitionism, but we cannot find a better word to describe the process we are proposing. We are by no means suggesting that anyone can do what he pleases. Precisely by means of articulating our principles, we believe that we will allow for the correction of the problem. Society will have knowledge of the *prima facie* factors physicians use to reach their decisions and will be free to accept or reject these standards. Morally responsible physicians will have a rational process to employ in making these decisions. In the final decision, the moment of clinical truth, the physician must choose which of several competing duties is his actual duty. In doing so, he must employ clinical intuition.

VII. THE JUSTIFICATION OF CLINICAL INTUITION

We recognize that our proposal contradicts the conventional wisdom of those who champion 'patient rights' and argue that the physician should honor every decision of a patient who has not been found legally incompetent. Nonetheless, we believe that the application of clinical intuition is justified even in those cases where it results in disobeying a critically, acutely ill patient's stated wish not to be treated. In such cases, it is our view that overruling the patient's refusal may accord most closely with the requirements of the profession of medicine, the demands of the law, and the expectations of patients and their families.

When acutely, critically ill patients expressly refuse to consent to treatment, physicians are faced with an emergency situation. Particularly in the current era of the 'malpractice phenomenon' ([14], p. xv), physicians are ill at ease with simply letting patients die, especially those patients who are not terminally ill. In addition to contradicting their professional training and code, this practice makes physicians vulnerable to the criticisms of families and the threat of civil and criminal liability.[3]

Notwithstanding the celebration of unlimited patient autonomy by some commentators on the medical scene, it is usually difficult to convince those more directly involved that the curable did not want to be cured, that the decision to refuse treatment, made in the midst of extreme pain, fear and anxiety, was authentic. Physicians who acquiesce in these decisions, or who request that acutely, critically ill patients sign papers releasing the physician and hospital from liability for nontreatment, know quite well that this provides inadequate protection from the anger of families, the disbelief of juries and the dictates of their consciences.

Even if the physician could be certain he was insulated from legal liability, he could not be certain of the authenticity of the patient's decision. When a physician is faced with a patient in acute pain, who perhaps seeks death as the only escape from an overwhelming fear of death, and when there is not enough time to get a legal declaration of incompetence, the physician – who knows that treatment will almost certainly permit the patient to survive the emergency – will often decide to overrule the patient's refusal. We believe this describes the practice of many physicians in this situation.

Modifications in the doctor-patient relationship have exacerbated the physician's dilemma. Until recently, decisions concerning treatment took place within a continuing, long-standing relationship. Physician and patient were often friends and neighbors. Relations between them were based on a mutually understood medical context. Today, however, an acutely, critically ill patient is often a stranger. The physician is forced to concentrate on the choice, because he has no existing frame of reference concerning the chooser.

The decision becomes not whether this choice of a particular patient is authentic, but whether a refusal itself can ever be considered an authentic decision.

Given these conditions of uncertainty and ignorance as to individual commitments and life-plans, the physician must decide whether a patient's refusal is 'authentic'. The physician must somehow determine that it is the patient who is deciding authentically, and not because of his treatable pain, anxiety, fear and confusion.

We want to emphasize that we do not rely on the common defense of medical paternalism based on the notion of role and responsibility. This defense argues that the role of the physician as defined by societal expectations generates specific obligations, such as the duty to preserve life in all circumstances, obligations that may not be applicable to other professionals. This argument seems unpersuasive when values and role responsibilities are in flux. It quickly becomes circular. The medical role is precisely what is in question. It is not helpful to argue that a particular notion of role legitimates a coercive intervention, for to do so begs the central question.

Faced with this situation, the physician must use the most general and commonly accepted rules of human behavior. Overruling the express refusal of an acutely, critically ill patient can be justified on the principle that all living things, and particularly all rational human beings, always seek to preserve their being ([9], I, 12). The physician who overrules a critically ill patient's stated refusal acts consistently with this principle of the will to survive. Even if a patient's refusal appears rational, this 'decision' is uncertain because it contradicts the 'natural law' of self-preservation. In view of this uncertainty, permitting the physician to overrule refusals made by acutely, critically ill patients with treatable illnesses constitutes a decision favoring the lesser of two potential evils. If pain and fear have led to an inauthentic refusal, the patient whose refusal is honored dies. But if a patient is treated successfully against his (authentic) will, he has at least the ability to exert legal retribution. He has regained freedom of action.

When a physician overrules the stated refusal of an acutely, critically ill patient, he does so analogically; the patient becomes similar to an unconscious patient, a patient from whom consent to life-saving treatment is *inferred* in emergency situations.[4] An assumption of implied consent in these and similar situations is based on the reigning public consensus that the *prima facie* 'best interests' of patients needing medical care are served by providing that care.[5]

This principle has been advanced, endorsed and elaborated in many states by the enactment of Good Samaritan legislation. Good Samaritan statutes permit physicians to treat critically ill or injured patients outside the hospital setting without fear of liability based on the absence of consent ([14], pp. vx–xvi). Consent is implied from the semi-conscious as well as the unconscious emergency 'patient' outside the hospital setting. Good Samaritan statutes will not meet the need they are designed to fulfill if they exclude those accident victims who, in acute pain but apparently rational, repeatedly state 'don't touch me' to the physicians who come to their aid.

We believe that the acutely, critically ill patient who refuses necessary, life-saving treatment more closely resembles the trauma victim and the profoundly irrational patient than a patient asked to consent to elective medical procedures. As we mentioned earlier, the implicit understandings of the doctor-patient relation are in a state of flux. Particularly now, when these 'social promises' of medicine are understood differently by different people, when a portion of the community remains committed to the traditional, paternal medical model, it is irresponsible for the physician always to assume that a patient means exactly what he says. A physician cannot know which mode of the patient-physician relationship this patient endorses.

This is why we advocate a public statement of the rules and application of clinical intuition. The prior acceptance of clinical intuition cannot completely protect a patient from unanticipated reactions to severe pain, fear and confusion; nor can it insulate the physician from subsequent criticism of his decision by a surviving patient or a deceased patient's immediate family. It does, however, provide better protection than the uncertain, idiosyncratic practice of the present. An announced and applied clinical intuition is far preferable to the current situation where no standards govern these decisions concerning refusals of treatment.

The position we are advocating is quite similar to the one proposed by Professor Hans Jonas. In a discussion of "The moral restraints on my freedom to decide against treatment for myself . . . ", Professor Jonas finds these restrictions essentially identical to those that ethically restrict our right to suicide. Jonas remarks:

> This, admittedly, is interference with a subject's most private freedom, but only a momentary one and in the longer perspective an act in behalf of that very freedom. For it will merely restore the status quo of a free agent with the opportunity for second thoughts, in which he can revise what may have been the decision of a moment's despair – or can persist in it. Persistence will in the end succeed anyhow. The time-bound intervention treats the time-bound act like an accident from which to be saved, even against himself, can be presumed as the victim's own more enduring, if temporarily eclipsed, wish (sometimes betrayed by the very fact of imperfect secrecy that made the intervention possible) ([10], p. 32).

It is evident that we do not support the principle of unfettered individual rights as a proper primary moral principle grounding the medical relation. Our defense of clinical intuition is based on a *balancing* of patient authenticity and physician responsibility – a subtle balancing which is not biased in advance in favor of the medical professional. We agree with the enthusiastic advocates of total autonomy that patients whose continuing existence depends on long-term medical treatment have both the capacity and the repose to make these decisions authentically. Patients who require renal dialysis or extensive and painful therapy, such as the severely burned patient (see Case 2), ought not to be coerced into accepting these treatments.

We hope that those who most avidly advocate patient autonomy would agree with us that a patient ought not to use a physician or medical treatment itself as a means to suicide. We believe it is clear that a patient ought not to cause his own death by withdrawing consent in the middle of certain interconnected medical or surgical treatments. For example, a patient who has consented to methotrexate chemotherapy ought not to be allowed to refuse the leucovoran rescue drug essential to neutralize the otherwise fatal toxicity of methotrexate (see Case 5). This particular concept has obvious 'slippery slope' implications and should be limited to those interconnected treatments that a physician would not begin *but for* the prior assurance that consent will not be withdrawn. The leucovoran problem is resolved by this minimal limit on patient autonomy – the more intricate considerations of clinical intuition are not required. But if it is appropriate for physicians to contradict a decision to refuse leucovoran rescue, then patient autonomy is never absolute. And if the leucovoran example reveals something unique about the medical relation, as we believe it does, it would be unfortunate if we failed to explore its implications.

Admittedly, our exploration of the best mode of the medical relation is colored by an increasing mistrust of the medical profession and the biomedical and natural sciences. Any theory that limits the decision-making rights of individuals is unpopular. An increasingly militant opposition to all forms of medical paternalism has resulted in legal decisions that have limited the authority of physicians to impose life-saving treatment on patients who expressly refuse such treatments. These decisions have been embraced by a few commentators ([20], pp. 116–163) as somehow establishing a general rule that physicians must obey any decision made by a patient, even a refusal of life-saving medical treatment. We believe these commentators have misread the legal precedents. It is our opinion that these decisions are correctly understood as specific exceptions to a general and abiding presumption in favor of life-saving treatment. Like all legal decisions, they must be interpreted on the basis of their specific facts. Thus interpreted, these decisions demonstrate some limitations on a patient's right to refuse life-saving treatments. A patient's refusals of life-saving treatments have been authorized in the following situations: (1) when the treatment indicated can at best prolong the life of a terminally ill [6] or comatose patient,[7] (2) when the treatment contravenes a recognised belief,[8] and (3) when the treatment destroys physical integrity, e.g., an amputation.[9]

The most frequently discussed precedent allowing a terminally ill patient to refuse life-prolonging treatment involved a proxy refusal made on behalf of an incompetent patient. *Superintendent of Belchertown State School v Saikewicz* involved the question of whether potentially life-prolonging treatment can be withheld without the judicially reviewed consent of an incompetent patient's legal guardian.[10] *Saikewicz* concluded that the presumption in favor of preserving life may be qualified when the question is one of prolonging the life of the terminally ill. When the illness is terminal and the patient is incompetent, a *subjective* 'substitute judgment' of what the *patient, if* he *could* make a competent choice would choose for his incompetent self is permitted.[11]

Saikewicz stated that a terminally ill incompetent patient can 'refuse' treatment to the same extent as a terminally ill competent patient.[12] *Saikewicz* says nothing about the ability of any patient legally to refuse *life-saving* treatments. The decision makes a clear distinction between a palliative and life-saving treatment:

> There is a substantial distinction in the State's insistence that human life be saved where the affliction is curable as opposed to the State's interest where, as here, the issue is not whether, but when, for how long, and at what cost to the individual that life may be briefly extended.[13]

And indeed, Massachusetts courts have three times prohibited the parents of a three-year old leukemia patient from refusing to submit their child to chemotherapy, a treatment that now holds out a significant chance not just of remission but of cure ([6], p. 269).

There are a number of legal decisions upholding the right of members of Jehovah's Witnesses to refuse blood transfusions. Few have involved actual refusals of life-saving treatments.[14] These decisions are distinctive because they are based on the preferred position of the First Amendment's guarantee of freedom of religion. But even this constitutional right is limited. The reliance placed on these cases by those who would use them as evidence of a general rule ignores their particular limitations and specific circumstances. These limitations include the patient's age and the existence of dependent spouse or children.[15] Circumstances that support the patient's decision include public knowledge that Witnesses believe infusions of blood and blood products result in eternal damnation.

Additional difficulties are raised by the Jehovah's Witness precedents. In some cases, the legal decision was made after the patient was successfully transfused, after the patient successfully recovered without needing the transfusion, or when the decision was rendered moot by the patient's so-called 'willingness to be coerced'.[16] This last is particularly troublesome; for if a patient has a right to refuse treatment, what right does the physician have to attempt to coerce that patient into foregoing that right? Moreover, those commentators who use the Jehovah's Witness precedents as the basis of a general right to refuse treatment attempt to extend the constitutional rights afforded religious freedom to every patient refusal, including those based on unarticulated personal beliefs.[17] For all these reasons, the physician faced with a patient who refuses life-saving treatment on grounds other than religious conviction receives no aid from the Jehovah's Witness precedents.

A third group of legal precedents permitting patients to refuse treatment is limited to unconsented destructions of physical integrity. These decisions involve the refusals of elderly patients to consent to the amputation of a limb. The need for amputation in such patients is caused either by an underlying disease or by a chronic, incurable and ultimately terminal disease.[18] Nonetheless, the degree of physical mutilation as well as the permanency of amputation do appear to provide some basis for a general rule allowing patient refusals to this kind of life-prolonging medical treatment.

Judicial precedents upholding the right of patients to refuse certain medical treatments in specific situations neither demonstrate nor provide a basis for inferring a general right to refuse life-saving medical treatment. While emphasizing that it is inappropriate to imply *any* general rule from these precedents, the very existence of these precedents reveals an underlying presumption in favor of overruling refusals of life-saving treatment. If the law favored patient autonomy in these instances, there would be no need for litigation to create specific exceptions.

The specific exceptions created by these precedents coincide with many of the considerations we propose as elements of clinical intuition, considerations such as authenticity, rationality, consistency and medical prognosis. The legal precedents are more restrictive than our principle of clinical intuition, because they impose additional conditions limiting patient refusals. These additional restrictions, such as patient responsibility for dependent spouse and children, are community considerations. Such third party interests may not be appropriate elements of a patient-physician relationship. Third party rights aside, our proposal of clinical intuition coincides with the traditional legal conception of the doctor-patient relationship as well as with developing trends in the law.

VIII. THE DEMANDING PATIENT

Throughout this paper we have been concentrating on the acutely, critically ill patient who refuses life-saving treatment. We have noted that the problem of the patient who refuses treatment has been exacerbated by changes in the DPR. Our proposal of clinical intuition is offered as a mediation between the traditional paternal model and an evolving libertarian model of the DPR. It is intended also to protect both physician and patient during a time of uncertain understanding and changing expectations. But even if our proposal were to be endorsed enthusiastically, we would not have resolved our concern with the potential consequences of a libertarian medical model.

We believe that discussions of a libertarian model have failed to consider one of its most significant consequences. It encourages the demanding medical consumer, the patient who demands medical treatment based on a personal determination of his needs and desires. Clinical medicine has always encouraged patients to present with a self-defined sense of dis-ease. But the patient who presents with symptoms and also demands specific treatment based on self-prognosis poses a different problem. Such patients view clinical medicine as one of the 'serving professions' and themselves as medical consumers. When this conception of the roles of medical practitioners and medical consumers is joined with the extreme importance most citizens place on health and medical care, treatment-of-choice becomes not only a product which can be consumed at will, but a right to which one is entitled on demand.

Perhaps this 'diagnosis' is too dismal, but the 'prognosis' is based on events of the last twenty years, beginning with a coincidence concerning patients' rights too pointed to ignore. Expanded legal requirements for informed consent to medical treatment were introduced in 1960;[19] it was also the first year in which the contraceptive pill was offered as a non-experimental, pharmacologic agent. Oral contraceptive medication was the first prescription drug that was (and is) in effect, a self-prescribed 'treatment'. Patients – i.e., 'medical consumers' desiring elective medication – demanded that physicians prescribe the contraceptive pill. Other popularly self-prescribed medications soon followed: tricyclic antidepressants, mood elevators and minor tranquilizers. Here patient demands were based at least in part on a belief that these medications were appropriate for self-diagnosed 'conditions' – not precisely diseases but rather perceived disadvantageous health states. Need was based on a belief that one was not feeling one's best and that medication would cure this malaise. Medication was requested and received for non-specific anxiety, for lethargy, for nervousness, for insecurity caused by a poor self-image. Medications and surgical procedures came to be seen as appropriate solutions or treatments for problems previously considered individual or social concerns, but in any case not biological abnormalities or specific diseases: problems such as alcoholism, hyper or hypo-activity, excessive appetite, a nose too large, hips too wide, hair too sparse.

Just when patients began to protect themselves from what they feared medicine and technology could do *to* them, they became entranced with what modern medicine could do *for* them. And what medicine can do for them, they have discovered, is not limited to medication and cosmetic surgery. By the early 1970's we were hearing of intestinal bypasses for marginal obesity, an invasive procedure that contradicts normal risk-benefit analysis for elective surgery. This procedure requires a substantial allocation of medical resources for a self-perceived need, and views a surgical treatment not as a curative procedure but as a mechanism for transformation of the self.

Physicians acknowledge the practice of surgeon-shopping for this and similar surgical procedures. Some surgeon will perform cardiac bypass surgery at the request of a patient with essential chest pain; or a cholecystectomy for a patient with functional abdominal pain, even when these self-styled patients are poor risks for elective surgery. Some doctors have praised the utility of CAT Scanning to reduce anxiety in patients with non-specific headaches. Here the CAT Scan provides the service of reassurance, a function traditionally performed by the physician as doctor, as teacher. Can CAT Scanning substitute for the physician? If the patient fears, for example, a 'brain tumor', the headache will most likely return. While the doctor can assure the patient why a tumor is unlikely, the CAT Scan can only show that no tumor has been detected – at least not yet. Because the physician has transferred the service of reassurance to the scanner, and because a machine is not, as is the physician, an experienced prognosticator, repeat scans are necessary for reassurance. Are the patient's medical needs adequately served by repeated scannings? Is this kind of service a legitimate medical practice, or is it a technological gimmick, a new and more marvelous version of the X-Ray machine in use thirty years ago that demonstrated how well children's shoes fit?

Most physicians are troubled by patients who demand treatment for self-defined conditions. Nonetheless, when treatment is available and the patient believes his sense of un-ease is 'curable' by means of physician-mediated treatment or medication, a physician willing to provide the demanded service usually can be found.

We believe the demanding patient presents a serious danger to clinical medicine. A patient who refuses treatment questions the relevance and importance of the physician's professional responsibility. He may even usurp the professional ethic that traditionally obligates the physician to maintain and to restore health, and to preserve life. But the demanding patient denies that the physician's responsibilities and expertise have any relevance except insofar as this coincides with the patient's desires. The demanding patient inverts the traditional model and makes the physician a passive agent. The patient proposes; the physician provides. The physician becomes a technician, practicing under the direction and control of his 'client'. We are not arguing that a person ought to have an enforceable legal claim to the medical procedures of his choice. Unless a patient presents with a life-threatening emergency, a physician may refuse to provide any service. But an evolving libertarian model is reinforcing a public understanding that demanded treatments can be obtained from some physician, at least so long as payment is assured.

Over 70% of all hospital costs are paid by Blue Cross, Medicare and Medicaid. Blue Cross negotiates with hospitals to determine what costs are to be reimbursed. Medicaid and Medicare limit coverage by administrative regulation. In some areas of care, such as length of hospitalization, need for hospitalization for particular services, and determinations of what medical services are necessary, the practice of medicine is already a regulated industry. This solution, and particularly the rapid rate of its expansion, is unsatisfactory to many patients and physicians. While limited financial resources and the spectre of bureaucratic control may be satisfactory practical reasons for opposing the trend towards patient-controlled clinical medicine, they are not sufficient philosophical reasons. If it is only money and the end of the exalted self-image of the physician that argue against patient control, those who favor the traditional medical model are already defeated.

One of the difficulties in making a theoretical argument against patient controlled medicine is that these arguments almost always seem 'élitist'. The knowledge and training necessary to become competent in both the science and practice of medicine require extensive specialized education. The physician faced with a patient-consumer who demands a certain medication has neither the time nor the pedagogical ability to make the patient his equal in knowledge concerning the specific drug and its biological potentialities. In some cases, the physician's hesitancy in prescribing medication may be based on an unarticulated clinical judgment. Moreover, the demanding patient often comes to the physician with a pre-existing distrust; he is more convinced by his perception of what the medication has done for his friends than the statistical risks, probable effects and possibly biased predictions of usefulness the physician offers.

IX. CONCLUSION

The charge of élitism may be inescapable; it is simply true that the physician is more capable than the patient of determining a specific diagnosis and prognosis, and of designing the most beneficial course of treatment. This is not to say that patients are uneducable or should be kept ignorant. The mistrust of physicians which is one of the causes of the demanding patient is in turn a result of the patient's relative lack of information about the science and practice of medicine. More than twenty years ago C. P. Snow said that the two cultures of the modern world were separated by the science of physics. A good argument can be made today that physics has been replaced by the biological sciences, particularly molecular biology and human genetics. Basic biological and medical knowledge could reduce the mistrust the public feels toward the physician, his motives and his intentions. It would also correct inappropriate, often misconceived understandings of what the wonders of modern medicine and medical technology can and should provide. Increased general biomedical knowledge could become the basis of an individual understanding and acceptance of responsibility for health maintenance and disease prevention. This would make the physician and patient partners as to goals and more nearly partners in health care procedures and curative medicine. Education would eliminate the too common belief that the 'magic bullets' of modern clinical medicine can replace or cure the medical effects of self-inflicted abuse. Patient education could also permit (and even require) the physician to start explaining why patients should do what they should do – not just telling them what they must do. Physicians are often disliked as well as mistrusted for their authoritarian approach, but so long as explanations must be exhaustive – and even then often only marginally understood – the brusque, authoritarian physician is an excusable if not sympathetic stereotype.

If the choice between the authoritarian and libertarian models of clinical medicine assumes an uneducated patient, we would propose the authoritarian model. But if this assumption is not necessary, it is possible that no such choice need be made. Clinical intuition, including most particularly the component of publicity and a before-the-fact awareness of its use, is an important step towards patient education. Another important step that need not await more comprehensive biomedical education rests within the power of the medical profession. The medical profession needs to attend to its own house: to encourage physicians not to perform unnecessary surgery; not to order or acquiesce in unnecessary diagnostic procedures; not to prescribe excessive medication. The medical profession should attempt to persuade both its members and those it serves that the ends of medicine do not include the ability to cure the human condition or to insure the physical and mental health and social and psychological well-being of any individual [11].

If patients had a more comprehensive biomedical background and physicians and patients had mutually known and consistent goals, there would be much less need for procedures such as clinical intuition. At present severe pain, fear of death and especially fear of a lingering and costly death can cause the acutely, critically ill patient to refuse to consent to treatment. Education and partnership would eliminate much of this fear and that aspect of pain that is caused by ignorance and anxiety. At present, we believe clinical intuition is the best approach to the problem of the acutely, critically ill but not profoundly irrational patient who refuses medical treatment.

University of Chicago
Chicago, Illinois

NOTES

[1] A notable exception to this is the work of Charles Culver, M.D., a psychiatrist at the Dartmouth Medical School, and Professor Bernard Gert of the Dartmouth Department of Philosophy. They have written extensively on the subject of the responsibility of physicians to patients who require but refuse psychiatric hospitalization. They have also specifically considered issues of physician paternalism and the justification of such paternalism ([7], [8]). Their work is represented in this volume by their paper, 'The Morality of Involuntary Hospitalization'.

[2] We have adapted a method that is parallel in many respect to the process described by W. D. Ross in his essay 'What Makes Right Acts Right?' ([16], pp. 16–29). Our method is described in greater detail later in this paper (see Section VI, *Further Thoughts on Clinical Intuition*). It is important to recognize that we are not merely applying Ross's principles to a medical situation. Rather, we are using his philosophical insights to develop a clinical method we refer to as clinical intuition.

[3] *Application of President and Directors of Georgetown College*, 331 F. 2d 1000 (D. C.

Cir., 1964); rehearing en banc denied, 331 F. 2d 1010 (1964); *Jones v. United States*, 308 F. 2d 307 (D. C. Cir., 1962).

[4] *In re Osborne*, 294 A. 2d 371 374–5 (D. C. Cir., 1972) "Where the patient is comatose or suffering impairment of capacity for choice, it may be better to give weight to the known instinct for survival which can in a critical situation alter previously held convictions. In such cases it cannot be determined with certainty that a deliberate and intelligent choice has been made".

[5] *Petition of Nemser*, 273 N. Y. S. 2d 624, 629 (Sup. Ct., N. Y. Cty., 1966).

[6] *Superintendent of Belchertown State School v. Saikewicz*, 370 N. E. 2d 417 (Mass., 1977).

[7] *Matter of Quinlan*, 355 A. 2d 647 (N.J., 1976).

[8] See Note 5. See also *Winters v. Miller*, 446 F. 2d 65 (2d Cir., 1971).

[9] *Matter of Quackenbush*, 383 A. 2d 785 (N.J. Super. Ct., Probate Div., 1978) (amputation of both legs); see *Petition of Nemser*, Note 5.

[10] See Note 6.

[11] See Note 6 at p. 430.

[12] See Note 6 at p. 428.

[13] See Note 6 at p. 426.

[14] See Note 4.

[15] *J. F. Kennedy Hosp. v. Heston*, 279 A 2d 670 (N. J. 1971); See also *Application of President and Directors of Georgetown College*, Note 3.

[16] *In re Estate of Brooks*, 205 N. E. 2d 435 (Illinois 1965); *In re Osborne*, 294 A 2d 372 (D. C. Cir., 1972); *United States v. George*, 239 F., Supp. 752 (D. Conn. 1965).

[17] *See Collins v. Davis*, 254 N. Y. S. 2d 666 (Sup Ct., N. Y. Cty., 1964).

[18] See Note 9. See also *Lane v. Candura*, No. M78–417, Mass, C. A., Middlesex Cty, May 22, 1978.

[19] *Natanson v. Kline*, 350 P. 2d 1093 (Kansas 1960).

BIBLIOGRAPHY

1. Cassell, E. J.: 1977, 'The Function of Medicine', *Hastings Center Report* 7, 16–19.
2. Culver, C. M. and Gert, B.: 'The Morality of Involuntary Hospitalization', in this volume, pp. 159–175.
3. Donagan, A.: 1977, 'Informed Consent in Treatment and Experimentation', *Journal of Medicine and Philosophy* 2, 307–329.
4. Dworkin, G.: 'Paternalism', *The Monist* 56, 64–84.
5. Feinstein, A. R.: 1967, *Clinical Judgment*, Williams and Wilkins Company, Baltimore.
6. George, S. L. *et al.*: 1979, 'A Reappraisal of the Results of Stopping Therapy in Childhood Leukemia', *The New England Journal of Medicine* 300, 269–273.
7. Gert, B. and Culver, C. M.: 1976, 'Paternalistic Behavior', *Philosophy and Public Affairs* 6, 45–57.
8. Gert, B. and Culver, C. M.: 1979, 'The Justification of Paternalism', *Ethics* 89, 199–210.
9. Hobbes, T.: 1651, *Leviathan* I, 12.
10. Jonas, H.: 1978, 'The Right to Die', *Hastings Center Report* 8, 31–36.

11. Kass, L. R.: 1975, 'Regarding the End of Medicine and the Pursuit of Health', *The Public Interest* 40, 11–42.
12. Ladd, J.: 'Physicians and Society: Tribulations of Power and Responsibility', in this volume, pp. 33–52.
13. Livy: *History of Rome*, Book XLIV, 22, 8. Transl. by George Baker, A. J. Valpy, London, 1834, pp. 326–327.
14. *Medical Malpractice*: Report of Secretary's Commission, 1973, p. xv, DHEW Publ. No. (OS) 73–88.
15. Rawls, J.: 1971, *A Theory of Justice*, Belknap Press, Harvard University Press, Cambridge, p. 20.
16. Ross, W. D.: 1930, *The Right and the Good*, Clarendon Press, Oxford, pp. 16–29.
17. Sidgwick, H.: 1874, *The Methods of Ethics*, MacMillan and Company, London, pp. 308–310.
18. Siegler, M.: 1977, 'Critical Illness: The Limits of Autonomy', *Hastings Center Report* 7, 12–15.
19. Szasz, T. S. and Hollender, M. H.: 1956, 'The Basic Models of the Doctor-Patient Relationship', *The Archives of Internal Medicine* 97, 585–592.
20. Veatch, R. M.: 1976, *Death, Dying, and the Biological Revolution*, Yale University Press, New Haven, pp. 116–163.

JOHN LADD

PHYSICIANS AND SOCIETY: TRIBULATIONS OF POWER AND RESPONSIBILITY

The subject of this essay is the social responsibility of physicians, that is, their responsibility to society as contrasted with their obligations to their patients or their duties to their colleagues. Before turning directly to this subject, however, I should like to make a few general remarks about what I intend to do here.

Any discussion of a topic like this must begin with the concept of role; for, since the time of Plato, the concept of role has been one of the organizing concepts of social ethics. Most contemporary discussions of the doctor's role, however, focus on the doctor-patient relationship rather than on the doctor-society relationship, which is my concern here. Accordingly, we find the usual answer to questions about the social responsibility of physicians to be that a doctor fulfills his obligations to society by being a good physician and taking care of his patients. In turn, society's part in this relationship (i.e., that of the government) is simply to provide legal protection for the doctor-patient relationship. Besides this, society's mandate to physicians is restricted to a few morally rather secondary matters like the licensing of physicians, issuing birth and death certificates, and prescribing drugs. (Economically and politically these legal powers may be important, but ethically they are secondary.)

Still, historically and from the ethical point of view, roles in general have always been considered to fulfill important social functions of one sort or another over and above the regulation of interpersonal relations among individuals. According, it has usually been held that the physician's role, considered as a social institution, performs important social functions of one sort or another; for example, the physician is said to be the guardian of the health of the community. Such an answer is obviously too simple-minded, but the point remains, namely, that it seems entirely reasonable to use the concept of role as the starting point of any discussion of the social responsibilities of physicians.

One more general remark is necessary. The kind of analysis that I shall undertake might be called a *socio-ethical* analysis. My general position is that questions about the physician's role and his social responsibility can only be seriously discussed within a historical-social framework: for what we are

S. F. Spicker, J. M. Healey, and H. T. Engelhardt (eds.), The Law–Medicine Relation: A Philosophical Exploration, 33–52.

interested in is how physicians ought to act in contemporary Western society and not how they ought to act ideally in a timeless Platonic world. Nor are we interested in finding some kind of universal cross-cultural physician type; for it is doubtful that we could find a meaningful ethical category of the sort we need here. After all, when we go outside our own culture we find the role, say, of the Navaho medicine man to be quite different from that of a medicine man in our own modern mass-industrial society. In order to avoid Platonism and empty generalities it will be necessary, therefore, to resort to some amateurish history and sociology: what one of my colleagues condescendingly calls *romantic sociology*. My conclusions may indeed turn out to be totally wrong in important respects, but I hope to have made my point if it becomes clear that no satisfactory ethical analysis of the kind required here can be made in a vacuum and that we need to turn to history and sociology for help.

I should point out, however, that my method will not be strictly empirical; for, after all, my ultimate purpose is ethical, not sociological or historical. For that reason, many of my hypotheses and conclusions are based on logical analyses of concepts. What I want to do is to trace out the logical and ethical implications of various concepts that pertain to the relationship of physicians to society. The models I shall examine are treated as ethical models generating guidelines for conduct and for the evaluation of certain activities. In other words, the sociological models I shall examine are of interest to ethics because they represent combinations of rules, ideals, rights and values that have served or might serve as organizing concepts for ethics.[1]

Finally, I hope that it will be understood that what I have to say is programmatic. It is also speculative. My purpose is to convince the reader that we need to try new approaches to the kind of problems discussed in this paper and that we must be ready to ask new kinds of questions. If my approach strikes some as radical: that is what it is supposed to be!

I. ROLE MORALITY AND ROLE RESPONSIBILITIES

Let me begin with a few remarks about role morality. The term 'role' has many different meanings. Here I want to use it as a moral concept rather than as a purely descriptive or explanatory concept. The concept of role, as intended here, is that of a 'cluster of rights and duties' owed by one person to another by virtue of occupying a certain social position ([9], pp. 15, 163); ([6], p. 128). Role morality, as Dorothy Emmett says, is concerned with how one should act in a certain capacity. A role provides a set of principles or rules that can be used to guide conduct and to justify and evaluate actions. Thus, for example, a physician (or a patient) is required to do *A* or to refrain from doing *B* simply because he is a physician (or patient); his having done *A* is right (or good) or his having done *B* is wrong (or bad) because that is what is demanded or, as the case may be, forbidden by his role; the role determines what may (rightfully) be expected of him, etc. It defines appropriate interpersonal conduct of a certain sort.

One especially noteworthy thing about a role is that it imposes certain constraints both on the person filling the role and on others dealing with him. Thus, a mailman is obliged to deliver mail to persons regardless of whether he likes them or not and others may not interfere with his delivering mail that they don't want him to deliver, say, to a particular person, etc. Roles typically require a certain degree of detachment or impersonality. That is a consequence of the fact that, at different times, different individuals can fill the same role.

The general problem we must first consider is the social import of role-morality. It is tempting to try to understand this aspect of role morality in utilitarian terms: thus, by analogy to rule utilitarianism we might have what could be called *role-utilitarianism*. As with the rules in rule-utilitarianism there are two sides to roles: first, roles determine what is right or wrong for certain individuals to do to each other, and secondly, the roles in question, like rules, are justified by reference to their social utility [33]. For it is generally assumed that it is good for society to have people playing certain kinds of roles.

The important point here is that, according to this analysis, roles point in two directions: to the individuals who are governed and served by them and to the society that benefits from having people perform the institutionally defined jobs associated with a role. Sometimes, of course, one side of a particular role is more obvious or more important than the other side. And, needless to say, there are roles in every society that are counter utilitarian, e.g., the role of the professional thief.

A more sophisticated, non-utilitarian version of this two-tier approach is to be found in Charles Fried's discussion of professionalism [12]. Fried distinguishes between two sorts of obligation: the obligation of the individual professional vis-à-vis his client and the social obligations of citizens and of bureaucrats, which is to work "socially – specifically, politically – for the establishment of just social institutions which will procure a fair share *from* and *to* everyone". The latter obligation, Fried says, is

the most particular devolution of the bureaucratic function. It is the sense in which we are all bureaucrats, the sense in which we are all responsible for realizing the abstract principles of justice ([10], pp. 186–87).

Rule-utilitarianism, role-utilitarianism and Fried's two-tier approach are all attempts to loosen the connection between social responsibility and private professional responsibility. The upshot is that a professional is absolved of "personal responsibility for (any unjust) result he accomplishes because the wrong is wholly institutional" ([10], p. 192).[2] One aspect of role morality that we must inspect carefully is its use to absolve role players of responsibility for the results of their actions. I shall return to the question of responsibility later.

Regardless of the specific kind of theoretical backing that is used for separating out these two sides of a role, there are a number of questions that still have to be asked about roles or rules. It is easiest to discuss them by pursuing our comparison of role morality with rule utilitarianism, although what I say will also apply to a view like Fried's. Turning then to rule or role utilitarianism, we must begin by asking whether the rules or roles that we have in mind represent the actual, accepted practices of our society or whether they represent ideal rules and roles that ought to be adopted or that would be adopted under certain favorable conditions.[3] If we opt for the first interpretation of rules and roles, then not only are we committed to a conservative approach to morality, but we are likely to end up with some duties and rights that are morally unacceptable. Role morality often calls for an endorsement of the status quo; and it is not always clear in rule utilitarianism how much we are committed to the status quo. The role of women and rules relating to the conduct of women provide a good example. (Hume, who was a rule-utilitarian of sorts, held that chastity was more virtuous in a woman than in a man.) [17] It is clear that we must be able to adopt a critical attitude towards any extant role or rule and be prepared to revise and even to reject it if it does not pass muster morally. There is no more reason to think that the physician's role today must be the same as it was in Hume's day than that the role of women is the same today as it was then. In any event, we must always be ready to reevaluate ethically all of the roles that we have inherited from the past, including the physician's role.

My thesis in this paper will be that certain aspects of the traditional, i.e. nineteenth-century role of the physician, are out of date and hence are no longer viable or acceptable. So the real title of this paper ought to be: *Old Model – New Realities*!

II. THE PROFESSIONAL MODEL: INDEPENDENCE AND AUTONOMY

In our society and in most Western societies, the occupational role of the physician is framed in terms of professionalism. Physicians belong to one of the so-called learned (or higher) professions, which traditionally comprise lawyers, ministers and professors, as well as physicians. Professionalism, in this sense, provides the key to understanding the physician's ideals and the role expectations that we associate with being a physician.

At the outset, we need to distinguish at least three different senses of 'professional'. First, there is the sense of 'professional' in which we speak of 'a professional baseball player'. Here 'professional' designates a person who engages in an activity for pay; he is contrasted with an amateur. A second sense of 'professional' applies to persons in occupations that require advanced specialized training, usually in a graduate professional school; in this sense, engineers, architects, accountants, and librarians are professionals. Finally, there is a sense of 'professional' that is restricted to the higher professions, so called.[4] The distinctive feature of the higher professions is what is generally known as 'professional autonomy'. It is this last feature that is of particular interest to us here.

Before proceeding, however, I want to point out a few characteristic attributes of professionalism in this last sense.[5] The basic concept of a profession is expressed in the statement: "A profession delivers esoteric services" ([16], p. 1). A professional person, such as a physician or lawyer, has had a long period of training during which he acquires a large body of esoteric knowledge and the skills of harnessing this knowledge for practical purposes. I use the term 'esoteric' advisedly, because the kind of knowledge acquired need not be scientific in the strict sense; all that is necessary is that it not be accessible to ordinary people without special training, perhaps an apprenticeship. Often there are rites of initiation into the profession to mark the successful completion of the training.

Secondly, professionals are expected to be motivated by the ideal of service, that is, they provide services to clients: their activities are supposed to be oriented exclusively to their clients' needs rather than to their own interests or to the interests of society. In this sense they are said to be 'altruistic', although a more accurate term might be 'referentially altruistic'. Professionals are "tied to the client by iron bonds of loyalty" ([12], p. 186).

Third, professions are autonomous in the sense that they are self-regulated and self-controlled: their control is 'collegiate'. [19]. The standards of competence and evaluation of services are set by the profession itself. Finally, in our country and England, at least, physicians and lawyers have traditionally operated as individual practitioners: entrepreneurs. The ideal has been that of the private practitioner. They have been economically independent and have been their own bosses, as it were.[6] I might note in passing that this aspect of professionalism has never characterized all the professions, for ministers and professors have hardly ever been private entrepreneurs and, of course, in other countries physicians and lawyers are frequently not private entrepreneurs, either. This aspect of professionalism is rapidly disappearing as physicians and lawyers become employees of organizations of one sort or another. As Freidson points out, the crucial issue for professionalism is the control over work and its outcome, the autonomy 'connected with skill', rather than the economic autonomy of being self-employed ([11], p. 36).

Let us now examine the notion of professional autonomy more closely. The idea is that the professional himself defines the needs of his client and the manner in which they are to be met ([19], p. 45). The physician determines whether you are sick and whether you need to be hospitalized, etc., just as the lawyer determines whether one of your rights has been violated and what should be done about it.[7] Secondly, fellow professionals are the arbiters of whether or not a professional has performed competently and, indeed, they determine what the standards of competence shall be.

Given these attributes of professionalism, it follows that the appropriate attitude of the client is trust. *Credat emptor*, as one writer puts it ([16], p. 3). By the same token, the client is supposed to be properly grateful for what the physician, lawyer, minister or professor does for him.[8] All this follows from the notion that the physician or lawyer is, as Fried expresses it, like a friend who takes care of you, whom you should trust and to whom you should be properly grateful for what he does. A somewhat more cynical way of describing the relationship is to say that old-fashioned professionalism encourages and even demands the psychological dependence of the client on the professional to whom he goes for service. In any case, the claim to 'moral' authority on the part of the physician or lawyer is built into a particular conception of the professional role.

If we look at the kind of autonomy that is accorded to and demanded by professionals from an analytical point of view, we can see that it has a certain logic. We will find that due attention to the logical side of professional autonomy is instructive. Let us consider the kind of service that physicians and lawyers traditionally had to offer, e.g., in the 19th century. The first thing to note is that their services extended to and included service to *losers*: thus, a physician could be accepted as having done his job satisfactorily even though his patient died, and a lawyer might do his job satisfactorily even though his client lost his case. Success in treatment and success in lawsuits are not regarded as essential to being a good physician or a good lawyer. (Perhaps the same could be said of professors and ministers; for, indeed, how could one measure their success?) Unlike businessmen and craftsmen, the services of professionals were not and could not be evaluated in terms of their end-results. Instead, the activities, processes and procedures they followed were evaluated 'for their own sake', as it were, and not for their products. Clearly a layman was (and is) unable to evaluate services in such terms; only a professional who knows what these processes and procedures ought to be is qualified to evaluate them. So for logical reasons evaluation must be by colleagues, i.e. collegiate evaluation, rather than by clients or other laymen, i.e. patron evaluation.[9]

III. BREAKDOWN OF THE OLD MODEL

A. *Loss of Independence*

The modern medical practitioner, like the lawyer, has lost a great deal of the professional independence that he had in the 19th century. There are many factors contributing to his becoming less of an entrepreneur. The enormous expansion of bio-medical technology has made the private practitioner increasingly dependent on other resources, e.g., for technical services. Furthermore, the dominant role of organizations in the delivery of medical care has severely limited his independence; in providing services to his patients he is dependent on hospitals, insurance companies, and other bureaucratic institutions. These institutions in turn determine and restrict his sphere of operations. There is no point in belaboring this obvious change on the medical scene.[10]

B. *The Loss of Professional Autonomy*

For our purposes, another aspect of the breakdown of the old model is more important, namely, the loss of autonomy in the sense described above. The reason for this development is simple; it is the consequence of the successes of modern medicine. Around the turn of the century physicians could not expect a very high success rate. In most areas there was little that they could do to cure a disease or to prevent a death. But now, with antibiotics and other new medical technologies, physicians may legitimately expect to cure their patients of many of their diseases.

As a result of this kind of success, then, the mode of evaluation has shifted to an external mode of evaluation – a product evaluation. But it should be obvious that when services are evaluated in terms of their end-results, their success or failure, the evaluation can be made by lay persons even though lay persons may not have the kind of specialized knowledge required to know why there was a failure or how to do what leads to the desired end-result. I may not know, for example, what is wrong with my TV set or how to fix it; but at least I know when it is not working. Similarly, when success can be used as a criterion for evaluating a physician's services, then there will be a natural shift from intra-professional (collegiate) evaluation to lay (patronage) evaluation. In Rhode Island, for example, there was recently a case in which a man who had had a vasectomy became a father a year later! You do not have to be a physician to know that something went wrong and that the doctor botched it! The man has the right, at the very least, to have his money back.

When, therefore, physicians bemoan the meddling of lay people in the evaluation of their services, the intervention of patients, families, lawyers and administrators, they are simply suffering from the symptoms of their own success. Their success brings them into the same category as professionals of the second type mentioned at the beginning, namely, engineers and architects, the 'new professionals', so-called.

For logical reasons, then, we can see that the physician is coming to be evaluated as a producer; as such he is subject to the demands and needs of consumers, his patients and society in general. This may be what people have in mind when they say that medical care has become a 'commodity'. The physician is no longer in a position to define the needs of his clients and to determine how they should be treated; the client, e.g., the patient or administrator, can now tell the doctor what he needs and what he must do. The ultimate control in medical matters has shifted away from the individual practitioners. As the success rate grows, this trend is bound to accelerate in the future.

IV. NEW REALITIES: SUCCESS AND POWER

Although he is no longer an entrepreneur and although he has lost his professional autonomy, the physician has vastly increased his power – both as a member of a group and as an individual practitioner. Much of this increase in power is due, obviously, to the new technology at his disposal. It also reflects the general 'professionalization' of society: the growth in power of persons and groups with professional expertise, the technocrats. Physicians have become decision-makers: they have the power to decide and to determine outcomes for individual patients that reaches far beyond anything imaginable a few generations ago. But even more important, perhaps, is the power of physicians as a group to determine the nature, availability and cost of medical and hospital care. The details are given in books like Victor Fuchs's *Who shall live?*[11]

The main point that I want to make is that the shift from the narrow professional model to the power model requires us to relate moral problems concerning physicians and society, not to an ethics of roles, but to the ethics of power. Physicians are no longer simply private entrepreneurs but have become part of what C. Wright Mills calls the *power èlite*. As such, they are determiners of our future and of the future of society. In order to understand their social responsibilities, then, we must turn to the ethics of power.

Power is the capacity to influence, control and determine the actions of others so as to affect significant outcomes. It is not only the capacity to make people do what they do not want to do or what they otherwise would be unlikely to do, but it is also the capacity to shape and to manipulate their wants so that they will not want what is in their real interest.[12] The point about power is that it is exercised over people and with respect to people. Thus, Lukes writes:

> To use the vocabulary of power in the context of social relationships is to speak of human agents, separately or together, in groups or organizations, through action or inaction, significantly affecting the thoughts or actions of others (specifically, in a manner contrary to their interests) ([28], p. 54).

There are two important points about the power of physicians that need to be emphasized. First, their power is group power, although not necessarily organized power. Perhaps no single individual physician is able to effect a social change or to prevent a social change, but when acting in concert with others he is in fact able to do so. In our society, most significant social action, whether organized or unorganized, is group action. Indeed, even formal decision-making is carried on by groups, e.g., by committees. It might appear that if a decision is made by a group that it is no longer made by individuals; for there is a sense in which the individual is lost in the group since it is usually difficult, if not impossible, to measure the amount and degree of any particular individual's contribution. Nevertheless, to assume that individuals do not count is a serious mistake. It is easy to assume that because group action is usually overdetermined in the sense that the action of no one single individual is necessary or sufficient to effect the outcome, that therefore the actions of individuals do not count. But ethically and from the point of view of moral responsibility, we must consider a group action to be the resultant of the actions of individuals acting in concert, consciously or unconsciously, so that the action of each participating individual can be attributed to him in the full-blown sense. Consequently, when anyone participates in a group action that action is an action for which he is accountable and he is responsible for its consequences.[13]

The second point is that medical power, like all power, is and can be exercised by inaction as well as by action and it can be used to prevent things from happening as well as to cause something to happen. It is easy to see that the medical establishment has the power to block projects, reforms, new ideas in the health care field, new ways of approaching personal and social problems arising out of situations where people confront sickness and death, and so on. I need not go into details. Physicians as a group tend, using Bachrach's and Baratz's words, to create and reinforce

> social and political values and institutional practices that limit the scope of the political process to public consideration of only those issues that are comparatively innocuous to them ([2], p. 7; [28], p. 16).

I might add that medical power often blocks consideration of alternatives that might serve the interests of particular patients better than some present practices.

In this regard, the decision of physicians to 'go along' with a present practice is itself an abuse of power, albeit of a negative sort. For the decision not to exercise their power is as much a decision as a decision to exercise it in the wrong way.[14] In cases like these, the non-exercise of power is sometimes as blameworthy as the wrongful exercise of power.[15]

V. POWER AND RESPONSIBILITY

The ethical side of power is responsibility. (I am using 'responsibility' here in the virtue sense, that is, in an ethical or normative sense rather than in a descriptive or attributive sense.)[16] Responsibility, in this sense, is contrasted with irresponsibility. Accordingly, power may be exercised responsibly or irresponsibly. What we are concerned with is the difference between a responsible and an irresponsible use of power. The difference is drawn by what I call *the ethics of power.*

There are two elements to the concept of responsibility in the virtue sense; first, the person involved must recognize his ability to choose and to affect the situation in which he finds himself and, second, he must be prepared to take fully into account the consequences of his actions or non-actions. Either the refusal to accept oneself as a moral agent with the capacity to make choices that influence outcomes or the refusal to take cognizance of the consequences of one's acts (or non-acts) is sufficient to qualify a person or an action as irresponsible.

Power and responsibility, as Lukes points out, are interrelated concepts. Wherever one's power extends, so also does one's responsibility and, in a sense, whenever a person has responsibility he does or ought to have the power to fulfill his responsibilities.

Power implies responsibility for what one has the capacity for doing but does not do as well as to do what one actually does. For example, if one has the capacity (power) to save a person from drowning then, other things being equal, he is responsible for saving that person and, if he does not, then he is culpable. Furthermore, his culpability is not lessened by the fact that he is unaware of his responsibility or denies it. (We have here an analogue of the legal concept of negligence. It might be called *moral negligence*.)

The most frequently neglected side of responsibility is the negative side, what one lets happen. We let people suffer, we let people starve, we let people die – when we could prevent all that. We let them go broke trying to pay their hospital bills for treatment that they do not want, etc., etc. Physicians as a group are in a position to prevent many of these things. Here I am not referring to particular physicians or to particular patients, but to what is called 'the system', i.e., what physicians in general do to patients in general and the practices they condone.

VI. THE ETHICS OF POWER

Since my concern in this paper is with what I have called the 'social responsibility' of physicians, let me end up with a few remarks on the ethics of power.[17] Freidson suggests that "there is a real danger of a new tyranny" resulting from the new power of the professions ([10], p. 381). What to do about it is partly a political problem and partly a moral problem. I shall conclude this paper with a brief discussion of the ethical dimensions of a responsible exercise of power.

There are three aspects of the ethics of power, of responsible power, that

I shall mention because they seem particularly relevant to the power of physicians as individuals and as a group.

To begin with, responsibility and power are public concepts; that is, power, if anything, is or ought to be an object of public scrutiny. The first aspect of the ethics of power is accountability, that is, the person who has the power ought to be prepared to explain, justify and defend his actions and non-actions. The exercise of power without accountability is ethically unacceptable. It is irresponsible. (Incidentally, the role ethics of physicians' conduct does not require, perhaps it does not even permit, public accountability. This is one point at which the two kinds of ethics diverge.) I do not mean to imply that in every particular case such an account must in fact always be given, but only that there must at least be the possibility that it can, under appropriate circumstances, be given. In Kant's terms, one's projects must be consistent with publicity. He calls this the *Principle of Publicity*.

Kant's formula is worth examining, for although it is directed against the kind of secrecy practiced by political tyrants, it applies equally well to other forms of tyranny, e.g. the tyranny of managers and of professionals:

> All actions relating to the right of other men are unjust if their maxim is not consistent with publicity .... A maxim which I cannot divulge without defeating my own purpose must be kept secret if it is to succeed; and if I cannot publicly avow it without inevitably exciting universal opposition to my project, the necessary and universal opposition which can be foreseen a priori is due to the injustice with which the maxim threatens everyone ([20], pp. 47, 48).

A second element in the ethics of power is that it obligates those in power to permit other interested and concerned parties to participate in decision-making.[18] Clearly there are many decisions in situations requiring medical attention where the physician ought to share his decision-making power with others.[19] In the wider context, medical decision-making and planning have crucially important consequences for society at large; accordingly, where such consequences are involved, the responsible exercise of power by the medical establishment necessitates sharing their power with other segments of society. We must not forget that one of the traditional bulwarks against tyranny has always been the sharing of power.

Finally, if the ethical requirements of responsibility are not met, i.e., if power remains irresponsible, then public intervention and control is called for – 'it is indicated', as the doctors would say! There are many sorts of control, ranging from the use of legal and governmental machinery to reliance on the market mechanism or the mobilization of public opinion. I do not want to suggest that any one of these types of control is more desirable than others or that such controls are always desirable. Obviously what measures are necessary depends on the particular issue that confronts us. But ethically the unrestrained abuse or misuse of power almost always justifies the institution of external controls of one sort or another. Medical power, which is our concern here, is surely no more morally exempt in this regard than other kinds of power. After all, what is at issue is our lives, our health and our fortunes, in sum, our welfare, which also includes our moral integrity, and these things ought not to be subordinated to the vested interests of the medical establishment and to its efforts to retain a monopoly of power over the health care system.

At this point, further elaboration would require getting into particularities. (I have listed some of the social problems connected with medical care in Appendix B.) My main aim has been to try to provide a general framework for asking questions about the physician's social responsibilities. To repeat what I said earlier: my purpose is ethical rather than historical or sociological. For that reason I am not interested in describing what is, was or will be, but in what ought to be in the context of late 20th century mass-industrial society. Furthermore, I have addressed myself specifically to the question of the physician's responsibility to society and have deliberately ignored his responsibility to the patient. (I have discussed the latter elsewhere [24].) My main thesis is that as far as a physician's social responsibilities are concerned, they can be understood better by relating them to his position in the power élite than by relating them to his role as old-fashioned family doctor. My position is summarized very well in the following passage from C. Wright Mills:

> The elite cannot be truly thought of as men who are merely 'doing their duty'. In considerable part they are the ones who determine their duty, as well as the duties of other men. They do not merely follow orders; they give orders. They are not merely bureaucrats; they command bureaucracies. They may try to disguise these facts from others and from themselves by appealing to traditions of which they imagine themselves to be the instruments, but there are many traditions, and they must choose which ones they will serve. And now they face decisions for which there simply are no traditions ([31], p. 41).

APPENDIX A: THE SERVICE IDEAL

Some questions have been raised about what is called the 'service ideal'. It may be of some interest, therefore, to try to define the 'service ideal' more precisely.

To begin with, it should be noted that the kind of service involved is a service *to individuals* rather than, say, to the community, to an organization or to society in general. It is, in other words, a personal service of some kind.

How, we may ask, does the service provided by professionals differ from the kinds of personal services provided by members of other occupations, e.g., servants, barbers, ski-instructors, and architects? A rough answer to this question might be that professional services are more basic, more essential or perhaps more necessary in some sense than non-professional services. It might be said, for example, that the services in question are connected to the vital interests or needs of the client, more so, than are some of the other services that we seek in order to satisfy some want or other.[20]

For our purposes, the significant difference between interests and needs, on the one hand, and wants, on the other hand, is that another person may often be a better judge than oneself of what is in one's interest or of what one needs. Thus, the professional, say, a physician or lawyer, might be considered to be better qualified to determine his clients' interests and needs than the clients themselves. He knows, or at least claims to know best 'what is good for them'. (Such knowledge, or knowledge claims, give rise to paternalistic attitudes on the part of the physician or lawyer.)

The suggestion that professionals may be compared to friends, a suggestion worked out in some detail by Fried, has somewhat the same kind of implications as the considerations just mentioned. For a friend is a person who is concerned with the other person's real interests and needs as contrasted with simply helping him to satisfy his immediate, perhaps even silly, wants. A true friend does not, for example, let his friend drive home alone after he has had too much to drink, even though he may want to do so.[21]

Perhaps this notion of real interests and real needs connects up logically with the concept of person. If so, in taking care of a person's real interests and real needs one might be said to be taking care of him as a person.[22] Thus, we can see why professional services are sometimes described as services to a client as a person.

Closely connected with the last notion is the concept of loyalty. For loyalty, as between friends, implies caring for another as a person, although perhaps in some exclusive sense [21]. That may be what Fried means when he says that the bonds of loyalty that bind the professional to his client (patient) are like the bonds of loyalty between friends.

It would appear to follow from such considerations that certain kinds of medical services provided by physicians reflect the professional 'service ideal' more completely than others. Where the service is a very specialized and technical one, e.g. that of a pathologist or radiologist, it might be more accurate to say that the physician is concerned, say, with treating an organ of a person rather than with treating the person himself, that is, he focuses on what is good for the organ rather than on what is good for the person.

In any case, I think that it is safe to say that physicians and lawyers, not to mention ministers and professors, usually claim to have special, expert knowledge of what is good for their clients and the service they provide is based on that special knowledge. That, according to the professional ideology, is why we need them. It should not be assumed, however, that we need to accept these claims; for, as I point out in various parts of this essay and particularly in Appendix B, the professional's claim must always be approached with a critical eye.

APPENDIX B: ISSUES WHERE MEDICAL POWER COUNTS

There are a number of areas where physicians, individually and collectively, have a social responsibility based on their power. A detailed discussion of these problem areas is outside the scope of this essay and, indeed, beyond my scholarly competence. So the items listed here are offered merely as examples of the kind of thing that I have in mind in this essay.

First, physicians can do something, individually and collectively, about the containment of the costs of health care. The rising cost of health care is a matter of concern to all of us. Estimates are that the rate of annual increase is around 15% and that the health care system will soon cost around 200 billion, that is, about one-tenth of the gross national product. According to all accounts, the same rising costs are taking place in other countries besides the USA. There is also common agreement that physicians have the power to control these rising costs, since they prescribe treatments, control access to hospitals, and determine the use of drugs, etc.[23] Furthermore, physicians are in a position to promote or to block the use of other health care personnel for routine medical care such as nurse-practitioners, midwives, and other kinds of paramedics.

Secondly, physicians exercise their power in setting priorities in the health care system. They impose their values on patients, nurses, administrators and society at large, either directly in their decision-making and by determining policy or indirectly through their 'authoritative' pronouncements on ethical and value issues in the medical context. In order to illustrate what I mean and to invite further comment, I shall construct two hypothetical value orderings, one that of a hypothetical physician and the other that of a hypothetical patient. Let us assume that the ranking is lexical, that is, like a lexicographic ordering, the first category (say a letter in the alphabet) must be completed before we proceed to the next category.[24] The lists might be as follows:

Hypothetical Physician's Ranking of Values:

(A) The preservation of life.
(B) The treatment of disease.
(C) The alleviation of pain and suffering.
(D) The maintenance of the patient's self-esteem.
(E) The preservation of the moral integrity of the patient and of his personal relationships to others, e.g., his family.

Hypothetical Patient's Ranking of Values:

(A) Moral integrity.
(B) Self-esteem.
(C) Alleviation of pain and suffering.
(D) Treatment and attempted cure where the prognosis is poor.
(E) Simply staying alive.

The point of these two lists, which are, of course, caricatures, is that the ordering of priorities is likely to be quite different as between physicians, patients, nurses, administrators, and ordinary people. In a pluralistic society, such divergence is to be expected; but in a progressive and liberal society one may hope, if not expect, that due consideration will be given to the values of others with whom one has to deal. According to almost any respectable theory of ethics, the imposition of a value scheme by one person or group on others is morally objectionable, other things being equal. In any case, insofar as physicians, individually and collectively, try to impose their priorities on others who are subject to their power, they are abusing that power, i.e., they are acting irresponsibly. (Irresponsible conduct is not infrequently the result of the best of intentions and the most idealistic of motives!)

There are a number of other areas, less specific than those just mentioned, where the medical establishment attempts to impose its own values and priorities on society. Examples are obvious: the stress on treatment rather than on prevention, the exaggeration of the importance of the so-called health care delivery system as the way to promote the health of society as contrasted with other possible ways of promoting better health. It is not necessary to dwell on these subjects any longer. I hope that I have made my point.

APPENDIX C: COMMENTS ON ETHICAL ANALYSIS AND METHODOLOGY

A few further comments on the purpose of the kind of analysis offered here and on the methodology followed may help to clarify some of the points made in this essay. The theoretical assumption behind my analysis is that moral decision-making and the moral evaluation of conduct require a body of what J. S. Mill called 'middle principles', that is, a body of rules, concepts, and principles that lie in the middle range between particular decisions or acts and very general principles like the principle of utility or the categorical imperative. (I call such principles 'super-principles'.) Traditionally, it was taken for granted that the 'received opinion' was the proper place to look for such principles.[25] Today, it would be impossible for any informed and reflective person to accept the received opinion as authoritative in the sense required. We are all aware of the multiplicity of factors, social, cultural, economic and historical that determine what is regarded as acceptable or unacceptable in the received opinion of any society, including our own. The facts of cultural diversity and relativity are sufficient to alert us to the limitations and provincialism of many of our accepted practices. We deny the relevance of these background conditions at our own risk: the risk of being bigoted, prejudiced, dogmatic, and intolerant. In any case, we can no longer afford to be uncritical in our acceptance of current moral beliefs and practices.

The first move in the critical evaluation of our own moral beliefs and of our society's moral practices is to compare them with other beliefs and practices. In order to do this, we need to examine the logical structure and relationships between various elements in the beliefs and ethical belief-systems that concern us; for I believe it is correct to assume that moral principles, practices and concepts come in clusters and are joined to each other by logical and ethical connections of various sorts. Hence, the examination of our own beliefs as well as those of others with whom we disagree is a logical and analytical undertaking of a very complex sort. The present essay is an attempt of that kind.

If, for the nonce, we adopt the term 'ethical discovery', we might conceive of the process in which we are engaged as analogous to scientific discovery as set forth in contemporary philosophy of science by those who espouse the so-called 'logic of discovery'. The key idea in the logic of discovery is that one starts one's inquiry by framing a number of hypotheses which are, in turn, evaluated and assessed comparatively by various logical and empirical means, instead of starting with a number of facts or observations and only after these have been collected moving to the stage of framing hypotheses. By analogy, in ethics we should perhaps follow the same procedure and start by comparing various 'hypothetical' ethical ideas, drawing out their implications and consequences, and evaluating them comparatively, so to speak.[26]

Underlying this methodology is a distinction, which needs, of course, to be elucidated, between *understanding* and *establishing* (=justifying or proving) a moral principle, rule, or concept. Understanding involves treating an ethical conception hypothetically as it were, without committing oneself either to the acceptance or to the rejection of it. This is what I have attempted to do with the concept of role morality and, in particular, with the idea of professionalism. I believe that an understanding of the 'logic' of professionalism is a necessary propaedutic to a critical evaluation and assessment of principles, rules and concepts relating to the social responsibilities of physicians. The same considerations apply to the other analyses in this essay as well as to many analyses that I have presented elsewhere.

Brown University
Providence, Rhode Island

NOTES

1 For further details, see Appendix C.

2 Fried argues that as long as the lawyer does nothing illegal or dishonest, he may "work the system for his client even if the system then works injustice" ([10], p. 193).

3 See [5].

4 It has been suggested that there might be a scale of professionalism with the higher professions at the top and the other 'professions' and semi-professions ranged on the scale according to whether or not they possess certain attributes of the higher professions. But this maneuver is not relevant to our present inquiry.

5 I have culled this list of attributes from some of the sociological literature on professionalism. See ([16], [32], [4], [19], and [27]).

6 See ([4], pp. 80 ff.), for a description of this aspect of professionalism in the United States and its social implications. To belong to one of the higher professions, according to Bledstein, was one way of joining the social élite. See also, [27].

7 "It is the practitioner who decides upon the client's needs, and the occupation will be classified as less professional if the client imposes his own judgment" ([14], p. 278).

8 "In the professional order of values, no client merited crueler fate, no client was quite so undeserving and detestable, as one who betrayed his patron by appearing to be ungrateful" ([4], p. 103).

9 Philosophers will recognize the distinction that Aristotle makes between *praxis*

(practice) and *poiesis* (making) [1]. There are important logical differences between the evaluation of the two kinds of activity. The physician and the lawyer are engaging in a practice, which is evaluated as an activity, whereas the manufacturer, engineer and architect are engaged in making, which is evaluated in terms of its products as distinct from the activity of the producer himself.

[10] See ([29], p. 115). For a detailed account of these developments, see [8].

[11] [13], see especially chapter 3, which is entitled: "The physician: captain of the team".

[12] Ivan Illich has emphasized this last point in [18]. He calls it the 'medicalization of society". I do not think that one has to agree with everything that Illich says to see that the medical establishment has succeeded in shaping our ways of looking at our health problems and our general sense of priorities in society.

[13] I have set forth this matter in more detail in [22].

[14] I have argued this question in more detail in my discussion of the alleged moral difference between letting a patient die and killing him ([25], chapter 8).

[15] The failure of various groups in pre-Nazi Germany that were in a position to oppose Hitler to come out against him provides a tragic example of the kind of abdication of power and responsibility that I have in mind here.

[16] An extremely useful discussion of responsibility as a virtue is to be found in [15].

[17] The ethics of power comes under what I have elsewhere called the 'ethics of responsibility' [24].

[18] I have explained the relationship between responsibility and participation in greater detail in [22]. Unfortunately, it is not possible to explain the relationship in greater detail here.

[19] This point is discussed in more detail in [7]. One often hears doctors say that in the final analysis the responsibility rests on the physician in charge and therefore he must be the one to make the decision. It is difficult to understand what this frequently asserted statement really means unless responsibility is given a purely legalistic meaning.

[20] Brian Barry gives us a useful discussion of the differences between interests, needs and wants, see ([3], pp. 47–49, 173–86).

[21] For a suggestive exposition of the friendship model of the doctor-patient relationship by Laín Entralgo, see [26].

[22] This line of thought might be pursued profitably by those who claim that physicians ought to treat their patients as persons.

[23] See [13].

[24] For an explanation of lexical ordering by Rawls, see ([34], pp. 42 ff.).

[25] For an illuminating discussion of this question see ([35], pp. 192–3).

[26] The views expressed here are presented in more detail in [23].

BIBLIOGRAPHY

1. Aristotle: *Nichomachean Ethics*, Book I.
2. Bachrach, P. and Baratz, M. S.: 1970, *Power and Poverty. Theory and Practice*, Oxford University Press, New York.
3. Barry, B.: 1965, *Political Argument*, Routledge and Kegan Paul, London.
4. Bledstein, B. J.: 1976, *The Culture of Professionalism*, Norton, New York.

5. Brandt, R. S.: 1963, 'Toward a Credible Form of Utilitarianism', in G. Nakhnikian and H. Castaneda (eds.), *Morality and the Language of Conduct*, Wayne State University Press, Detroit.
6. Downie, R. S.: 1971, *Roles and Values*, Methuen and Co., London.
7. Duff, R. S. and Campbell, A. G. M.: 1979, 'Social Perspectives on Medical Decisions relating to Life and Death', in J. Ladd (ed.) *Ethical Issues relating to Life and Death*, Oxford University Press, New York.
8. Ehrenreich, B. and J.: 1971, *The American Health Empire*, Random House, New York.
9. Emmett, D.: 1966, *Rules, Roles and Relations*, MacMillan, London.
10. Freidson, E.: 1970, *Profession of Medicine*, Dodd, Mead and Company, New York.
11. Freidson, E. (ed.): 1971, *The Professions and their Prospects*, Sage Publications, Beverly Hills.
12. Fried, C.: 1978, *Right and Wrong*, Harvard University Press, Cambridge, Mass.
13. Fuchs, V. R.: 1974, *Who shall live?*, Basic Books, New York.
14. Goode, W. J.: 1969, 'The Theoretical Limits of Professionalization', in Amitai Etzioni (ed.), *The Semi-professions and their Organization*, Free Press, New York.
15. Haydon, G.: 1978, 'On Being Responsible', *The Philosophical Quarterly* 28, 46–57.
16. Hughes, E. C.: 1965, 'Professions', in K. S. Lynn (ed.) *The Professions in America*, Houghton-Mifflin, Boston.
17. Hume, D.: *Treatise of Human Nature*, book III, part II, section xii.
18. Illich, I.: 1976, *Medical Nemesis*, Pantheon Books, New York.
19. Johnson, T. E.: 1972, *Professions and Power*, MacMillan, London.
20. Kant, I.: 1957, *Perpetual Peace*, Beck, L. W. (trans.) Bobbs-Merrill, Indianapolis.
21. Ladd, J.: 1967, 'Loyalty', in Paul Edwards (ed.) *The Encyclopedia of Philosophy*, MacMillan, New York.
22. Ladd, J.: 1975, 'The Ethics of Participation', in J. Roland Pennock and John Chapman (eds.) *Participation in Politics*, Atherton-Lieber, New York.
23. Ladd, J.: 1977, 'Egalitarianism and Elitism in Ethics', *L'Egalité* V, 297–323.
24. Ladd, J.: 1978, 'Legalism and Medical Ethics', in Davis, J. W., Hoffmaster, B., and Shorten, S. (eds.), *Biomedical Ethics*, Humana Press, New York.
25. Ladd, J. (ed.): 1979, *Ethical Issues Relating to Life and Death*, Oxford University Press, New York.
26. Laín Entralgo, P.: 1969, *Doctor and Patient*, McGraw Hill, New York.
27. Larson, M. S.: 1977, *The Rise of Professionalism*, University of California Press, Berkeley.
28. Lukes, S.: 1974, *Power: A Radical View*, MacMillan, London.
29. Mills, C. W.: 1951, *White Collar*, Oxford University Press, New York.
30. Mills, C. W.: 1956, *The Power Elite*, Oxford University Press, New York.
31. Mills, C. W.: 1959, *The Causes of World War Three*, Simon and Schuster, New York.
32. Moore, W. E.: 1970, *The Professions: Roles and Rules*, Russell Sage Foundation, New York.
33. Rawls, J.: 1955, 'Two Concepts of Rules', *Philosophical Review* 64, 3–32.
34. Rawls, J.: 1971, *A Theory of Justice*, Harvard University Press, Cambridge, Mass.
35. Schneewind, J. B.: 1977, *Sidgwick's Ethics and Victorian Moral Philosophy*, Clarendon Press, Oxford.

WILLIAM J. CURRAN

CLINICAL INVESTIGATIONS IN DEVELOPING COUNTRIES: LEGAL AND REGULATORY ISSUES IN THE PROMOTION OF RESEARCH AND THE PROTECTION OF HUMAN RIGHTS

INTRODUCTION

An essay of this sort presents a problem of scope. Legal systems are essentially parochial. Each relates to a particular country and its jurisdiction, and each is based in the history and culture of a particular nation. When considering issues of legal regulation of clinical medical and behavioral research, a thorough survey would require detailed review of the laws and administrative regulations (or ministerial decrees, departmental decrees, legislative delegative instruments, etc.) in each developing country under consideration.

It also must be realized that a legal analysis concerned with the establishment and interpretation of protective guidelines for the use of human beings in research must include review of what are often considered ethical principles and ethical justification for human research, as well as so-called ethical review mechanisms. What may start out as an ethical issue rather quickly evolves, in this field, into a legal requirement with all the trappings of law, legal enforcement, and punishments.

PART I: STATE OF THE ART IN REGULATORY SYSTEMS

There is a great deal of variety in the legal-regulatory systems concerned with clinical investigation [5], [4]. The most sophisticated systems are quite complex and involve a number of different regulatory mechanisms and policy-setting agencies. The tendency around the world has been for the industrial nations to move closer and closer together in regulatory policy. The less industrialized nations (in terms of biomedical research activity and therapeutic drug industrial growth) are unable to install or to implement such policies as their own. However, it is common practice for these countries to expect importers and foreign-supported research groups to meet the standards of their home countries and to apply these standards wherever they go in the developing world. For example, a developing country may not have the resources or personnel to inspect and pass upon the quality, safety, and/or efficacy of a therapeutic drug or medical device produced in a foreign country. Before allowing the product to enter, however, the developing country may

S. F. Spicker, J. M. Healey, and H. T. Engelhardt (eds.), The Law–Medicine Relation: A Philosophical Exploration, 53–74.

demand proof that the product has already – in the same form and dosage recommended – been inspected, approved, and licensed in the home country of the corporation. This is often called a "Certificate of Free Sale" and the import country may require the Certificate (signed by a national or state regulatory agency) and submission of a sample of the product as sold in the home nation plus all labels and other consumer-provider literature expected to accompany the sample at the point of sale. There are, of course, many nations which require less than the above for importation of new drugs or medical devices, or for the installation of any type of medical care innovation, whether developed within their own borders by their own investigators, or imported from abroad.

In the various countries of the world the currently operating regulatory systems may be classified generally into four groups:

(1) the regulatory process related to the national funding of clinical, biomedical studies;

(2) the regulatory process related to therapeutic drug and device development, mainly in private industry;

(3) the legal and regulatory standards of clinical practice and related clinical research (with unclear lines between the two), including medical professional malpractice law, professional licensure controls, and other protective health and welfare laws, often local or state law, rather than national law or policy;

(4) the ethical, moral, social and cultural standards which underpin all of the above. Much of this last category is often unwritten and even rarely expressed openly. It can be found in the social and educational background of the scientists, physicians, academics, and research administrators who populate the research establishments and clinical facilities where the clinical medical research is done. Slowly, however, a great deal of what has been seen as 'ethical' becomes law as it is adopted and enforced, or is enforced without ever being consciously adopted, under any of the three regulatory mechanisms noted above.

1. National Medical Research Funding

The most comprehensive means, or potential means, of regulation of biomedical research under conscious national policy is through the nationally supported funding agency for such research. In most industrialized countries (and in some developing countries) these are known as National Research Councils (NRC) [11]. In many countries these Councils are part of a wider group of scientific and cultural councils which may operate under a single national policy board. Such councils function in some developing countries because of their earlier colonial relationship, their current relationships (such as to the British Commonwealth), or because the governments and the scientists, often trained in Europe or America, have found such bodies to be of sound, proven value in promoting scientific and medical research.

Referring to these NRCs as 'regulatory mechanisms' may, in fact, offend some people in the research establishments and even in the government itself. These Councils are often referred to as only quasi-governmental, or as acting independently of government control, even though most function primarily to distribute public moneys of the central or federal treasury. Some, however, also distribute or influence distribution of funds from industrial sources. Most of the research support from NRC goes to university-based research facilities based upon grant applications from research scientists and physicians who hold academic appointments. In the West German Federal Republic, a so-called 'dual system' of medical research is in operation. It is composed of

(1) a group of independent research institutes, the Max-Planck-Gesellschaft and others, of which about a third of their programs are in the biomedical field;

(2) university-based medical research supported from a variety of sources including funding for research from the *Deutsche Forschungsgemeinschaft* (German Research Society) which has funds from the Federal and State (*Länder*) Governments and from industry.

There is no centralized planning of scientific and biomedical research in West Germany which covers all of the systems of research support.

In the United States the equivalent national or federal agency is the National Institutes of Health. The NIH is composed of a number of specialized institutes along with general programs. It has both an intramural (research in its own laboratories and clinical facilities) and an extramural (funds distributed to universities and other research establishments) program. The funds of NIH are exclusively federal. It operates under the policies of the U.S. Public Health Service and the Federal Department of Health and Human Services.

In my opening remarks I used certain descriptive terms for the National Research Councils or their equivalent in other nations. I would like to explain these references. I called the Councils 'the most comprehensive' means of regulation. By this I meant that they cover all types of biomedical research from the most basic scientific and biomedical to the most specialized and advanced clinical applications. On the other hand, the pharmaceutical industry and drug regulatory agencies are concerned only with drug trials. (Device regulation has also been expanding during the 1970's, usually under the same regulatory body concerned with drugs.) The close relationships of the NRCs and the NIH to the medical academic community, often with overlapping committee structures, makes comprehensive coverage feasible.

Also, I called the NRCs a 'regulatory mechanism'. This description seems clearly justified to me, though the degree of regulatory authority held and exercised differs from country to country and even from time to time in the same country, depending both on national policy and the administrative style of different chairpersons and members on the Councils. The Councils operate, however, within an academic tradition. This is true in the NIH as well as in the Council systems, as I have noted elsewhere [3]. Within the academic tradition a great deal of freedom is given to the clinical investigators. They must describe their methodology in detail in order to receive a grant, but they are allowed to make adjustments in the best interest of the research objective during the project itself. The reviewing bodies of the funding agencies are usually free to apply a combination of standards in approving or rejecting projects and in setting ranking-priorities among them. This means that they may consider, in addition to (1) the reputation and status of the chief investigator and his facility and (2) the quality of the research design, the following three factors:

(3) the funds available to be spent and the type of distribution plan adopted; – for example, small grants versus large projects, grants versus contracts, geographic and institutional distribution of an equitable nature;

(4) the national objectives of the biomedical research plan; – for example, the Council may have established policies for certain special areas of research, or for selected research disciplines. These are rarely rigid requirements and applicants in these fields must meet the other standards as well;

(5) the ethical standards accepted by the reviewing bodies; – in earlier years, these standards were rarely articulated. More recently, written criteria have been adopted and ethical review mechanisms have been installed.

It should be understood that from the viewpoint of a law-trained observer, the last three points noted above are all regulatory in character and effect, even though none of them (except the budget, or public part of the budget) may be set forth in a 'law' considered and passed by a legislative body. These criteria essentially make up the national policy on medical research.

2. *Drug Industry Regulation*

In most industrial countries, at present, a complete examination of the state of the art on legal and ethical standards for clinical medical investigation requires the review of a dual system – that related to national funding and that related to regulation of the drug and therapeutic device industry. It has been the habit of many commentators in the past to be concerned with only one of the two systems, virtually ignoring the other [10]. The commentators on ethical standards and human rights protection have tended to follow this same practice.

In some nations, including the United States, the funding and drug regulatory agencies on the national level are part of the same overall central department or ministry of health. In others, they are quite separate, in keeping with the semi-independence of the research councils; the councils also may be part of, or report to, an educational ministry in keeping with their academic support role.

The drug regulatory agencies are very clearly regulatory and very clearly governmental. Their role is to protect consumers of drugs. Nevertheless, they must realize that they cannot be so heavy-handed on regulation as to virtually destroy the industry or defeat or discourage drug development, to the extent that it exists in their countries. These are often difficult lines to follow consistently.

There is an international character to drug industry regulation and regulatory policy which is not as easily found in other areas of this subject. This is due to the international character of the industry itself. There is a conscious tendency to follow the lead of certain national regulatory bodies such as the U.S. Food and Drug Administration (FDA) and similar agencies in Sweden and the United Kingdom. This does not usually mean reciprocity of application and licensing. It means that standards adopted in a leading industrial country are apt to be considered and separately articulated, formulated, and promulgated in the administrative codes or degrees of other nations, without attributing the new regulations to the source. Usually, the new decrees are changed, substantively or procedurally, to accommodate the other nation's drug industry and its regulatory system.

Earlier, in considering the criteria applied by the public funding agencies, I mentioned five factors. These were as follows: (1) reputation and status of the investigators and their research facilities; (2) quality of research design; (3) funds available and pattern of distribution; (4) national objectives and policy on biomedical research; and (5) ethical standards. I considered the last three to be the areas where the Councils and NIH tended to perform regulatory functions and set policy. In the drug regulatory agencies, the first two areas are considered of greater importance.

France seems to place emphasis and scientific confidence on the first criterion – the competence and reputation of the investigator. France has a special, rigorous licensing system for investigators. Other nations place greater emphasis on the second criterion – control of the actual design – though they weight the competence of investigators also. The combination of the first two criteria makes up most of the formal regulatory codes. In the public funding agencies, on the other hand, these first two factors are less formally articulated. In fact, there may be no formal rules in these areas. The review panels or committees, usually made up of academic researchers, are expected to 'know' the 'personal reputation' and 'research design' factors and to apply them without formal guidance. We noted earlier that the public funding agencies seem to permit the researcher greater freedom to vary the research design after the funds are appropriated. They rarely do much 'monitoring' of on-going projects, though this practice may be changing.

The drug regulatory agencies do not apply Factors (3) and (4). These are the concern of the separate, private industrial firms under regulation. During the early 1960's, when the public funding agencies were first considering and adopting ethical standards (Factor (5) above), the reaction of the drug regulatory bodies was to leave this domain untreated as well. To a considerable degree, they considered these issues as either already covered by regulations on safety, or local law, or the 'ethics' of individual investigators.[1] It was not until the 1960's or the 1970's that drug regulatory agencies began to adopt ethical standards and to write them directly into their own regulatons. These have taken two forms:

(1) substantive regulations regarding the rights and welfare of research subjects and patients;

(2) required prior review and approval of clinical drug trials by ethical review bodies, usually the same bodies originally set up to comply with the policies of the public funding councils or NIH for biomedical and behavioral research.

When the second form of regulation is adopted, it often makes it unnecessary to adopt the first form. That is, whatever ethical standards are applied by the ethical review bodies, or Institutional Review Boards (IRB) in the United States, are automatically applied to drug trials. Nevertheless, many of the drug agencies do adopt substantive ethical standards. In many agencies, the 'ethical decrees' are intertwined with other standards.[2] In some, however, a sub-set of regulations may be labelled 'professional ethics'. These regulations often repeat, word for word, the provisions of the *Helsinki Declaration.*[3] Some regulations refer to the Declaration, thus incorporating its substance by reference, a rare practice by such agencies, as noted earlier.[4] It is often not clear whether the 1975 amendments of Tokyo to the WMA Declaration are included by this method. Even more unclear would be the significance of any later changes in the WMA Code, if made *after* the incorporation of the Declaration into a national drug law.

3. *National Legal and Ethical Standards*

In my opening remarks I referred to four regulatory systems in the various nations. Two of these I called 'processes' and these have been outlined above. The last two were referred to as 'standards'. These are drawn from legal sources and the ethical, moral, social, and cultural practices of the people of the countries in general and the academic-professional groups in particular.

These two sets of standards are closely related. The legal criteria are drawn from the professional practices in most instances, though basic principles of law and justice are also applied. The legislatures may add additional rules not drawn from practice and may set up procedural mechanisms. Furthermore, these two sets of standards inevitably find their way into the 'process systems' described earlier. The funding agencies apply these standards almost unconsciously. The drug regulatory bodies are much more formal but they utilize these standards nevertheless.

Some current principles which seem to be purely ethical are actually legal, at least in their detailed formulation. The most important of these is the concept of 'informed consent' of the research subject. This concept is borrowed completely from the legal-medical malpractice field where it was developed for clinical medical situations involving patient consent. This developmental legal history has been described in England and in the United States and it can be found in West German and Japanese law as well [9], [14]. Of course there are ethical or philosophical aspects of the 'informed consent' rule implicit in the requirement of truth-telling and the ideal of autonomy of the individual [1]. However, the substance and standardization of the concept is found in law. The requirement of consent of the patient is not found in ancient medical ethical codes.

Other principles treated as if they were developed by ethicists or available in older ethical codes are the distinctions in handling different types of research subjects such as children, pregnant women, prisoners, the mentally ill, or other mentally incapacitated or handicapped persons. On the contrary, these distinctions were *not* included in either of the two major ethical codes in this field: the Nuremberg Code of 1947 and WMA Code of 1964. Most of these distinctions derived from legal traditions in the "Law of Persons" or personality law (both in the Roman Codes and the English Common Law systems). It is only very recently (and in the most sophisticated ethical-legal regulations in such countries as the United States, Sweden, the United Kingdom, and the Federal Republic of Germany) that these special research subject areas have been given particularized treatment. They were first mentioned in the 1975 Amendments to the *Helsinki Declaration* where reference is made in the code to national legal provisions, if not to ethical norms.

The restrictions on the participation of pregnant women are particularly found in drug regulations due to the experience with Thalidomide in the 1960's. Research on 'children' (minors under the law) is restricted in nearly all countries. The use of prisoners or mental patients was rather universally prohibited in Europe after World War II because of the Nazi atrocities with both groups, even though the Nuremberg Code was specifically intended as an ethical standard under which prisoner-subjects could be used in medical research. Surprisingly, this prohibition, so clear and so universal, was not to be found in the formal rules of either regulatory processes discussed above. It has now appeared in the new drug code of West Germany.[5] The European prohibition has only recently moved rather solidly into the United States after decades of the application of the *Nuremberg Code* in Europe.[6]

4. *International Ethical-Legal Codes*

Part of the underpinning of the regulatory processes of the public funding bodies and drug agencies in regard to human rights and the protection of the welfare and safety of subjects is provided, not only by national legal and ethical standards, but by internationally sponsored ethical codes. These are the *Nuremberg Code*, adopted in 1947 at the Nuremberg War Crimes Trials [12] and the *Declaration of Helsinki*[7] of the World Medical Association (WMA) of 1964.[8] The latter was substantially amended by the WMA at its meeting in Tokyo, in 1975, making it very largely a new Code of Tokyo, though it is still called the *Declaration of Helsinki* (see Appendix).[9]

Both of these Codes can properly be called professional ethical formulations. *Nuremberg* was actually promulgated in a legal case (The Medical Case, Nuremberg WCT) but it was intended as an articulation of existing ethical and legal practices. It was put together for the Tribunal by a medical group of advisers headed by Dr. A. C. Ivy of the United States. Since the Tribunal was a special international court, the Code has never entered the legal systems of the world as a judicial precedent. It has been accorded largely 'ethical status' in the decades since the end of the War.

Nuremberg is perhaps best known for its statement on consent of the subject – Principle One of the Code. It begins, "The voluntary consent of human subject is absolutely essential". It goes on to develop the concept of free choice which must not contain any "force, fraud, deceit, duress, over-reaching, or other ulterior form of restraint or coercion". Then the draftsmen went on to describe the informational part of an enlightened consent. The subjects should be told:

> the nature, duration, and purpose of the experiment; the method and means by which it is to be conducted; all inconveniences and hazards reasonably to be expected; and the effects upon his health or person which may possibly come from his participation in the experiment.

Lastly, the principle deals with the personal responsibility or duty by the investigator, a very necessary part of all regulatory provisions. The Code makes the obtaining of proper consent the duty of the chief investigator. The duty cannot be delegated to another with impunity.

Even though this concept was developed by medical advisers, the strong and able hand or hands of lawyers can be seen in the actual wording of Principle One. The key words used are terms of art in law, terms such as 'fraud', 'deceit', 'over-reaching', 'hazards reasonably to be expected', 'duties and responsibilities', 'delegation', and 'impunity'.

The other principles of *Nuremberg* are still critically important in all regulatory programs for clinical investigation, including drug trials. Some of the principles were eventually modified. Some apply more to the use of healthy volunteers than to patient-subjects where the research relates to their illness.

The principles which are most generally accepted are the requirements that animal experimentation come before and serve to justify any use in humans, that the investigation be adequately designed to produce fruitful results, and that all efforts be taken to avoid all unnecessary harm to the subjects. Also, Principle Six contains a basic risk-benefit statement by providing that the risk to subjects should never exceed the humanitarian importance of the problem to be explored. Notice that this latter principle applies primarily to volunteer subjects. Later commentators view the wording as too liberal toward research risks. Direct benefit to subjects who are patients is not mentioned in the *Nuremberg Code*.

It should also be noted that much of *Nuremberg* may have no application in the U.S.S.R. where it is claimed that no medical research is allowed on healthy volunteers.[10]

The World Medical Association *Declaration* was developed specifically to fill the alleged gap in an ethical code which had to cover both clinical and non-clinical medical research. The *Helsinki Declaration* is directed at *physicians* as investigators. It is not considered applicable to other types of researchers, though most other professionals respect its principles. In the original *Declaration* of 1964, it was specifically asserted that the Code was *ethical and not intended as law*. Physicians were admonished that they must also follow the law in their local jurisdictions.

The most important change in the WMA *Declaration* from *Nuremberg* was the suggested difference between what was called 'clinical research combined with professional care' and 'non-therapeutic clinical research'.

Most important, the therapeutic category allowed some modification of the strict *Nuremberg*-type informed consent. The investigator was required to obtain patient consent after a 'full explanation' was given but only 'if at all possible' consistent with patient psychology.

In the Amendments of 1975, the requirement regarding consent appears in a section on 'basic principles'. It is not the first named principle as in *Nuremberg*; it is listed as the ninth of twelve principles. It requires that the subjects be adequately informed of the aims, methods, benefits, hazards and discomforts of the proposed study. The subject must be able to withdraw consent at any time without reprisal or restrictive conditions. It is then suggested that 'the doctor' obtain the person's 'informed consent', preferably in writing. Thus the WMA Code again places responsibility on 'the doctor' (presumably the chief investigator) to obtain consent. The more legal term 'informed consent' is used and the largely North American practice of obtaining *written* informed consent, or an informed-consent *document*, is suggested.

The most noted new provisions in the Amendments of 1975 are those related to means of enforcement. These are found in Basic Principle 2 and Basic Principle 8. In Basic Principle 2, researchers are required to 'transmit' their research designs to "a specially appointed independent committee for consideration, comment and guidance". It is generally understood that this committee will be an ethical review panel[11] [13]. As finally accepted by the WMA, the provision does not require that the recommendation or recommendations of such a committee be binding on the chief investigator. Nevertheless, this Principle is critically important as an international endorsement of the movement toward ethical review mechanisms.

Basic Principle 8 admonishes professional journals (and other formal publications) not to accept for publication any papers reporting the results of investigations which are not conducted in accordance with the principles of the *Declaration* of 1975. This acceptance into the revised *Declaration* is significant because it supports the relatively recent decision of professional journals to employ this criteria in accepting articles for publication. The two principles are interlinked, since a convenient means for journal editors to assure compliance with the standards of the *Declaration* is to require proof from the author that the project was passed and was monitored throughout by an appropriate ethical review panel.

The high quality and ethical sophistication of the *Declaration* of 1975 was largely due to the work of the Nordic Committee of the WMA which conducted a very thorough review of world experience in this field prior to preparing its recommendations to the WMA.[12] In completing its work the Nordic Committee consulted the staff of the World Health Organization in Geneva, among other groups and authorities.

5. *Ethical Review Mechanisms*

One of the most significant developments in this field over the past decade has been the establishment of ethical review panels on local, regional, and national levels in many countries of the world.

The United States was first in providing the impetus for the establishment of local ethical review panels composed of peers or colleagues of the researchers. An essay by L. G. Welt [15] and a research survey project by the Law-Medicine Institute of Boston University in the 1950's helped to call attention to the potential for such a mechanism.[13] After the NIH, in the early 1960's, required the establishment of ethical review boards for extramural grants, the same standard was applied to applications from abroad. This requirement led directly to the establishment of such review groups in some European nations, notably the United Kingdom[14] and Sweden [8],[15] and also at the World Health Organization in Geneva [7].

A number of other European countries have since moved to set up some form of ethical review system. These countries include Denmark, Norway, Finland, Switzerland, France, the Irish Republic, and the Federal Republic of Germany. There are also ethical review committees, some of long standing (1950's and 1960's), in Australia and New Zealand.[16] A preliminary survey indicates that there are ethical review committees in India and Thailand.[17]

Procedurally and in composition of membership there is some degree of similarity in the operation of these review mechanisms. Most of the panels are composed of research scientists and clinical investigators, with lawyers, ethicists or clergy being the most common non-scientists represented. The panels generally consider proposals directly submitted by principal investigators prior to submission to national research funding agencies or filed by those conducting drug trials. Although the decisions of the panels may be legally binding in some countries, notably the United States, the panels tend to function informally, making suggestions to the investigators, and very rarely actually disapprove a project. Rather, they are able to persuade the investigator to modify the project (or, most frequently, justify his method of securing or expressing the content of informed consent documents) or, in instances of impasse, to withdraw his proposal temporarily or permanently.

Except in the United States, there have been no efforts to impose procedural requirements on these panels or committees at the local level (hospitals, research institutes, and medical schools). In the United States, the IRBs operate under guidelines issued by the Federal Department of Health and Human Services. Proposed regulations have been issued by both the Department (for NIH) and the FDA. It is reported that the two agencies are collaborating to try to issue similar or at least non-conflicting 'final' regulations.

There are distinct benefits to be gained from establishing local or regional ethical review mechanisms. Most important, the system decentralizes decision-making and provides for self-regulation in the universities, hospitals, and research institutes. These local committees or panels are seen not as 'legal' bodies but as mechanisms for clarifying the ethical issues ingredient in research protocols which employ human subjects. A central committee or federal body would be far more critically viewed as a governmental-legal system imposing its will on local situations. Cooperation within local or regional panels or IRBs has been uniformly quite good according to what information is available.

As a matter of substantive due process or substantive justice, the local panels, if adequately trained and experienced, can function to provide specific interpretation to principal investigators on their proposed projects, thus adding to the general principles available through the more broadly worded ethical codes such as *Nuremberg* and *Helsinki.*

Lastly, the ethical review panels are a preventative mechanism, acting *before* the project is initiated and patients or subjects are put at risk. In this respect they exercise what in law is called licensing rather than adjudicatory functions. That is, they grant or allow an activity to be performed rather than determine a controversy or the guilt or innocence of a person. This distinction has many consequences. It allows for a negotiating process since the seeker of the license for permission to do research can modify his proposal to accommodate the requirements, if he wishes the permission. Also, the decisions are less apt to need written opinions or discussions and are less likely to require appeals to higher authority or courts. Of interest is the fact that these panels usually perform a licensing-like function prior to another licensing or granting function, i.e., the financial award process performed by the National Research Council or the National Institutes of Health.

The major activity which may affect the procedural and substantive role of IRBs in the United States in future years has been the excellent work of the National Commission for the Protection of Human Subjects of Biomedical and Behavioral Research. The numerous reports of the Commission are quite good in exploring the many aspects of the ethical issues ingredient in human research, and many new Federal regulations will result from the Commission's work.

PART II: INTERNATIONAL ETHICAL-LEGAL RELATIONSHIPS

In the numerous fields of law it is not common to find major concepts and substantive provisions which have international origins or which are generally applied across national boundaries. Although law is nationally parochial, we are dealing here with a field where international development has been very much in evidence. We may question why the domain of ethical-legal standards for human experimentation, including clinical medical research, has grown on such an international basis. I would cite the following:

(a) The field of clinical research is essentially scientific. Scientific progress has always been promoted internationally, and scientists have a strong interest in eliminating international barriers to scientific communication. This is also true of the drug industry which is characteristically international in scope and interest.

(b) Since World War II there has been an international abhorrence of 'crimes against humanity' and the violation of basic human rights. The Nazi 'experimentation' on humans in the concentration camps was appropriately judged a crime against humanity as well as part of the program of genocide. This historical fact has continued to tie medical experimentation, especially on confined, institutionalized persons, to possible serious abuse of human rights on an international scale.

(c) The world-wide health and medical organizations have maintained a strong interest in high standards of ethics and law in clinical research. In particular, we can cite the World Medical Association, the World Health

Organization, and the Council for International Organizations of Medical Sciences. Other United Nations agencies have also been important in this movement, especially UNESCO.

From a more specific or positive law and ethics standpoint, the international character of this field has been built upon the following:

(a) the *Nuremberg Code* promulgated in 1947 by an international tribunal;

(b) the various international declarations and other instruments of the United Nations after World War II which concerned human rights and torture, the latter including dangerous 'experimentation' on humans;

(c) the various Declarations (borrowing a term of international law, not ethics) of the World Medical Association beginning with the *Declaration of Geneva* (the revising of the *Hippocratic Oath*) and continuing through various specific field Declarations and particularly focusing on the *Declaration of Helsinki* of 1964. (There were earlier drafts circulated world wide.) The WMA has also continued to articulate other ethical principles in its international Declarations in such areas as the brain criteria definition of death and human organ transplantation;

(d) the international application of regulations on clinical research of the drug regulatory agencies. These regulations are particularly important in two areas:

(1) controls imposed on domestic drug companies concerning the clinical research they do abroad;

(2) controls or standards imposed on clinical research undertaken abroad by corporations seeking license of a 'new drug' in a country other than their own.

Points (a), (b) and (c) require no further elaboration. They were examined earlier. These three are generally treated as ethical pronouncements, though they are very strongly rooted in legal doctrine as well. The fourth and last point (d) – drug regulation – is clearly legal. The subject is too complex and varied from country to country to be explored here, but, as pointed out earlier, there are generalizations which can be found and appropriately applied: The first is the tendency to follow the regulatory leadership of the larger industrial countries. The most frequently cited and emulated agency – whether in Asia, Europe or South America – is the FDA. This does not mean that the FDA is always the strictest and most critical regulator. In some areas the Swedish regulators are even more demanding. The British agency is also very critical. The West German Federal Republic's new regulations are extremely far-reaching.

It has been stated by officials of the Federal FDA that the strictness of its own laws and regulations has, in the past ten years, driven some domestic drug developers, including clinical investigators, into foreign countries. In 1975, Dr. J. Richard Crout [2] remarked that most of the new drug applications then being presented to the FDA were already under clinical study or actually marketed in other countries. He gave as the reasons for the departure from U.S. based development:

(a) the Investigational New Drug (IND) regulations controlling the conduct of clinical research; and

(b) the operation of our local IRBs.

The FDA has, like NIH, moved to require that clinical research conducted outside the United States, but offered in support of an application for a new drug license, be conducted in accordance with scientific standards similar to those in the U.S. and in accordance with some set of ethical standards. Both agencies have seen ethical review mechanisms in the country where the research is conducted to be a means of enforcement and proof of ethically proper conduct of clinical research. Despite these developments, it still seems to be to the advantage of many corporations to conduct and support clinical investigation outside the U.S. The increasing strictness and detail of ethical standards in the U.S. in the 1970's, in such areas as fetal, genetic and psychiatric research, could result in an acceleration of this trend in the 1980's.

PART III: GUIDELINES FOR THE CONDUCT OF CLINICAL RESEARCH IN DEVELOPING COUNTRIES

It seems clear at the present time that international ethical and legal standards, designed to protect the safety and welfare of human subjects and to protect their human rights, should be applied to clinical research in any developing country where the research is supported by public funds. In all fairness no distinction should be made between funds which are clearly governmental, such as NIH grants or contracts, and funds provided by large foundations of a charitable nature.

In short, it is feasible to require that proper ethical-legal standards be observed in clinical research in developing countries, even though some of these countries may not currently have established their own standards. It is feasible because *international* standards are available which can be adapted to local conditions. These international standards could be a combination of the principles of the *Nuremberg Code*, the United Nations *Declarations* regarding human rights, children, women, handicapped persons, plus the

Declaration of Helsinki as revised (1975) in Tokyo by the World Medical Association.

These international principles should be adequate as a general foundation for the ethical dimensions and support of clinical research conducted in developing countries, without imposing further substantive requirements from the U.S. regulatory system of NIH and the FDA.

I would further suggest that the granting bodies from the U.S. require that, in addition to following international ethical standards, the principal investigator or group be responsible for having their project reviewed by a locally based ethical review committee, either by way of the regular mechanism of review established in that country, or by a specially established committee for that project. The main responsibility of this review body would be to interpret and apply the ethical principles of the codes to the particular situation in the country, with considerable range for variation.

The establishment of an ethical review mechanism should be in accordance with the requirements of the WMA *Declaration* (Basic Principle 2), not under the regulations for IRBs as is the case in the U.S. The application of the WMA principle should afford considerable leeway to the country in how the members of the committees are to be selected, their actual composition, and their procedural operations.

The ethical review bodies in the developing countries should be concerned with the following:

(a) *Assuring compliance with the specific laws and administrative decrees of their own countries pertinent to particular projects.* These laws would be important in such areas as age of consent for children, parental rights, special restrictions on use of other population groups, confidentiality, and access to patient records.

(b) *being aware of the general reputation of the investigators (or having access to such information), and having within the committee or available to it a general knowledge of the resources for carrying out the project.* This area of concern may seem to overlap with the technical or merit review in the U.S. system. However, experience has shown that locally based ethical review committees must have this sort of knowledge and interaction-potential with the investigator and the research institution. Otherwise, the committee is too remote from the realities of the research environment to exercise its initial review responsibilities and its continuing relationship to long-term projects. In some countries technical-merit review may be closely related to or take place within the same establishment as the ethical peer review. This may now be the case in India and Thailand.

(c) *being aware of the special dangers and inconveniences that subjects or patient-subjects may experience in certain local environments or research institutions involved in the project.* Here, as in (b) above, the importance of on-scene knowledge is stressed. The issues here concern the safety and welfare of the subjects in the particular geographic area of the developing country, a matter which cannot be judged well from afar.

(d) *formulating and assessing the 'risk to benefit ratio' of the particular project.* This is one of the most sensitive ethical issues – that of overall ethical justification of the project under international standards. The local review committee should measure the direct benefits, if any, to the patients or subjects (as in an immunization-agent trial where the individuals are not sick, yet may receive personal benefit) and the indirect or community benefit of the project and weigh that potential benefit against identified or reasonably expected dangers and inconveniences.

(e) *formulating and assessing the nature, content, and methodology of 'informed consent' of subjects and any limits on these requirements in the particular project within the context of the social, cultural, and legal environment of the country concerned.* This is also a sensitive area. The principle of informed consent is often called the touchstone of the ethical issues in human experimentation. Yet the application of this rather sophisticated doctrine has been inadequately explored in the developing nations. The international medical ethical codes do require informed consent. However, the WMA *Declaration's* Amendments of 1975 (II, Section 5) in clinical research allows the principal investigator to dispense with individual, informed consent of patient-subjects, or to vary the form of the consent where it is considered 'essential' to do so. However, the investigator-clinician must transmit the reasons for decision to dispense with individual consent to the independent (ethical) committee required under Basic Principle 2. The assumption is that the committee will review the reasons and give the investigator guidance on whether the deviation from the regular requirement is justified under the special circumstances.

(f) *providing a form of monitoring of the performance of the project, once approved, and giving guidance to the investigator, the research institution and to individual subjects who may have questions or complaints about the project.* This is an important protective role that only a locally based group can perform. No specific rules should be applied to the monitoring process. It should be allowed to develop on a case by case basis.

These guidelines should be helpful to locally established ethical committees, whether *ad hoc* in nature or an actual part of a regular system. It would be erroneous, however, to assume that these committees in developing countries will always relax the more demanding interpretation of the international ethical and safety standards. On the contrary, these nations may impose stricter standards in some situations, especially as they relate to the population groups. Most countries, whether industrial or developing, tend to adopt stricter rules in these areas than were common in the U.S. in the past two decades.

The areas where interpretation may be expected are particularly in regard to points (d) and (e) above. In part (d), the risk to benefit ratio, some developing nations may be more prone to use community benefit for measuring gain from publicly supported research. They may be more likely to feel that the people will support research for community interests and long-term benefit more solidly than the more present-oriented people of the industrial world. Next, it can be expected that the medical research community of many developing countries will be small, closely knit, and enjoy close relations with individuals and bureaucrats in their national government. They will therefore tend toward similar views about the seriousness of particular health hazards and diseases in these countries. There may be strong leadership in selecting priority areas for clinical research, either with strong guidance from the Ministry of Health or from authority figures in the health community establishment, e.g., persons in a few key hospitals, or Ministry Laboratories. These views on the most important health hazards and on the priorities for clinical research will influence the 'benefit' component in subtle, informal ways in the process of favoring particular investigators, selecting the problems to be explored, and giving weight to national and community benefits to be expected from the results of the research.

In point (e), which concerns 'informed consent', there can be many problems in developing countries, and the consensus approach identified with point (d) may not appear. Some countries and ethical committees may be very strict on requiring consent from all subjects. The prohibition against the use of prisoners, mental patients, and children in biomedical and behavioral research often relates to lack of assurance of free consent. However, where large populations of patients and other local people may be without formal education, there may be less reliance on 'informing' all subjects of the details of a proposal for research. The subject-patients may be aware of the research in a general way, but not fully informed. 'Community consent' may also be sought for some types of projects. The leadership of a community, or of a school system, may be solicited to provide a general approval for a project. The subjects may then become aware of the project and eventually participate, but the consent for involvement may be thought to be community-derived rather than grounded in each citizen's will. In any situation like this, the risk-to-benefit ratio must be closely examined, and the populations would have of necessity to be protected against being brought into projects where risks and dangers to their own health and welfare exist.

If these guidelines were to be followed, research projects in the developing countries would be carried out properly and remain within international ethical standards. The stress is upon strengthening the opportunity of the developing countries themselves to interpret the substantive requirements in relation to the relative social and health conditions which prevail in their own countries. One should avoid suggesting procedural structures and underscore the substantive principles which apply to the developing countries of the world. Upon these principles, the United States should be able to base its decision to support clinical research in developing countries with reasonable assurance that the safety, welfare, and rights of persons participating in biomedical and behavioral research are being protected.

Harvard Medical School
Boston, Massachusetts

APPENDIX

DECLARATION OF HELSINKI 1975

I. *Basic Principles*

1. Biomedical research involving human subjects must conform to generally accepted scientific principles and should be based on adequately performed laboratory and animal experimentation and on a thorough knowledge of the scientific literature.

2. The design and performance of each experimental procedure involving human subjects should be clearly formulated in an experimental protocol which should be transmitted to a specially appointed independent committee for consideration, comment and guidance.

3. Biomedical research involving human subjects should be conducted only by scientifically qualified persons and under the supervision of a clinically competent medical person. The responsibility for the human subject must always rest with a medically qualified person and never rest on the subject of the research, even though the subject has given his or her consent.

4. Biomedical research involving human subjects cannot legitimately be carried out unless the importance of the objective is in proportion to the inherent risk to the subject.

5. Every biomedical research project involving human subjects should be preceded by careful assessment of predictable risks in comparision with foreseeable benefits to the subject or to others. Concern for the interests of the subject must always prevail over the interests of science and society.

6. The right of the research subject to safeguard his or her integrity must always be respected. Every precaution should be taken to respect the privacy of the subject and to minimize the impact of the study on the subjects's physical and mental integrity and on the personality of the subject.

7. Doctors should abstain from engaging in research projects involving human subjects unless they are satisfied that the hazards involved are believed to be predictable. Doctors should cease any investigation if the hazards are found to outweigh the potential benefits.

8. In publication of the results of his or her research, the doctor is obliged to preserve the accuracy of the results. Reports of experimentation not in accordance with the principles laid down in this Declaration should not be accepted for publication.

9. In any research on human beings, each potential subject must be adequately informed of the aims, methods, anticipated benefits and potential hazards of the study and the discomfort it may entail. He or she should be informed that he or she is at liberty to abstain from participation in the study and that he or she is free to withdraw his or her consent to participate at any time. The doctor should then obtain the subject's freely-given informed consent, preferably in writing.

10. When obtaining informed consent for the research project the doctor should be particularly cautious if the subject is in a dependent relationship to him or her or may consent under duress. In that case the informed consent should be obtained by a doctor who is not engaged in the investigation and who is completely independent of this official relationship.

11. In case of legal incompetence, informed consent should be obtained from the legal guardian in accordance with national legislation. Where physical or mental incapacity makes it impossible to obtain informed consent, or when the subject is a minor, permission from the responsible relative replaces that of the subject in accordance with national legislation.

12. The research protocol should always contain a statement of the ethical considerations involved and should indicate that the principles enunciated in the present Declaration are complied with.

II. *Medical research combined with professional care* (*Clinical research*)

1. In the treatment of the sick person, the doctor must be free to use a new diagnostic and therapeutic measure, if in his or her judgement it offers hope of saving life, reestablishing health or alleviating suffering.

2. The potential benefits, hazards and discomfort of a new method should be weighed against the advantages of the best current diagnostic and therapeutic methods.

3. In any medical study, every patient – including those of a control group, if any – should be assured of the best proven diagnostic and therapeutic methods.

4. The refusal of the patient to participate in a study must never interfere with the doctor-patient relationship.

5. If the doctor considers it essential not to obtain informed consent, the specific

reasons for this proposal should be stated in the experimental protocol for transmission to the independent committee (I,2).

6. The doctor can combine medical research with professional care, the objective being the acquisition of new medical knowledge, only to the extent that medical research is justified by its potential diagnostic or therapeutic value for the patient.

III. *Non-therapeutic biomedical research involving human subjects (Non-clinical biomedical research)*

1. In the purely scientific application of medical research carried out on a human being, it is the duty of the doctor to remain the protector of the life and health of that person on whom biomedical research is being carried out.

2. The subjects should be volunteers – either healthy persons or patients for whom the experimental design is not related to the patient's illness.

3. The investigator or the investigating team should discontinue the research if in his/her or their judgement it may, if continued, be harmful to the individual.

4. In research on man, the interest of science and society should never take precedence over considerations related to the well-being of the subject.

NOTES

[1] See [3].

[2] This is the case in the Austrian law on clinical drug research. See *International Digest of Health Legislation* 22, 18–24, 1971.

[3] This is the case in the Costa Rica law and in Tunisia.

[4] The draft law on clinical investigation in Poland takes this approach.

[5] Division 6, Sections 38 and 39.

[6] Many states have now prohibited non-beneficial medical research on prisoners. The Report of the National Commission for the Protection of Human Subjects of Biomedical and Behavioral Research suggests strict controls on such research and suggests guidelines for programs which could be approved. The FDA has not yet taken action on so-called 'phase 1' testing of drugs in prison settings.

[7] Published by the World Medical Association.

[8] The WMA prepared various earlier drafts which were circulated. See [3].

[9] Published by the World Medical Association.

[10] Personal correspondence with Dr. John Dunne, World Health Organization, Geneva, who visited research organizations in the U.S.S.R. recently and reported this situation to me in June, 1979.

[11] This is the position of the head of the WMA headquarters at the time. In another paper I have analyzed this provision, pointed out its careful wording, a compromise in language over possible stronger wording. See [6].

[12] Personal interview with Dr. Paul Riis, June 1978.

[13] Research grant, NIH, No. 7039, 1960.

[14] See [3]. Also see the Report of Royal College of Physicians, London, 1967.

[15] See the unpublished speech of G. Giertz, Swedish Society of Medical Sciences, November 13, 1973.

[16] See the excellent survey reports on these two countries prepared by Dr. Craig D.

Burrell, Sandoz Foundation, U.S.A., January 1979, for the WHO-CIOMS research efforts in this field.

[17] Correspondence to CIOMS in current research efforts indicated above. See [2].

BIBLIOGRAPHY

1. Bok, S.: 1978, *Lying: Moral Choice in Public and Private Life*, Pantheon Books, New York.
2. Crout, J. R.: 1976, 'New Drug Regulation and Its Impact on Innovation', in *Impact of Public Policy on Drug Innovation and Pricing*, Mitchel and Link (eds.), American University, Washington.
3. Curran, W. J.: 1969, 'Government Regulation of the Use of Human Subject in Medical Research: the Approach of Two Federal Agencies', *Daedalus* 98, 542–595.
4. Curran, W. J.: 1975, 'Legal and Practical Requirements for the Registration of Drugs (Medicinal Products) for Human Use', *International Fed. of Pharm. Manufacturers Associations* (*IFPMA*), Zurich, Switzerland.
5. Curran, W. J.: 1978, 'International Survey of the Regulation of Human Experimentation', *Report to Fogarty Center*, Washington, D.C., (unpublished survey).
6. Curran, W. J.: 1978, 'Evolution of Formal Mechanisms for Ethical Review of Clinical Research', *Lisbon Conference on Medical Experimentation and the Protection of Human Rights*, 12th Round Table Conference, CIOMS, 30 Novermber–1 December.
7. De Moerloose, J.: 1976, 'WHO Experiences on Ethical Aspects of Research Involving Human Subjects', 10th Session General Assembly, CIOMS.
8. Giertz, G.: 1978, 'The Work of the Ethical Committees' [English translation], Swedish Medical Research Council.
9. Hosokawa, I.: 1975, 'A Physician's Duty of Disclosure: A Comparative View of the Law in the United States, Japan, and West Germany' (Master's Thesis), Harvard Law School.
10. Kay, D. A.: 1975, 'International Regulation of Drugs', *Amer. Society of International Law*, Washington, D.C.
11. 'Medical Research Systems in Europe', *Wellcome Trust-Ciba Foundation*, London, 1973.
12. Nuremberg Military Tribunal, *The Medical Case*, 181–183, 1947.
13. Refshange, W.: 1977, 'The Place of International Standards in Conducting Research on Humans', *Int. Conf. on Role of the Individual and the Community in the Research, Development, and Use of Biologicals*, WHO, Geneva.
14. Skegg, D. D. G.: 1975, 'Informed Consent to Medical Procedures', *Medicine, Science and Law* 15, 124–131.
15. Wolt, L. G.: 1961, 'Reflections on the Problems of Human Experimentation', *Connecticut Medicine* 25, 75–79.

ROBERT M. VEATCH

FEDERAL REGULATION OF MEDICINE AND BIOMEDICAL RESEARCH: POWER, AUTHORITY, AND LEGITIMACY

With federal regulators probing every nook and cranny of what used to be the decision-making domain of the private health care practitioner and medical researcher, it is understandable that the power, authority, and legitimacy of such regulation would be questioned. Three separate questions need to be addressed. The first is the most general: Is it legitimate in general to regulate any decisions in medicine? The second narrows the focus substantially to a rather small sub-set of medical decisions – those made by medical professionals. Is it legitimate to regulate decisions in medicine made by health professionals? Finally, it will be necessary to ask a question of a different order. Assuming it is legitimate to regulate some decisions made in medicine or at least regulate some decisions made by health care professionals, is it prudent to do so?

I. THE RIGHT TO REGULATE MEDICAL DECISIONS OF THE CITIZENRY

The first question may turn out to be deceptively difficult, even the hardest of the three: Does the federal government have the power, the authority, and the legitimation necessary to regulate any medical decisions at all? It is crucial to realize that the vast majority of medical decisions are not the ones that are normally thought of first as stereotypical medical decisions. The vast majority of medical decisions are made by citizens who are trained in medicine only in a rudimentary way. They are decisions made by lay people in an effort to improve, restore, or maintain their own health or the health of significant others who are family, friends, or acquaintances. When I take aspirin for a headache, apply a band-aid to my son's cut knee, or advise a next-door neighbor to avoid breathing the exhaust from his father's car, I make medical decisions. In fact, if one defines medicine as the institution in a society incorporating the beliefs, values, and practices in a society related to health and illness into social patterns and roles ([15], pp. 36–58), then countless decisions made daily by every citizen are appropriately seen as health decisions. When I decide to jog before breakfast, abstain from medicating myself with the nitrites in bacon, or help my child with his health education homework,

S. F. Spicker, J. M. Healey, and H. T. Engelhardt (eds.), The Law–Medicine Relation: A Philosophical Exploration, 75–91.

I make medical decisions. Only the smallest fraction of medical decisions are thus made by individuals with any special medical training or skill. That has been true since the beginning of societal institutionalization of medical practices and is still true in highly technologized, professionalized cultures such as our own.

Federal regulation of medicine, then, raises the most fundamental questions of political philosophy about the power, authority, and legitimacy of the government to control the lives of individuals. The power of a well-organized, stable government to regulate personal decisions seems beyond real doubt, but also quite uninteresting from the point of view of political philosophy. I am not going to address this question of sociology or political science. The questions of authority and legitimacy are quite another matter, however ([22], pp. 324–86). If consideration of pure power is excluded – whether that be physical or psychological or economic power – we are still left with the question of whether there is a legitimate basis for governmental intervention into our daily medical decisions: our decisions to self-medicate, refuse blood transfusions, use laetrile for our cancers, use penicillin for our viral influenzas, or conduct physiological research studies on our fellow human beings without gaining the permission of some federally legitimated review mechanism such as an institutional review board.

It is not obvious why a federal Food and Drug Administration should have the right to prohibit access to drugs simply because it has not found them to be adequately safe and effective by whatever definition of those terms and whatever set of values it has used to make such judgments ([11], pp. 507–11). Safety and efficacy are sometimes erroneously thought to be purely scientific questions to be resolved by the best pharmacological science available. No compound, however, is ever proved totally safe. At most we insist that it be safe enough given the purposes envisioned, the alternatives available, and the value of the effect anticipated. It is logically impossible to judge adequate safety without making value judgments. An experimental chemotherapeutic agent for a cancer does not have to meet the same safety requirements as a cold remedy. Safety is necessarily an evaluative judgment comparing benefits and harms envisioned.

Efficacy, likewise, is necessarily a value judgment. A compound is found effectively useful (as opposed to effectively harmful) only when the effect is a desired one. It is reported that the Spanish Pharmacopia describes estrogen-progesterone combinations as effective in regulating menstrual cycles, but as having a serious side effect of preventing pregnancy.

It is not easy to see why a federal agency, especially if it is staffed with professional scientists with their own sets of values and commitments, should have the authority to limit an individual citizen's right of access to such a compound simply because there is a disagreement about the value of the effects produced or the justifiability of the risks.

Federal regulation of drug use and other medical decisions by the citizen is not easy to justify. The legitimation of such regulation must be rooted in some fundamental societal understanding of the basic principles for the structure and function of the society. Every society will exist with some such set of principles. To the extent they are rooted in morality rather than mere power, they will reflect what has come to be called the moral point of view ([2], pp. 90–92). Rational people would agree to abide by some basic set of principles for organizing the society. Such contractual models for the establishing of a set of basic principles differ substantially over whether the task is the generation *de novo* of a set of principles that are an acceptable set or whether the task is the discovery of a set of pre-existing moral principles. In either case, the most basic principles are socially constructed, whether the construction is believed to reflect some underlying transcendent reality or not ([5], pp. 179–188). Traditionally, in both religious and secular thought, the rights and responsibilities making up the basic principles have been seen as discovered – rights that humans are endowed with by their Creator or that exist in the moral laws of nature.

Regardless of the underlying metaethical assumptions, members of the society are metaphorically seen as contracting or covenanting together to abide by some basic norms or principles. In modern thought, they include principles of liberty ('compatible with like liberty for all'), equality, and the duty of promise- or contract-keeping.

It is to these basic principles that one must turn if one is to discover if any legitimate basis for governmental regulation of medical decision-making exists. To the extent that liberty is one of those principles, the burden of proof is on those who favor federal regulation to constrain medical decisions of individuals or medical agreements among mutually consenting adults in private. If patient and physician agree among themselves that a service is to be performed at an agreed upon fee, it is difficult to see why the federal government should intervene. If a private practitioner wants to purchase a CAT scanner for his office, on what grounds can a government legitimately constrain the purchase? If adult medical lay people agree among themselves to share in providing abortion, counseling, or other 'self-help' services, on what grounds can a government legitimately constrain such agreements?

But to view such societally structured medical decisions as free choices by or among isolated individuals is naive. Necessary to any plausible contractarian view of social institutions is a recognition that the society pre-exists any individual in it and shapes the very values, preferences, and opportunities available. Moreover, many, perhaps all, decisions have enormous impacts on other parties. Externalities of decisions can be great. At the very least governments are justified in constraining individual medical decisions when they have significant detrimental impacts on other. Equality of liberty requires such governmental regulation. Thus parents are given great latitude in making day-to-day medical decisions for their children, but are not given unlimited discretion. They may choose to take certain risks with their child's health. They may decide not to have an infected wound examined by a medical professional or to tolerate a child's consumption of an unhealthful diet. They may not, however, refuse a medical treatment which, if offered, would restore the child safely, simply, and surely, to reasonably normal health ([17], especially pp. 183–90; [9], pp. 135–57).

Protection of the liberty and welfare of others provides the most obvious rationale for legitimate governmental intervention. It is supported by utilitarians and libertarians alike [14]. It easily justifies controls on the consumption of medicinals which, if ingested, would predictably put other parties at risk. If amphetamine consumption led predictably to violent behavior, it could justifiably be controlled. Alcohol could legitimately be controlled on account of its enormous deleterious impacts on innocent parties. Tobacco could be controlled because of its impact on passive smokers or the health insurance money pools of public or quasi-public groups, but not, on this basis, for purely paternalistic reasons. Very few other drugs, however, have such predictable, direct, harmful effects on others. Their regulation on the grounds that the liberty or rights or welfare of others will be jeopardized is implausible.

Another way in which individual liberty can have a detrimental impact on others is by conveying false or misleading information. Trust is essential in the contractual relationships among individuals of a society. Federal regulations which attempt to assure truthfulness in advertising and labelling are justifiable on these grounds. Regulation to assure that information is available that reasonable people would find in deciding to use medicinals also can be seen as furthering liberty and welfare of individuals. This still does not, however, provide a basis for controlling by federal regulation access to drugs and devices for individual use provided they will not have predictable, harmful impacts on others and provided they have been labelled with information that is truthful and information that reasonable people would find important. Federal regulation of the use (not the labelling) of laetrile, penicillin, morphine, or anti-depressants is indeed hard, if not impossible, to justify. Control of the practicing of medicine and related services such as psychotherapy without a license is hard, if not impossible, to justify. Those who are critical of the regulation of medical professionals in clinical and research settings stand in an important libertarian tradition out of which it is very difficult to justify federal regulation for reasons other than protection of the liberty and welfare of others.

Since basic liberties may be infringed by placing constraints on individual lay people to make medical decisions for themselves and other consenting parties, one way of preserving personal liberty while still assuring adequate information for making decisions would be to replace licensure of professionals with a certification process that provides reliable information to individuals about the qualifications (or lack thereof) of any person who wants to engage in medical practices. Under the basic principle of liberty, individuals would be able to make choices about how they want to be treated, and by whom, while still having a source of information necessary for making the choices. If one wanted to choose neurosurgery from someone trained only in hog butchering and knew what he was choosing, that decision would be permitted.

Serious problems with the replacement of licensure with certification may outweigh any of these advantages. For one, contraints would still have to be placed on practicing medicine on those who cannot consent. But if everyone had indiscriminate access to potent pharmacologicals, it would be extremely difficult to control their use on children, the mentally ill, and other non-consenting parties. Furthermore, if the privilege of practicing medicine were elevated to a right by shifting from licensure to certification, other privileges might quickly require the equivalent of licensure. The privilege of being reimbursed through governmental insurance mechanisms or obtaining the use of a governmentally funded operating room presumably should go only to those who will use the public's resources in ways acceptable to the public. Thus, while the principle of liberty might militate against licensure for purposes of self-medication and medical treatment among consenting adults at their own expense, the equivalent of licensure would be required for non-paternalistic reasons whenever the public interest or the interest of non-consenting parties was at stake.

Other basic principles of the society may also be a source of legitimation for regulation of lay medical decisions. Some principle of equity in distribution of social goods will necessarily be incorporated into a social contract that provides the basic principles of the society. In the name of providing equality of liberty, or in the name of equity more generally, some constraints on decisions by lay citizens may be justified. Some classes may have to be constrained in their medical behavior in order to prevent their choices from impacting on the medical liberties, welfare, and claims of justice of others. Society is so integrated that the isolated individual decision-maker is a mere fiction. Principles of justice may justify regulation that the principle of liberty would not.

Even pure paternalistic actions may be appropriate in certain situations. Prudent individuals would accept paternalistic actions on their behalf if, at some future time, they were found by some reasonable process to be incapable of acting freely, if, for instance, they became comatose or were judged by due process to be insane. They would insist on rigorous procedures so that their liberty would not be compromised when they possessed the capacity to choose in cases where only their interests were at stake. This seems to me to be one serious flaw in Siegler's and Goldblatt's essay. By the same token, prudent individuals would acknowledge the legitimacy of paternalistic actions on those who have been found by rigorous due process never to have been competent to act freely and competently.

Justification of federal regulation of individual medical decisions by citizens will be difficult. It may not be impossible. Protection of the claims of liberty and equity of others and protection of the welfare of those who do not possess the capacity for competent decision-making, may legitimate controls on medical decisions by lay people. A society might even exercise its liberty to contract with certain groups, identified by profession or by socialization into special roles, to provide certain functions seen as essential to the common good or required by the basic principles of the society.

II. THE RIGHT TO REGULATE MEDICAL PROFESSIONALS

A second social contract might be established – one between the society and professional groups [21]; for earlier suggestions of this contractual basis for the relation between the society and a profession see Veatch [20], Pellegrino [16], Magraw [13], and May [12]. While the first contract establishes the basic principles for ordering social institutions, the second would establish a relationship between the citizenry and a profession. In an exchange freely negotiated, the two groups might exchange pledges of mutual obligation in return for certain benefits that might accrue. From the liberties possessed by individuals and with the protection of the duty to keep contracts, citizens, professional and lay, may contract with one another, individually and collectively, binding one another with responsibilities and rights. These responsibilities and rights can be said to be acquired, that is acquired through individual or group action rather than derived directly from the more basic principles (cf. [8], pp. 5–9). Society, beginning in about the late Middle Ages, began to recognize professional groups, vesting them with substantial autonomy and monopolistic authority in exchange for certain responsibilities assumed by the professional group and certain benefits that would be gained by the society ([1], p. 28). Provided the second social contract does not violate any of the basic principles that are the basic constitutive elements of the society itself, such private arrangements can legitimately be transacted. In the name of liberty and the right to negotiate contracts such arrangements may be made. The rights and responsibilities of the professional group are thus derived from a second level of contract created by the society within the framework of its constitutive principles. Neophyte professionals, as they are socialized into the profession, are simultaneously socialized into the social contract establishing their rights and obligations vis-à-vis the society. The fact that each professional gains very concretely and very materially from the privileges granted by the society in the funding of medical education and the protection of the exclusive right to practice the craft reinforces the basic social contract between the profession and the society as a whole. Any professional student who accepts the benefits offered by the society and the privileges of licensure explicitly affirms his acceptance of the pre-existing professional contract.

If this is the basis of professional rights and responsibility rather than some internal, more particularistic self-generated professional moral code, then the legitimation of federal regulation of medical professionals may turn out to be much easier than the legitimation of federal regulation of medical decisions made by lay people. Lay people are governed by the first social contract and the practices and regulations growing out of it, while medical professionals are justifiably constrained as well by their explicit commitment to practice within the framework of regulation created by the broader society in exchange for the privileges that come from being a publicly licensed professional.

Since the right to regulate licensed professionals (as opposed to lay people or merely certified professionals) derives from this second social contract freely entered into by professionals (collectively and individually), it seems there are only two possible constraints on society's right to regulate professional medical behavior. First, the contract between the society and the profession is generated within the framework of the basic principles of the first social contract. If there are any restraints on individual and collective decision-making implied by that first contract – and we have seen that it is quite hard to defend such constraints – they would place limits on the content of the contract with professionals. For instance, it is often argued that commitment to the principle of liberty makes a contract to sell oneself permanently into slavery illegitimate. If that constraint exists, a profession and the broader society would be enjoined from any contract giving the society the right to regulate professional behavior in a way that was comparable to enslavement. Permanent societal regulation of the terms, location, fees, and specialty of practice might not be an acceptable condition of the second contract if these were tantamount to having professionals sell themselves into slavery. In reality the profession is not about to agree to arrangements with the society that permits this degree of federal regulation. Lesser stipulations by society, in exchange for the rights and privileges of practicing medicine, however, are not at all incompatible with our basic commitment to liberty, equality and contract-keeping which presumes that free individuals will have the right to contract, as individuals and as groups, in such a way that regulation constrained their terms, location, fees, and specialty of practice. Physicians, when they agree to the terms of licensure, pledge to be bound by the regulations accompanying that license and the procedures established for changing those regulations.

A second limit on the right to regulate might be imposed by the nature of the contract between the society and the profession itself. If I am right in seeing this as a second level of social contract, then contractual agreements made between the profession and the society giving certain freedoms to the profession, might themselves constrain regulation. A society could include within its contractual agreement with the profession the right to regulate fees under certain circumstances. It could also contract in such a way that it surrendered any such right during the period of the contract. Should it concede any authority to regulate in its understanding with the profession, this would remain as a limit on the right to regulate for the duration of the agreement subject only to the prior constraints on the right to contract. If society suddenly decides it wants to regulate but foolishly concedes its right to regulate a particular area, it may find itself in an unfortunate position of having made a bad deal.

Thus there are only two limits on society's right to regulate licensed professionals. First, society cannot violate its own basic constitutive principles. Second, it cannot renege on previous promises made to professionals. Other than these constraints any regulation in exchange for licensure is legitimate. Of course, if licensure were replaced by simple certification of the training and skills of citizens, society's right to regulate through the contract between the society and the profession would disappear. No contracts granting privilege and monopoly would exist, and individuals, certified or not, would be able to engage in practices limited only by the first contract.

If this is the proper understanding of the limits on the right of the government to regulate, then it will be crucial to understand the time frame of the various contracts. The rights and obligations of the original social contract appear to be without time limit. Furthermore, if society is such that all participate in the complex social institutions and the privileges of citizenship before they have the capacity to accept or reject the contract, then each individual backs into the basic principles accepting them and acting within their framework before he ever has the chance to reflect on them. Such an individual has limited chance to reject the principle by surrendering his citizenship, but excluding such limited opportunities for renegotiating, he is bound in perpetuity.

Other contracts arrived at within the context of the basic, enduring principles are quite another matter. Private contracts are bound by certain limits. Some kinds of commitment in perpetuity are unacceptable. It seems like similar limits must be placed on the contract between the society and a profession. Renegotiations may be seen as taking place once in a lifetime as new professionals enter the field. This would explain the widespread use of grandfather clauses giving established professionals the right to practice in spite of the fact that they do not meet requirements of education or skill imposed on newly licensed professionals. Some pharmacists practicing today have had no more than two years of college training in spite of the fact that five years or more is now required of those being licensed today.

Another point for possible renegotiation would be at the time of license renewal. Licenses to practice are increasingly being seen as limited grants of privileges subject to renewal with imposition of re-examinations and other requirements. Possibly renegotiation which would give the society the right to regulate what it had previously surrendered might take place at the time of recertification.

Regardless of how the specific problems of renegotiation of the contract between society and the profession are solved, the notion of a second social contract entered into freely by professionals provides a very different basis of federal regulation than the basis that may exist for federal regulating of lay medical decisions. The right to regulate professional decisions in clinical and research settings seems to be very broad indeed, limited only by the constraints placed on individuals and groups to contract with one another and accepted, acquired rights and responsibilities.

III. THE WISDOM OF REGULATING MEDICAL PROFESSIONALS

The thesis that professionals are in a social contractual relationship with the larger society bound by the most basic principles of the society, provides a basis for understanding the *right* of society to regulate legitimately, but it does not answer the more critical question of whether it is *prudent* for a society to regulate its professionals. Assuming at least some such regulation is prudent, it does not reveal when and how such regulation would be wise. Since our basic societal principles emphasize liberty subject to the constraints of justice, promise-keeping, and other fundamental values, it would be understandable if, whenever possible, society chose not to regulate – that is, chose not to exercise its right to regulate. It will regulate only when basic principles require it or when necessary for the general welfare.

Consider as an example the contemporary debate about the definition of death and governmental efforts to regulate some aspects of medical professional decisions vis-à-vis the definition of death ([19], pp. 21–76). As part of the traditional arrangements between society and the profession, professionals had both the exclusive right and the responsibility for pronouncing death. Individual professionals have been given substantial discretion for determining exactly when a person ought to be called dead and what measures ought to be used for determining that death ought to be pronounced. As long as there was virtually no debate of any practical significance, practitioners were left much to their own to make such judgments without regulation. Common law did, however, impose certain restrictions. The physician was obligated to pronounce death when, and only when, the judgment was made that all vital functions had ceased irreversibly.

The decision to call a person dead and to initiate all of the social behaviors that accompany death pronouncement was essentially a social decision, not one based on medical facts. If someone had proposed to call a person dead when his brain function had irreversibly ceased even if other functions continued, there would be no biological basis for favoring one social policy over the other. No one raised that possibility; at least no one pressed it, perhaps because the distinction made no practical difference.

Once it became possible, however, to maintain other vital functions of a person whose brain had ceased functioning, the social policy choice became important. Society could have left physicians unregulated, permitting them to choose to call a person dead either when the brain ceased or when all vital functions ceased. That would have led to policy chaos, however. Society could have left to the profession the task of making the social policy choice. If so, the profession would have been acting as a surrogate for the society, not making a judgment about which its training gave it any special expertise, but acting as society's agent for the purpose of choosing among two rather plausible options for deciding when to call a person dead.

We are left with the question of when it is prudent for society to leave such judgments to the professional group, trusting it to make a choice that society can accept, and when it should take matters into its own hands establishing statutory law, case law, or other regulation that specifies that a person shall be called dead when certain functions cease irreversibly.

Since it is generally easier to leave matters to individuals exercising common sense than to attempt to force their behavior by regulation, it is often prudent to forego acting on the right to regulate. Two conditions make it particularly prudent for society not to regulate professional behavior. If the question at stake is believed to be one in which the profession as a whole or practitioners as individuals will reach the same decisions that the society would incorporate into regulations, then society might decide not to regulate. Unless lay people particularly want to be involved in the actual decision-making, they might cede their authority to professionals. The same decisions would result. In an earlier day, no regulation of death pronouncement was necessary because the overwhelming consensus of wise physicians differed not at all from the consensus of prudent lay people. Individual practitioners, to be sure, might deviate just as individual people did. But it was in the profession's interest to control such deviants. Aggressive societal intervention was unnecessary.

Now, however, there is an enormous range of views on the subject [7]. Some argue the shift to a concept based on loss of brain function is too liberal ([10], pp. 132–40), while others claim that it is too conservative. They argue that it would permit some people to be considered alive who really ought to be considered dead ([6]; [19], pp. 13–30). Furthermore, since the question is one not answerable with biological or neurological evidence, disagreement also exists among medical professionals. If the distribution of the views in the medical profession followed the same pattern as that in the rest of society, then society might reasonably still leave the question to the professional group. The only thing given up by society in that case would be the right to make the decision about social policy directly.

But the pattern of distribution of views in any professional group is often not the same as in the society at large. Those choosing to enter any profession hold values that do not reflect the values of the larger society. In this case, it appears that neurologically trained people are more willing to consider the functions of the brain to be the essentially significant functions for deciding a person ought to be treated as alive. Regardless of how the values held by the professional group differ from those held by the rest of society, the delegation of policy-making authority by the society to the profession on important issues when there are value differences makes no sense. It is plausible and prudent for society to regulate through its publicly legitimated authority. If physicians really hold the values expressed by Siegler and Goldblatt – and I'm afraid some do – society would be foolish to trust physicians' clinical intuitions on matters literally as crucial as life and death and personal freedom.

Even if there are values held by the profession that differ from those of the broader society, the society might choose to forego regulation when the issues at stake are trivial. In an earlier day, it could have required that two physicians jointly pronounce death, that an entire team of practitioners take on the task, or that certain specific procedures be used for measuring the irreversible cessation of vital functions. Although the decisions at stake were critical – literally life and death – the variation in pronouncing death that would result from imposing such regulations was not. The differences in techniques for measuring the cessation of functions would lead to differences in death pronouncement that were trivial. Society, in its wisdom, chose not to regulate such decisions. When the results will be trivial, society would often be wise not to regulate even if the professional holds values that differ from the lay person.

If, however, there is a good reason to believe that the professional group will base its decisions on a different set of values or beliefs than those held by the broader society and the differences in behavior will not be trivial, then it is foolish for society to fail to exercise its right to regulate.

This is why it makes no sense for society functioning through governmental agencies to endorse professional self-regulation and professional enforcement of their own codes of ethics. Some states regulate through licensure requiring that licenses can be suspended for unprofessional conduct. If society rather than the profession defines what is unprofessional conduct, that is reasonable, but the term implies that the limits of acceptable behavior will be defined by the profession and its code. Some states mistakenly turn over to the professional organization or to members of the profession, adjudication of questions of professional misconduct. It is essential to a profession that it generate its own code based on values and commitments internal to the profession ([3], pp. 669–88). A professional code is, thus, radically different from a contract or covenant negotiated between the society and the profession ([16], pp. 29–31). A code is an autonomously generated summary of the standards embraced by a group based on its own, often particularistic values. No justification to the broader society is necessary. It is not even possible according to many views of professional ethics.

To the extent that a professional code is based on professionally held values rather than publicly held ones and to the extent the value differences are significant and the resulting behavioral differences are not trivial, society is foolish if it legitimates enforcement of the profession's code rather than the social contracts providing the basic principles for organizing the society's institutions and the relationship of lay people with professionals.

Under these circumstances it is a mistake for society to cede to the professional group the authority to determine the concept of death used for pronouncing a person dead. It is especially foolish if there is any evidence that the professional group as a whole holds philosophical, religious, or other evaluative positions that differ from the broader society.

There is substantial evidence that on many crucial philosophical and ethical value questions the profession does differ from the broader society. Since decisions, if left to professionals, would impact directly on non-professionals, we have precisely the circumstances where society ought to regulate the profession in mandating the concept of death to be used by professionals. No professional need be bound by such societal regulation. He has the option, under normal circumstances, of ceasing to be bound by the contract by the society and the profession. But then he must surrender his privileges as well as his obligations.

A similar analysis explains why society has the authority to impose regulations on professionals in the prescribing of drugs. Society does not permit a physician to prescribe heroin – no matter what we may think of society's judgment and no matter what individual practitioners may think about the humaneness of using heroin in caring for terminal cancer patients. If society holds values that it considers central and if it believes individual practitioners or the profession as a whole holds different values, it has the right to regulate medical practitioners. It also would be wise in doing so.

If society would be wise in regulating the behavior of professionals, it would be foolish to delegate to those professionals or some of their group the authority to make the key evaluative choices. The FDA, for example, should be seen as an arm of social policy. To the extent that it imposes restriction on the behavior of lay people who are citizens, it must confront the arguments against the right of the society to regulate the medical decisions of individual citizens. Its legitimacy in regulating health professionals' decisions to use unapproved drugs or use approved drugs for unapproved uses is a totally different matter. It has the right to control practitioners' behavior and is wise in doing so whenever there is reason to fear that practitioners will act on values that differ significantly from those of the larger society and when the consequences will be other than trivial.

At the same time if the FDA is an agency of society that may legitimately regulate professionals and possibly may even legitimately regulate the behavior of lay citizens, it is a mistake to turn over the decision-making of such an agency to professionals used to staff it. The FDA is, and ought to be, a political animal regulating professionals and lay people in ways based on societally held values within the constraints of the basic principles of the social contract. Society as a whole may hold different values about risk-taking in the use of saccharin or level of certainty in evaluating evidence about the use of laetrile. They may hold different values regarding the benefits and harms of the alternatives to these chemicals.

Federal regulations requiring consent for the use of human subjects for medical research can be defended on the same basis. All ought to recognize that there are disutilities of requiring consent. They exist especially in those rare cases when researchers believe they have good reason for not obtaining consent. It seems, however, that the fact that a researcher believes consent should not be obtained is not enough reason for society to forego a regulation requiring consent. The difference in perception regarding a requirement of consent may be accounted for on a number of bases.

Some may argue that medical professionals cannot be trusted to act with good will in the absence of regulation. There is some evidence that some researchers are lacking in good will ([4], p. 51). That by itself, however, does not seem to be an adequate reason for justifying regulation. In the first place, the number of researchers lacking good will is small. Almost never have I encountered outright evil intent on the part of either researchers or clinicians. Even if practitioners lacking good will did exist, the interests in the profession in controlling those that were so outrageously malevolent might be great enough to motivate intra-professional regulation. That mechanism has worked successfully in dealing with a small number of seriously malevolent practitioners. If lack of good will were the problem, elaborate regulations requiring consent or other standards of professional conduct might be expendable.

That is not the problem, however. The real problem is a difference in basic value commitment. Clinicians are traditionally committed to doing what they think will benefit their patients. Researchers are uniquely committed to doing what they think will produce the greatest good. With some exception both groups have a good record of acting in good faith on those commitments. But neither value commitment corresponds with the values of the broader society committed to liberty, equality, fidelity to promises, and a set of values quite alien to traditional professional ethics.

The alternative to federal regulation on questions such as consent is reliance on the well-intentioned intuition of a group whose individual judgments may, to some extent, be based on values that differ significantly from those who value self-determination. If the lay population relied on professional judgment of those not seeing self-determination as inherently critical, the citizens' right to self-determination would be violated, at least in certain cases. It would be violated in all clinical cases where physicians were committed to serving the patient's interest and believed it was in the patient's interest not to obtain consent. It would also be violated in all research cases where researchers were committed uniquely to the principle of producing the greater good on balance and thought that on balance greater good would be served by not getting consent. The only prudent course when professionals are given authority to act and yet are believed to hold values differing from those upon whom they must act, is for society to enact regulations requiring behaviors valued by lay people such as getting consent.

The final stand for those who oppose federal regulation might well be a retreat to the fact/value distinction claiming that at least in technical areas of medicine, regulators ought to refrain from regulating. Sophisticated professionals might concede that many FDA decisions are really judgments based on values or on commitments to ethical principles such as liberty. They might concede that obtaining consent in problematic cases will depend on whether one values self-determination or wants to maximize benefits to the patient or society. They might concede that the basic conceptual questions about when to call a person dead are essentially philosophical; that no medical training helps one decide whether to call a person dead when his neurological function or circulatory function ceases irreversibly. They might accept the legitimacy of regulation in these areas.

They might still hold out, however, for freedom from regulation in more technical areas such as deciding whether there is any evidence of tumor regression after laetrile testing, whether there will be psychological harm from informing a patient he is in a cancer chemotherapy protocol, or whether in using an electroencephalogram for measuring the irreversible loss of brain function the period of testing ought to be 24 hours or whether it can be reduced to six hours or one hour or even dispensed with entirely. These, at least, they argue, are purely scientific questions that should remain outside the grasp of the federal regulators safely tucked into the protecting arms of the professional group with scientific expertise in the area.

The prudent society will normally leave such technical questions free from regulation. But even these questions are not totally outside the rational oversight of the broader society in situations when significant social policy decisions must be made based on such seemingly purely scientific or technical questions. It is increasingly recognized that no scientific questions totally escape evaluative, ethical, metaethical, and metaphysical assumptions. Occasionally, although I believe it is quite rare, basic questions of value or world view, basic philosophical assumptions or underlying systems of theory and belief, will significantly impinge on judgments that at first seem purely technical. It is impossible to prove that laetrile does not cure cancer, only that evidence at an acceptance level of confidence seems to reasonable people to lead to the conclusion it is useless. Judgments based on philosophical and other beliefs and values will necessarily enter these evaluations at the point of deciding what level of confidence is acceptable, what constitutes reasonableness, and what outcomes are useless. The broader society should be aware that if it defers judgments, even in these technical matters, to professional experts, there is a risk that a judgment will be made that would not have been made by lay people if, by some miraculous transposition, they were to gain the knowledge of the experts and retain the values they now hold as lay people. Fortunately, this need not often be a problem. The risks of public intervention in such areas through federal regulation may produce more harm than good. The same criteria emerge, however, as in instances when a decision must be made by society whether to regulate professionals in their policy making roles. If the basic values differ significantly and the questions being asked are not trivial, then the public should be concerned about the possibility that even on apparently technical matters judgments may be made that would not have been made by lay people holding differing values. In such cases federal regulation may turn out to be a prudent protection. The risks of such intervention, especially in the areas normally thought of as the scientific domain, are great. It is not illogical, however, for the public to insist on such regulation as part of its social contract with the profession.

Georgetown University
Washington, D. C.

BIBLIOGRAPHY

1. Amundsen, D.: 1978, 'The Physician's Duty to Prolong Life: A Medical Duty Without Classical Roots', *Hastings Center Report* 8(4), 23–30.
2. Baier, K.: 1965, *The Moral Point of View*, Random House, New York.
3. Barber, B.: 1963, 'Some Problems in the Sociology of the Professions', *Daedalus* 92, 669–88.
4. Barber, B., *et al.*: 1973, *Research on Human Subjects*, Russell Sage, New York.
5. Berger, P.: 1967, *The Sacred Canopy*, Doubleday, Garden City, New York.
6. Brierley, J., *et al.*: 1971, 'Neocortical Death After Cardiac Arrest', *The Lancet* (Sept. 11), 560–65.
7. Charron, W.: 1975, 'Death: A Philosophical Perspective on the Legal Definitions', *Washington University Law Quarterly* (No. 4), 979–1008.
8. Feinberg, J.: 1970, *Doing and Deserving: Essays in the Theory of Responsibility*, Princeton University Press, Princeton, N. J.
9. Holder, A.: 1977, *Legal Issues in Pediatrics and Adolescent Medicine*, John Wiley, New York.
10. Jonas, H.: 1974, 'Against the Stream', in *Philosophical Essays*, Prentice-Hall, Englewood Cliffs, N. J., pp. 132–10.
11. Lasagna, L.: 1976, 'Drug Discovery and Introduction: Regulation and Overregulation', *Clinical Pharmacology and Therapeutics* 20(5), 507–11.
12. May, W.: 1975, 'Code, Covenant, Contract, or Philanthropy', *Hastings Center Report* 5(6), 29–38.
13. Magraw, R.: 1973, 'Science and Humanism: Medicine and Existential Anguish', in Roger J. Bulger (ed.), *Hippocrates Revisited*, Medcom Press, New York, pp. 148–57.
14. Mill, J.: 1956, *On Liberty*, The Liberal Arts Press, New York.
15. Parsons, T.: 1951, *The Social System*, The Free Press, New York.
16. Pellegrino, E.: 1973, 'Toward an Expanded Medical Ethics: The Hippocratic Ethic Revisited', in Roger J. Bulger (ed.), *Hippocrates Revisited*, Medcom Press, New York, pp. 133–47.
17. Swinyard, C.: 1978, *Decision Making and the Defective Newborn*, Charles C. Thomas, Springfield, Illinois.
18. Veatch, R.: 1975, 'The Whole-Brain-Oriented Concept of Death', *Journal of Thanatology* 3(No. 1), 13–30.
19. Veatch, R.: 1976, *Death, Dying, and the Biological Revolution*, Yale University Press, New Haven, Connecticut.
20. Veatch, R.: 1976, *Value-Freedom in Science and Technology*, Scholars Press, Missoula, Montana.
21. Veatch, R.: 1979, 'Professional Medical Ethics', *Journal of Medicine and Philosophy* 4(1), 1–19.
22. Weber, M.: 1964, *The Theory of Social and Economic Organization*, The Free Press, New York.

SECTION II

CAUSATION AND RESPONSIBILITY: SCIENCE, MEDICINE AND THE LAW

KENNETH F. SCHAFFNER

CAUSATION AND RESPONSIBILITY: MEDICINE, SCIENCE AND THE LAW

I. INTRODUCTION

The topics I shall address – causation and responsibility in medicine, science, and the law – represent a most interesting set of concepts which I believe have important areas of overlap. Unfortunately, to discuss all of these topics would require far more space than is available. I will attempt to draw on what scholars – who have thought deeply about causation in the law and in science – have written, and will argue for a *unitary* conception of causal explanation in medicine, in science, and in *some* legal contexts. I shall treat the issue of responsibility only briefly but I will argue that my unitary thesis has some interesting implications for a theory of error in medicine, and accordingly, for notions of responsibility and for malpractice law.

My argument will require a review of some of the past and recent literature on causal explanation in law, in science, and in everyday contexts. Occasionally I shall resort to technical philosophical language, and one biomedical example, but I hope that I also provide sufficient translation of the language and the example so that the central ideas will be salient and clear.

II. HART, HONORÉ, AND MACKIE ON CAUSATION AND CAUSAL EXPLANATION

For reasons which will become clearer I shall outline a position defended by H. L. A. Hart and A. M. Honoré which has been influential in the legal area, and then consider a recent alternative to that position, one which is proposed by John Mackie in *The Cement of the Universe*.

In 1959, Hart and Honoré, in their scholarly and seminal study, *Causation in the Law*, began by noting that lawyers

> have rejected philosophical theories [of causation] usually with the insistence that the lawyer's causal problems are not 'scientific inquests' but are to be determined 'on common-sense principles'. Similar dissatisfaction with what the philosopher has hitherto tendered as an analysis of the meaning of causation is often expressed by saying that this analysis, although doubtless adequate for the *scientist's* causal notions, distorts what the historian does, or attempts to do, in identifying the causes of particular events ([16], p. 8).

S. F. Spicker, J. M. Healey, and H. T. Engelhardt (eds.), The Law–Medicine Relation: A Philosophical Exploration, 95–122.

Though Hart and Honoré view Hume, and especially John Stuart Mill, as offering helpful suggestions, they believe they can provide a more realistic account of causation in the law. Essentially they argue for a *typology* of different analyses of causation since, in their view, causality is a "cluster of related concepts" ([16], p. 17).

The central notion of causality is one which Hart and Honoré believe is a generalization of our primitive experiences in the world:

Human beings have learnt, by making appropriate movements of their bodies, to bring about desired alterations in objects, animate or inanimate, in their environment, to express these simple achievements by transitive verbs like push, pull, bend, twist, break, injure. The process involved here consists of an initial immediate bodily manipulation of the thing affected and often takes little time ([16], p. 26).

These experiences lead to a realization that secondary changes as a result of such movements can occur, and for such (a series of) changes "we use the correlative terms 'cause' and 'effect' rather than simple transitive verbs . . . " ([16], p. 27). The root idea of cause for Hart and Honoré arises out of the way human action intrudes into a series of changes and *makes a difference* in the way a course of events develops ([16], p. 27). Such a notion, these authors maintain, is as central to causation as is the notion of constant conjunction or invariable sequence stressed by Hume and Mill. The concept of cause is also generalized by analogy to include not only active elements, but also static, passive, and even negative elements, such as the icy condition of the road causing an accident, or the lack of rain causing a crop failure ([16], p. 28–29).

Hart and Honoré agree that the concept of causation and the concept of explanation are often closely associated:

The use of the word 'cause' in ordinary life extends far beyond the relatively simple cases where 'effects' are deliberately produced by human actions: it is also generally used whenever an *explanation* is sought of an occurrence by which we are puzzled because we do not understand why it has occurred.

An explanation of this facet of causation leads Hart and Honoré to analyze (1) the distinction between causes and conditions, and (2) the types of generalizations that are involved in singular causal statements. Such distinctions as exist between causes and conditions (which are also necessary to produce an effect) are subtle and complex, but seem to depend on two contrasts: "between what is abnormal and what is normal, and between a free deliberate human action and all other conditions" ([16], p. 31).

Causes tend to be identified with abnormal conditions, and to the first approximation Hart and Honoré suggest that normal conditions are usual conditions. Such a judgment, however, is often context-dependent. A special laboratory from which oxygen is normally excluded suggests that the presence of oxygen will be construed as a *cause* of fire rather than a condition. Practical interests including controllability may also dictate which element is identified as the cause, i.e., what 'makes the difference' in a series of conditions. Furthermore, the distinction between cause and condition is often strongly affected by 'human habit, custom, or convention'. 'Normal' conditions may be established by law, for example, so the cause of a measles epidemic may be seen as the *failure* of a number of parents to have their children immunized. The identification of a cause in a series of necessary and/or sufficient conditions may also be the consequence of a search for an explanation. For example, if a death (or injury) occurs, many elements could be cited as the cause, such as heart cessation or lack of oxygen in the brain. The focus of interest may be not on those universal elements but rather on why this death (or injury) *occurred rather than* that a healthy human continued to exist.

Hart and Honoré also maintain that 'voluntary human action' plays a special role in causal inquiries:

> because . . . when the question is how far back a cause shall be traced through a number of intervening causes, such a voluntary action very often is regarded both as a limit and also as still the cause even though other later abnormal occurrences are recognized as causes ([16], p. 39).

Hart and Honoré's position on causal generalizations raises several important points:

First, Hart and Honoré importantly depart (as does Mackie) from a regularity theory of causation such as we find in Hume and Mill. In a regularity theory, the central idea is the analysis of causation as one of an invariable sequence of events in nature. This implies that a causal claim involves a tacit generalization which asserts such an invariable sequence. Hart and Honoré note, however, (*contra* Mill) that often a *singular* causal statement is made with a degree of confidence which we would *not* attribute to any exceptionless generalizations of which it was an instance. They also do not think that relaxing the 'exceptionless' qualification to one that holds in 'most cases' will provide the clarification needed. Mill's position, that we single out a cause from a complex set of conditions which *invariably* produces an effect, is seen as *a radical misrepresentation* ([16], p. 42). Rather what occurs, Hart and Honoré contend, is that we begin with 'rough rubics of common experience' when we ascertain that a cause has produced an effect, for example when we discern that a blow caused a child's broken leg. We need not have detailed scientific knowledge of the effects of impacts on bones of varying thickness, unless we need to *predict* the effect. But prediction is not usually demanded, since legal and common-sense interests in causal claims are primarily inquests that occur *after* an event has happened. It is sufficient that there exist some broad generalizations that cover the particular case of interest as well as "similar cases differing from it in detail" ([16], pp. 43–44).

The generalizations to which one appeals to provide explanatory but not predictive force do not necessarily involve high probabilities. Hart and Honoré cite the example that "diphtheria now very *rarely* causes death" ([16], p. 45).

A causal inquiry often does make use of generalizations from the applied sciences as part of a defense against counterexamples or rival, alternatively possibly causal claims. This is an important point which reveals the main function of generalization in Hart and Honoré's thesis.

> The generalizations implied in singular causal statements are not statements of 'unconditional and invariable sequence' and the sense in which the cause is sufficient to produce its consequence is not defined in this strict way. The generalizations involved are statements of general connection between broadly described types of event which are brought to bear on particular cases distinguished from counterexamples ... ([16], pp. 105–106).

Such a comparative inquiry designed to rule our rival explanations is distinguished, however, from the deductively organized explanation, more akin to Mill's position, which one might find in, for example, an account of the cause of a machine's failure.

Hart and Honoré distinguish causal analyses of the type discussed thus far (where physical interactions are involved and what Mackie calls the 'physical' type, even though a human action may be a component), from a *different type* of causal notion involving *purely* human interaction. In this latter type, which is termed 'interpersonal transactions', we have to deal with "the concept of *reasons* for actions rather than *causes* of events ... " ([16], p. 48). Examples of inducement, temptation, and ordering illustrate this class of interactions. Hart and Honoré do admit, however, that the distinction between causation and interpersonal transactions becomes vague in certain cases. Generalizations, Hart and Honoré claim, though they do have a place in such 'interpersonal' analyses, are 'less central' than in the previous type of inquiry. In addition they distinguish another "class of relationships between persons which have analogies with interpersonal transactions", namely providing "an opportunity for doing something".[1]

In a defense of a 'unitary' theory of causation as against Hart's and Honoré's at least dualistic schema, John Mackie contends that the main distinction which Hart and Honoré perceive between 'physical' and 'interpersonal' causation is due to their conceding too much to Mill in the physical sphere. Recall that Hart and Honoré admit the significance of generalizations in an analysis of causal sequences in their first type of causality, but stress the lack of such generalizations in the interpersonal area. Mackie, to an extent following C. J. Ducasse [7] before him, argues that "it is only in very tenuous senses that any singular causal statements are implicitly general" ([20], p. 121). For Mackie, and to some extent for Hart and Honoré, elliptical generalizations are not *part* of causal claims, rather they are better conceived of as *evidence* or background information that "will sustain the counterfactual conditionals involved in [a specific] singular causal statement" ([20], p. 121). Mackie wants to go further than Hart and Honoré and maintain that causal claims do not even *need* such evidence: "the elliptical generalization can be discovered and (tentatively) established by the observation of the very same individual sequence the conditionals about which it may be said to sustain". The role of elliptical generalizations for Mackie is perhaps more importantly to "inform us of the *irrelevance* of various other changes in the spatio-temporal neighborhood of the observed sequence . . . " ([20], p. 122).[2]

Mackie's account begins with Hume's problem of causality: how can we distinguish causal from non-causal (or accidental) sequences: if Y follows after X, under what conditions and with what warrant can we claim that X caused Y? One common-sense way of analyzing such causality is to say that X caused Y if Y would not have happened if X had not happened. Unfortunately this will not do, at least without further qualification, since there might be *other* causes of Y.

Mackie goes on to provide an analysis of these qualifications, and pauses to discuss the distinctions between causes and conditions which are already encountered in the review of Hart and Honoré. Basically Mackie agrees that *necessary in the circumstances* plus another relation, that of *causal priority*, are the appropriate qualifications. Appeal to specific circumstances allows him to outflank difficult issues involving causal overdetermination. The notion of causal priority means "that the world has some way of running on from one change to another" ([20], p. 51). This notion has to be unpacked further if it is to be helpful, and Mackie does this by arguing that X can be shown to be *sufficient* in the circumstances in a weak, i.e., non-counterfactual sense, *and* causally prior, by a straightforward experiment in this world: we put X into the world and then Y occurs ([20], p. 51). However, "necessity and sufficiency in a strong sense plus causal priority involve counterfactual claims", i.e., these more important concepts require appeals to "how the world *would have* run on if something different *had been* done and this type of appeal involves reference to an alternative possible world(s)" ([20], p. 52). We construct these alternative worlds in both unsophisticated ways, by imagination and analogy, and in a more sophisticated manner by using general propositions with appeals to inductive and deductive reasoning. It is this need for an alternative world, however, which reveals the central importance of Mill's *method of difference*. This method is a codification of the need for contrast cases that, according to Mackie, "contribute most to our primitive concept of causation" ([20], p. 57).

In an attempt to determine the extent to which (as well as the manner in which) generalizations are involved in causal claims, Mackie reviews some of the advances due to Mill, but in addition goes beyond him. Mill recognized the complication of a plurality of causes by which several different assemblages of factors, say *ABC* as well as *DGH* and *JKL*, might each be sufficient to bring about an effect *P*. Let us now understand these letters to represent types rather than tokens. Then if (*ABC* or *DGH* or *JKL*) is both necessary and sufficient for *P*, how do we describe the *A* in such a generalization? Such an element is for Mackie an *insufficient* but *non-redundant* part of an *unnecessary* but *sufficient* condition – which Mackie kindly decides to call an *inus* condition. Using this terminology, then, what is usually termed a cause is an *inus* condition. But our knowledge of causal regularities are seldom *fully* and *completely* characterized: we know some of the *inus* conditions but rarely all possible ones.

Causal regularities are, according to Mackie, "*elliptical* or *gappy* universal propositions" ([20], p. 66). One can represent this using Mackie's formalism invoking Anderson's notion of a cause field of background conditions, *F*, which focuses our attention on some specific area and/or subject of inquiry, and note that:

> In F, all ($A \ldots \bar{B} \ldots$ or $D \ldots \bar{H} \ldots$ or $\ldots$) are followed by P and, in F, all P are preceded by ($A \ldots \bar{B} \ldots$ or $D \ldots \bar{H} \ldots$ or $\ldots$).

The bar above *B* and *H* indicates that these types are functioning as negative causes in this generalization.

Though such an account of causal regularities on the surface looks quite unhelpful, Mackie argues, and I agree with him, that such "gappy universal propositions [or] incompletely known complex regularities, which contribute to . . . [causal] inferences will sustain, with probability, the counterfactual conditionals that correspond to these inferences", and also that the gappy universal will "equally sustain the subjunctive conditional that, if this cause occurred again in *sufficiently similar* circumstances, so would the effect . . ." ([20], p. 68, my emphasis). Mackie leaves open what the notion of "sufficiently similar circumstances" might mean.[3]

III. THE DEBATES CONCERNING UNIVERSAL GENERALIZATIONS AND PREDICTION IN SCIENTIFIC EXPLANATION

Those acquainted with contemporary philosophy of science will recognize in what has been presented thus far several often discussed themes. A debate concerning the nature of explanation in general and scientific explanation in particular began in the forties. Issues such as the necessity of generalizations in historical and everyday explanation, whether explanations have to be predictive, and also whether reasons are causes, have been the central concern of an immense number of books and articles in philosophy of science and philosophy in general. The writings of Gallie [9], Dray [6], Gardiner [10], Scriven ([28], [29]), and Hempel [17] are perhaps the most prominent in the domain of the philosophy of science.

I shall now turn to a review of some of these issues, tending to agree with Hempel's position as elegantly argued in his *Aspects of Scientific Explanation*.

A. *The D-N, D-S, I-S, and S-R Models*

The extant models of scientific explanation include the deductive-nomological or D-N model, the deductive-statistical or D-S model, the inductive-statistical or I-S model, and the statistical-relevance or S-R model. I will concentrate on the I-S and S-R models.

The deductive-nomological or D-N model is probably the ideal form of scientific explanation. There are foreshadowings of it in Aristotle's *Posterior Analytics* and it is discussed, though not under that name, in Mill's *A System of Logic*. Today it is closely associated with the work of Hempel and Oppenheim, who about thirty years ago argued for it in an extremely clear and influential article [18]. Hempel has also been its principal exponent and defender [17].

Schematically, the deductive-nomological model can be presented as follows:

$$\frac{\begin{array}{l} L_1 \ldots L_n \\ C_1 \ldots C_k \end{array}}{E}$$

where the L's are universal laws and the C's represent initial conditions. E is a sentence which describes the event to be explained. In this model E follows *deductively* from the conjunction of the law or nomological premises and the statements describing the initial conditions.[4] This type of explanation can be found in the science of mechanics and in physics in general.

If the premises involve *statistical* generalizations the model changes. If the generalizations are operated on deductively to generate an explanation sentence, as in population genetics with infinite populations, we have an instance of deductive-statistical or D-S explanation. Far more interesting, however, are those situations in which one wants to explain an event in which the sentence describing that event only follows *with probability* from a set of premises. For example, following Hempel, if we wish to explain John Jones's recovery from a streptococcus infection, we might refer to the fact that he had been given penicillin. There is, however, no general, *universal* exceptionless law which requires *all* individuals who have been given penicillin to recover from such an infection. At most we can schematize the logical relation under the I-S model as:

> The statistical probability of recovery from severe streptococcal infections with penicillin administration *is close to 1.*
>
> John Jones had severe streptococcal infection and was given penicillin.
>
> ═══════════════════════════════
>
> John Jones recovered from the infection.

Here the double line does not stand for a *deductive* inference but means: "makes practically certain (very likely)". The double line accordingly represents *inductive* support, thus the appellation "inductive-statistical model". A very large percentage of explanations in the biomedical sciences has this inductive-statistical character.

The I-S model has several peculiarities not usually associated with the D-N model. For example, it should be obvious were John Jones severely allergic to penicillin that his recovery would not have been close to 1 – he might have died due to anaphylactic shock. This consideration points up the need to place John Jones, or any individual entity that is named in an I-S explanation, into the *maximally specific* reference class about which data is available

([17], pp. 394–403). Any "information . . . which is of potential explanatory relevance to the explanation event . . . " must be utilized in "formulating or appraising an I-S explanation" ([17], p. 400).

Reflection on some of these considerations and on certain counterexamples to the D-N model has recently led Wesley Salmon to propose an alternative to the models discussed thus far. For Salmon, an explanation is *not an argument* and thus does not require us to appeal to either deductive or inductive logic in analyzing the relation between premises and conclusion. Rather, according to Salmon, an explanation of the sentence 'why does this X which is a member of A have the property B' is 'a set of probability statements'. These represent the probability of members of various *epistemologically homogeneous sub-classes* having a particular property A, say A & C_1, A & C_2, . . . , also possessing another property B. Also necessary to the explanation is "a statement specifying the compartment to which the explanandum event belongs" ([25], pp. 76–77).

Thus the S-R model is really a partition of a class into *epistemologically homogenous sub-classes*, made on the basis of any available, statistically relevant information.

In addition to the difference with Hempel over the non-argument status of an explanation, Salmon contends that there is no reason that a probabilistic statement involving a *very low* probability cannot be utilized in an explanation. If the statistically relevant class (e.g., the class of atoms of radioactive U^{238} which will decay into lead) is such that the probability of decay is very low, that is all that can be said in response to an explanation of why this atom of U^{238} decayed into lead.

I shall return to the S-R and I-S models, but for the moment let us turn to an application of these models with respect to the issues of causal explanation.

B. *Causal Explanation Using the D-N, I-S, and S-R Models*

For Hempel, "causal explanation conforms to the D-N model" ([17], p. 348). Causal connection can be represented in general laws (e.g., Lenz's law of the direction of current induced in a wire near a moving magnet). Initial conditions, the C's cited earlier, can function as the causal *antecedents* in a D-N schema, so that the C's constitute a sufficient condition in the light of the L's for an effect, the explanandum E.

Hempel has applied his models of explanation to sequences of events, sometimes referred to as 'genetic explanations'. The sense of 'genetic' employed here needs to be distinguished from the sense of that term in Mendelian genetics. Here 'genetic' refers to a developmental sequence of events, a genesis.

For Hempel, an historical explanation to account for the fact that popes and bishops came to offer indulgences is

> basically nomological in character ([17], p. 448). In a genetic explanation each stage must be shown to 'lead to' the next, and thus to be linked to its successor by virtue of some general principles which make the occurrence of the latter at least reasonably probable, given the former ([17], pp. 448–449).

A genetic explanation, then, for Hempel, is a chain of either D-N or I-S sub-explanations, the explanandum of the previous explanation functioning as one of the premises in the next sub-explanation.

Salmon's views concerning the relations of causal explanation and the S-R model have very recently undergone a significant amplification. Salmon writes:

> If we wish to explain a particular event, such as death by leukemia of GI Joe, we begin by assembling the factors statistically relevant to that occurrence – for example, his distance from the atomic explosion, the magnitude of the blast, and the type of shelter he was in. We must also obtain the probability values associated with the relevancy relations. *The statistical relevance relations are statistical regularities, and we proceed to explain them. Although this differs substantially from things I have said previously, I no longer believe that the assemblage of relevant factors provides a complete explanation – or much of anything in the way of explanation* [my emphasis]. We do, I believe, have a bona fide explanation of an event if we have a complete set of statistically relevant factors, the pertinent probability values, *and* causal explanations of the relevance relations. Subsumption of a particular occurrence under statistical regularities – which, we recall, does not imply anything about the construction of deductive or inductive arguments – is a necessary part of any adequate explanation of its occurrence, but it is not the whole story. The causal explanation of the regularity is also needed. This claim, it should be noted, is in direct conflict with the received view, according to which the mere subsumption – deductive or inductive – of an event under a lawful regularity constitutes a complete explanation. One can, according to the received view, go on to ask for an explanation of any law used to explain a given event, but that is a different explanation. I am suggesting, on the contrary, that if the regularity invoked is not a causal regularity, then a causal explanation of that very regularity must be made part of the explanation of the event ([26], p. 699).

What is required, then, is a *causal* explanation of those statistically relevant factors superadded to the earlier S-R models: the fundamental importance of explicating causal explanation now cannot be seen as the task of the S-R model *per se.* [5]

C. *The Hempel-Scriven Debate*

In several articles Michael Scriven independently raised some of the objections to the Hempel models (primarily the D-N model) that Hart and Honoré and Mackie directed against regularity theories of causation. Against the need for generalizations or laws in explanation, Scriven has argued that laws are better conceived of as 'role-justifying grounds' for an explanation [28], and *not* as part of the explanation itself. Scriven also maintains that we can sometimes be quite certain of a given explanation *without* being able to justify it by reference to any specifiable laws ([28], p. 456).

In reply, Hempel has noted that it is not clear why only laws and not additional initial conditions should not function in role-justification. Furthermore, Hempel argues, we should distinguish an *analytical* account of what might be involved in explanation (or causation) from our preanalytic use. But Hempel also provides what I think are stronger arguments against Scriven. First, which concrete *events* are selected and cited in a causal sequence or genetic explanation will be a function of what is perceived as relevant – and this cannot be decided without appeal to some general principles. Also, such explanations as Scriven cites which *look* primeval, such as explaining an ink stain on my rug by citing my knee knocking the desk on which an open bottle of ink rested, *are* affected by changing scientific knowledge. A child would be surprised to see opaque mercury spilling on a rung *not* producing a stain. Explanation, argues Hempel, will only be present if there are certain (tacit) nomic connections.

Scriven [29] also criticized Hempel on the *thesis of structural identity*, i.e., that every explanation is a potential prediction, and *vice versa*. Hempel has now distinguished two subtheses (still defending the first subthesis that every explanation is a potential prediction), but does not require the converse that every prediction is an explanation. (Recall that Hart and Honoré maintained that causal explanations are often inquests, and that what is cited in a causal explanation could not in most circumstances have been used to *predict* the occurrence of the event.)

Scriven cited an example of a request for an explanation as to why an individual has paresis. The explanation, Scriven argued, was that the individual has syphilis, and that syphilis is a necessary condition for paresis, even though very few of those afflicted with syphilis will experience its sequela, e.g., paresis. One *could not* have predicted the paresis, though one could *explain* it by citing the precondition of syphilis.

Hempel's response to this is correct to a point, namely that the syphilis does *not* explain the paresis any more than a man's purchasing a ticket in the Irish sweepstakes *explains* why he won ([17], pp. 369–370). However, Hempel does not in connection with this case note that the syphilis is a '*partial* explanation' (though he does later discuss this concept [17], pp. 415–418). What we find here, as in many cases of partial explanations, is one of Mackie's gappy or elliptical generalizations which can function as a partial rationalization of a causal claim but which requires additional information in order to guarantee an explanation.

Scriven [29] and Toulmin [30] have cited Darwin's theory of natural selection as an example in which explanations of evolution are offered but for which predictions could not be given. I will not deal with this example except to note that evolutionists themselves realize they need to modify their theory to make it more predictionist. (See [19]).

Finally Scriven has adduced several examples in which we only know that certain conditions were fulfilled *because* the effect occurred. One example Scriven cites is the explanation of the collapse of a bridge due to metal fatigue. Another is the explanation of the murder of his wife by a husband due to his jealous rage: unless the murder occurred we do not know the rage was sufficiently strong.

Hempel admits these cases, terming them 'self-evidencing', but argues that though they pose interesting methodological problems, they do not vitiate the thesis of structural identity. Since jealous rage and metal fatigue and the like may sometime become independently verifiable, it is only a pragmatic, and not a logical difficulty. Explanation still is by reference to laws and initial conditions, and thus the *potential* prediction thesis, albeit in a counterfactual sense, is rescued.

IV. THEORIES, EXPLANATIONS, AND ERROR IN THE BIOMEDICAL SCIENCES

Having explored certain received views of causal explanation, I wish now to examine those distinctive features of theories and generalizations which have a bearing on causal explanations in the biomedical sciences and which also have implications for a theory of error in medicine.

A. *The Nature of Theories and Generalizations in the Biomedical Sciences*

Consider the thesis (which I have discussed elsewhere) that basic biomedical science typically contains not theories or laws of a universal character, but rather theories of the 'middle range'. This notion was originally introduced into sociology by Robert Merton ([22]). In my approach it denotes those theories in embryology, neurology, immunology, and certain areas of genetics which are often species-*specific*. Theories of the 'middle range' are 'mid-way' between biomedical universals and the universal truths of population genetics; they are *not* perceived to be universal in the sense of biochemistry and population genetics, and they have the logical character of an *overlapping series of interlevel temporal models*.

By 'interlevel temporal model' I mean to point out that biomedical theories often use idealized entities (e.g., genes or cells) abstracted from their complex environment; they may also interact with other higher or lower level entities, (e.g., organ or molecule) along a temporal dimension. By an 'overlapping series' I intend to refer to the similarity but not identity that exists between physiological mechanisms among members of a group of organisms. Even genetically closely related organisms will exhibit variation in basic mechanisms due to mutations, genetic recombinations, and subtle environmental differences.

One way that the relation between closely related organisms vis-à-vis some well-characterized physiological mechanism can be visualized is to picture a three dimensional graph (dimensionality greater than three might provide more realism but would sacrifice familiarity). Suppose that the x axis represents a subtly changing genome, say $g_1^x \ldots g_{100}^x$, and the y axis a different genome $g_1^y \ldots g_{50}^y$. (These variations could be graded by the similarity to the 'wild type', say g_1, via activity of the product, e.g., ability to catalyze a specific reaction.) Let the z axis represent the number of organisms in some selected experimental population. Then some organisms will probably possess identical genomes (say the clones O_1 and O_2 (both $= g_{20}^x g_{12}^y$)). Some organisms will be closely related and partially overlapping, for example an O_3 ($= g_{20}^x g_{13}^y$), and some are likely to be quite different, for example an O_4 ($= g_{100}^x g_{45}^y$), even though O_4 may be a 'sibling' of O_1, O_2, and O_3. Each of the O's could be analyzed as possessing the 'same' basic mechanism, though the efficiency of the catalyzing enzymes which are the products of the hypothetical genes might be quite different. Such an abstract example is often realized in biological organisms for example in connection with i and o mutations in the operon theory (see [27]).

Such variation generates polytypic classes and is also one of the reasons why both (1) statistical methods are often necessary for analyzing biological experiments (since it is often impossible to separate the organisms into pure subclasses) and (2) statistical generalizations are more appropriate than universal generalizations in the biomedical sciences.

One example of a 'middle-range' theory from the biomedical sciences is what has often been termed the "two component theory of the immune response".

B. *The Two-Component Theory of the Immune Response*

The rudiments of this theory had two (or possibly three) independent origins which were first clearly articulated in the 1960's. The theory culminates in the important cellular distinction between *T* (or thymus derived) cells and *B* (or bursa or bursa-equivalent) cells and the synergistic interaction between them in the immune response. The theory continues to be further elaborated at all levels and there is sound evidence that a full understanding of its various components will lead to more rational therapies in the areas of organ transplantation rejection, cancer, and autoimmune diseases, such as rheumatoid arthritis. Already the theory has allowed a clearer interpretation of a wide range of immune deficiency diseases, and has served as the intellectual source for successful life-saving thymus and bone marrow transplants.[6]

The theory had its 'protosource' in a chance finding of Glick [11] that a hindgut organ in birds known as the bursa of Fabricius had an important immunological function. This had been overlooked by numerous investigators because bursectomy only affects the immune system if it is performed *very* early in life. Glick's work was further developed in Wolfe's laboratory at Wisconsin, and the same principle – early or neonatal organ ablation – was then applied to the thymus, another organ with a then unknown function, in the early 1960's, by Archer, Pierce, Good and Martinez working in Good's laboratory at the University of Minnesota. Independently, J. F. A. P. Miller was working along a different line of research, attempting to determine the effects in mice of thymectomy on virus-induced leukemia. Miller [23] noticed a wasting effect of neonatal thymectomy in his mice, and quickly discovered by additional research that the thymus played an important immunological role in both graft rejection and lymphocyte production. A third possibly independent line of research which culminated in a determination of the immune function of the thymus was pursued by Waksman and his colleagues at Harvard. In late 1962 Warner and Svenberg ([31], [32]) proposed the 'hypothesis' of "dissociation of immunological responsiveness", which suggested that the thymus was responsible for homograft immunity, and the bursa for the production of antibody producing cells. This notion was further clarified by other investigators, the primary work taking place in Good's laboratory, and later labeled the "two component concept of the immune system" by Peterson, Cooper and Good [24]. The importance of synergistic interaction of the two systems and their cellular components was discovered by Claman, Chaperon, and Triplett [5]. The theory as recently conceived is outlined in Figure 1. At this writing no bursa equivalent in mammals has been discovered, and some investigators believe that bone-marrow derived cells can become *B* cells without a bursa equivalent.

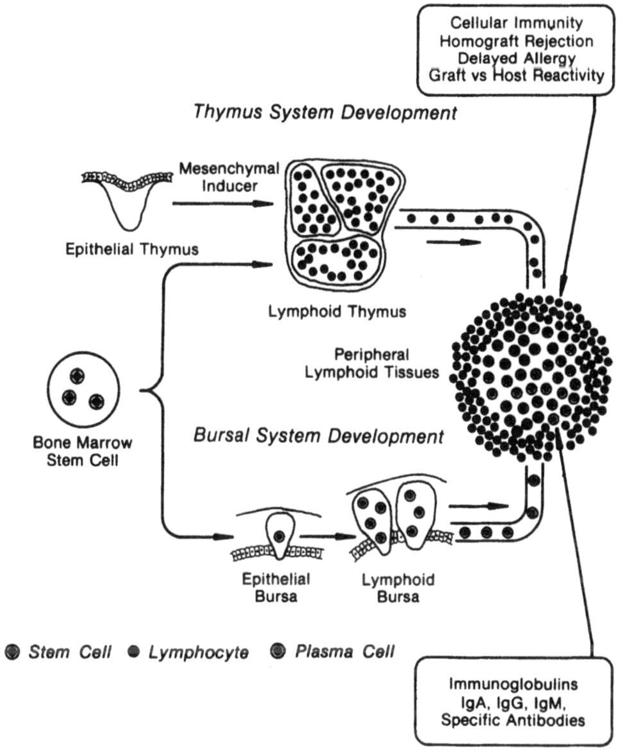

Fig. 1. The two-component theory. The two branches of the immune mechanism are believed to develop from the same lymphoid precursor. The central thymus system starts as an epithelial structure arising from third and fourth embryonic pharyngeal pouch and becomes a lymphoid organ under stimulation by a mesenchymal inducer. The bursal system develops by budding from the intestinal epithelium. After release from the central organs into the bloodstream, the lymphoid cells reassemble in peripheral lymphoid tissues. Here the lymphocytes – thymus dependent in origin – control cellular immunity, while bursa-dependent plasma cells synthesize serum antibodies (fig. and legend from Good ([12], p. 9) modified for reasons of space).

The two component theory is confirmed both by a wide range of experiments in the laboratory and by clinical findings. By 1970 it resulted in a reconceptualization on the part of the World Health Organization [8] of immune deficiency diseases in humans. (See Table I)

TABLE I

Classification of primary immunodeficiency disorders

Type	Suggested Cellular Defect		
	B Cells	T Cells	Stem Cells
Infantile X-linked agammaglobulinemia	+	...	...
Selective immunoglobulin deficiency (IgA)	+[a]	...	...
Transient hypogammaglobulinemia of infancy	+	...	...
X-linked immunodeficiency with hyper-IgM	+[a]	...	...
Thymic hypoplasia (pharyngeal pouch syndrome, DiGeorge)	...	+	...
Episodic lymphopenia with lymphocytotoxin	...	+	...
Immunodeficiency with normal or hyperimmunoglobulinemia	+	+[b]	...
Immunodeficiency with ataxia telangiectasia	+	+	...
Immunodeficiency with thrombocytopenia and eczema (Wiskott-Aldrich)	+	+	...
Immunodeficiency with thymoma	+	+	...
Immunodeficiency with short-limbed dwarfism	+	+	...
Immunodeficiency with generalized hematopoietic hypoplasia	+	+	+
Severe combined immunodeficiency:			
Autosomal recessive	+	+	+
X-linked	+	+	+
Sporadic	+	+	+
Variable immunodeficiency (largely unclassified)	+	+[b]	...

Source. – From Fudenberg *et al.* [8].
[a] Involve some but not all B cells.
[b] Encountered in some but not all patients.

The theory illustrates some of the philosophical points concerning theory structure in the biomedical sciences. First it should be noted that this theory is vigorously interlevel and contains entities which are biochemical and molecular (antibody molecules for which a full sequence of amino acids has been worked out), cellular (lymphocytes and plasma cells), tissue level (peripheral lymphoid tissue), organ level (thymus), and systemic (lymphatic system, circulatory system). Secondly, the evolutionary *variation* associated with the theory should be noted: the thymus is present in all organisms evolutionary distal to the Lamprey eel, but the lack of a bursa in mammals also underscores variation at the organ level. The range of diseases cited in Table I illustrates the more extreme types of variation that can occur in humans. There is also a fine but significant structure variation in the HL-A system (i.e., in those genes and antigens which control self versus non-self recognition, and which is responsible for organ transplanation rejection). In addition to these features, it should be noted that there is both an ontogenetic and a phylogenetic aspect to the theory. The ontogeny is illustrated in Figure 1, and the continuing process of stem cell differentiation has been confirmed in the adult life of irradiated mice. The ontogenetic and phylogenetic roles of the thymus and the cellular immunity as a defense against neoplasms has figured extensively in the literature. Finally it should be pointed out that this theory is closely integrated into immunology as a whole and also into general biology. It is difficult to separate this theory from (1) an analysis of antibody structure, (2) the clonal selection theory, (3) the role of the HL-A system in immunogenetics, (4) the role of other cells as macrophages, and so on, not to mention the connection to (1) genetics, (2) a theory of protein synthesis, and (3) a theory of evolution.[7] The theory in its multiple interconnections illustrates in a rather different biomedical discipline Beckner's and Arber's point (see [4], p. 160 and [1], p. 46) that theory in biology is 'less linear' and 'more reticulate' than is physical theory. In point of fact the two component theory displays 'reticularity' in two different dimensions: *horizontal* in its interconnection with other biological theories and fields at the same level, e.g., cell biology within and without immunology, and *vertical*, in its interconnection with systems at different levels of aggregation as depicted in Figure 1.

C. *Biomedical Theories and Elliptical Generalizations*

The variation which leads to the 'overlapping series' character of such biomedical theories often necessitates (in my view) the use of gappy or elliptical generalizations, and the statistical character of biomedical generalizations introduces a probabilistic element into any 'causal' explanation in many areas of the biomedical sciences. Along with Mackie I agree that the non-universal character of such models is no bar to using them in a legitimate causal manner, i.e., with counterfactual force. Here it is important to make several distinctions which help clarify my thesis. First, we should distinguish *generalizations* into (1) universal or exceptionless (with further subsenses to be specified below) and (2) statistical. Second, we can distinguish 'universal' generalizations into two subsenses: (1) universal generalizations_1, which refers to organism scope, i.e., to the extent to which a physiological mechanism will be found in all organisms, *and* (2) universal generalizations_2, which refers to the property illustrated by the phrase "same cause (or same initial conditions and mechanisms), then same effect". This second sense of 'universal' is roughly equivalent to a thesis of determinism. With these distinctions, we can reformulate our position and its differences with Mackie more precisely.

Biomedical theories employ many generalizations which though they are *not* universal generalizations_1 are universal generalizations_2. As such, they possess counterfactual force. In addition, largely because of biological variation, system complexity, and the inability to fully specify (recall the gappiness of generalizations) and control for all relevant initial conditions, biological theories often have to employ statistical generalizations. These also have a type of counterfactual force, but it is probabilistic, *i.e.*, one can assert with confidence that if X had not occurred Y *probably* (at some level of probability ± an error range) would not have occurred. Such statistical generalizations also take care of part of the problem to which Mackie alludes when he refers to the necessity to allude to 'sufficiently similar circumstances' in order to provide subjunctive conditional force for generalizations.

I consequently disagree with Mackie, and to a lesser degree with Hart and Honoré, in that the linguistic elements of such models are generalizations, although they are restricted and often statistical generalizations. I also maintain that it is by virtue of the generalization character that (causal) explanations in the biomedical sciences occur.

D. *Filling in the Gappy Generalizations*

Under this view the gappy universals or generalizations which Mackie introduces also have to be interpreted, vis-à-vis their completion, in two different ways. An increase in knowledge can result from (1) additional information at the same level, or it can come from (2) moving to a deeper level where more precise information can be obtained.

To illustrate these two directions of further completion of a gappy restricted generalization we may refer again to the example of the two-component theory.

The articulation of the two-component theory of the immune response and the developing reconceptualization of immunodeficiency diseases cited in Table I led to a realization that immunodeficient patients might have their immune system 'reconstituted' via transplantation. In the late 1960's several thymus and bone marrow transplants (the latter for reconstruction of missing stem cells) were performed, with variable but often dramatic results. Good who was closely involved with these and earlier developments has written extensively on immunological reconstitution. It is worth quoting him at some length:

During the First International Workshop on Immunodeficiencies, it was the opinion of several participants, including us, that, since SCID [severe combined immunodeficiency disease] involves gross deficiencies of the two basic immunity systems, an essential defect in the disease must represent a perturbation located proximal in differentiation to the separation of the development into two distinct systems. We postulated that correction of the genetic or developmental anomalies underlying SCID and perhaps other immunodeficiencies, would require that cells from immunologically normal persons be provided. Further, we argued that these cells should be given in a form that had not yet undergone differentiation along the two separate lines taken normally by immunologically competent cells. Several theoretically sound approaches were proposed: (1) the injection of fetal liver cells either alone or together with a fetal thymus implant; (2) the injection of bone marrow cells either alone or together with a fetal thymus. Further, it was proposed that matching donor and recipient at the major histocompatibility complex in man (HL-A) as discussed at that conference, should be used in an effort to avoid a fatal GVH [Graft Versus Host] reaction.

These discussions led to the performance in 1968 of the first two matched bone marrow transplants: one for SCID in Minneapolis, and one for the Wiskott-Aldrich (WA) syndrome in Madison, Wisconsin.

On returning to Minneapolis from the conference and being confronted with a child with the certainly fatal SCID syndrome, Hong and his co-workers tried to reconstitute the patient by using fetal liver from a 12-week-old embryonic donor. The fetal liver was given together with a fetal thymus from the same abortus. Although humoral and cellular immunological functions were reconstituted by the transplant, the recipient soon developed evidence of a severe GVH reaction which proved fatal. Although it could have been that a small fresh blood transfusion was responsible for the GVH reaction, discouragement with the use of stem cells to SCID set in, particularly because others at the same time had tried marrow transplants and had produced fatal GVH.

Another set of experiences changed this discouragement to a hopeful perspective when we realized from our own experimental work and from studies of Simonsen and Silvers that in mice and rats a fatal GVH reaction was not induced unless antigens of the recipient differed from those of the donor cell in characteristics controlled at the so-called major (H-2) histocompatibility complex. From this reasoning it was possible to postulate that marrow transplantation to correct SCID would require matching of donor and recipient according to major (HL-A) histocompatibility determinants. Studies in man by Amos and Bach, and by Bach and Amos, had already shown that vigorous rejection of allografts, as well as *in vitro* mixed leukocyte culture (MLC) reactions, were determined by the major histocompatibility system in man – HL-A. Each of us had independently reached the conclusion, from studies of the animal systems cited above coupled with clinical observations, that fatal GVH reactions in man should not be a problem if matching of the major histocompatibility determinants were achieved. We knew from work in our laboratories that seemingly perfect matching between siblings eliminated positive MLC reactions in almost all instances ([13], pp. 78–79).

A male infant with SCID of the *X*-lined type was subsequently treated with a bone marrow transplant from three out of four of his HL-A matched and MLC compatible eight-year-old sister. After an initial but happily short-lived GVH reaction, the child's immune system was completely reconstituted. As of last report [13] the child was in vigorous, good health, though interestingly he is now a hematopoietic chimera with bone marrow cells of a female (*XX*) karyotype.

This example illustrates several themes concerning gappy generalizations employed in supporting causal analyses, and also points toward an important issue in medical error. First, as a result of the experimental therapy cited it should be noted that stem cells can now be interpreted as bone-marrow derived cells, thus clarifying the nature of two component theory at the cellular level. Second, the role of the HL-A system in the immune system is highlighted by the experiment. During the past ten years knowledge about this system and the genetic locus (the major histocompatibility locus or MHC) which controls it has increased dramatically. The relation of this system to the immune response, not only in transplanation but also in disease susceptibility and resistance, is now the focus of a number of vigorous research programs. Accordingly we now can appreciate the various ways in which the gappy or incomplete generalizations which function in medical knowledge can become further completed.

E. *Gappy Generalizations and a Theory of Error in Medicine*

The fact that causal sequences displayed in clinical diagnosis, prognosis, and therapy rely on incomplete generalizations underscores the important issue of error in medicine. In their article, "Toward a Theory of Medical Fallibility", Samuel Gorovitz and Alastair MacIntyre argue that medical error is "inherent in the nature of medical practice" and that injury is "unavoidable not merely because of the present limitations of human knowledge . . . but rather because of the fundamental epistemological features of a *science of particulars*" ([15], p. 71).[8]

The inherent and subtle statistical variability to which I alluded is, I believe, at least a significant source of such injury. At any given time it represents a *then*-irreducible, uncontrollable source of medical error and, accordingly, is beyond the responsibility of the clinician (but not necessarily of society – (see [15], pp. 66–70)). As the gaps in the generalizations become filled-in or more clearly circumscribed, however, such error can be decreased. Obviously this is one of the major rationales for medical research, continuing medical education, and physician recertification programs. In a legal analysis of a 'malpractice' claim, then, appeals will be made to causal accounts of an injury as well as to the proper standard of care. Both of these will depend, crucially, on the state of incompleteness and inherent variation in biomedical theories and generalizations.

V. CAUSAL EXPLANATION IN BIOMEDICINE AND THE LAW

It is time to bring together a number of the issues and factors in causal explanation by way of an abstract model. The model, though expressed in quasi-formal terms, reflects a pragmatic approach to the problem as will be evident after elaborating the quasi-formal schema.

As argued thus far, a principal feature of causal explanations is the availability of gappy causal generalizations. Since these are usually of a statistical form, we can represent such a statistical, causal generalization as follows:

$$C_1^1 \,\&\, C_2^1 \,\&\ldots\&\, C_m^1 \overset{(P^1)}{\Longrightarrow} E$$

or more succinctly by:

$$\bigwedge_{i=1}^{m} C_i^1 \overset{(P^1)}{\Longrightarrow} E$$

Here the *C*s refer to descriptions of antecedent conditions and the *E* to a description to the event to be explained. The double arrow represents *causal implication*, but *not deterministic implication*: the (P^1) value represents the probability of *E* following from the conjunction of the *C*s.[9]

The superscript 1 refers to one possible explanation of *E*. An *alternative*, usually competing generalization, could be represented by

$$\bigwedge_{i=1}^{n} C_i^2 \overset{(P^2)}{\Longrightarrow} E$$

The explanation is then particularized by asserting $C_i(a_i)$ to obtain *E* with probability P^i.

The question of the reference class(es) to which a_i most appropriately belongs is one which has occasioned considerable debate in the literature of statistical explanations ([17], [25]). In the present account, it seems wise to follow Salmon's suggested modification [25] of Hempel's "requirement of maximal specificity" [17]. Salmon introduces what he terms a "requirement of the maximal class of maximal specificity". In such a requirement, one utilizes the probability P^i that is associated with the "broadest homogeneous reference class", i.e., that class of C's that lead to E's for which we have epistemically available no further subclass partition that alters the value of P^i.

To incorporate the likelihood of further explication of the conditions in terms of additional detail at the same, lower, or even 'higher' levels these Cs could be written as

$$C^j_{i\,\vdots\,\cdot\,\cdot}$$

where the subscript dot notation serves as a mnemonic of the provisional and gappy nature of the generalization. (For similar reasons, E could also be represented as $E\vdots\ldots$)

In the model I favor, *all* explanation, including as limiting case deductive-nomological and deductive-statistical explanations, is ***elliptically comparative***. The comparative aspect of causal explanation is usually implicit in an explanation sketch. Rival explanations tend to function as background elements, which usually involve lower probability generalizations. In an analytical account of causal explanation, however, it would be wise to introduce such rival explanations explicitly as their presence clarifies certain perplexities concerning causal explanation. This comparative element in causal explanation can be represented formally by using a generalization of the schema outlined thus far as:

$$\bigvee_{j=1}^{n}\left\{\begin{array}{l} \bigwedge_{i=1}^{m} (x)(y)(C^j_{i}\vdots\ldots(x) \overset{(P^j)}{\Longrightarrow} E\vdots\ldots(y)) \\ \bigwedge_{i=1}^{m} \quad C^j_{i}\vdots\ldots(a_i) \\ \qquad\quad y = a_{m+1} \\ \hline\hline E\vdots\ldots(a_{m+1}) \end{array}\;[P^j]\right\}$$

and where $\sum_{j=1}^{n} P^j = 1$ for reasons of normalization.

What this schema represents, then, is a disjunction of j rival causal explanations each with inductive statistical force P^j, almost all of which remain covert in actually stated explanations. In my view making explicit these comparative, competing causal explanations is not dissimilar to Salmon's partitioning of a class into various subclasses and the specification of *one* of those as *the* subclass. His alternative subclasses function as the analogue of the competing explanations in my account.

In general, however, this schema is only a *component* of an even more complex account involving a *series* of such explanatory schemas, with the $E \vdots ..$ of one explanation function as a $C \vdots ..$ of a subsequent explanation. If we represent the temporal (and causal) succession by *left* subscripts such as ${}_1E$, ${}_2E$, ${}_1C$, ${}_2C$, ... we then arrive at a reiterative model in which an ${}_iE \vdots ..$ could function as a $C^j_{m+1} \vdots ..$ in a succeeding explanation component. This would be similar to Hempel's account of genetic explanation.

It is important to stress that what this way of construing the matter yields is a series of tacit and (at least partially) competing genetic explanations in which the probability of the last event ${}_nE \vdots ..$ is the product of the P^js of the component sequences. These P^js may not be independent, so conditional probabilities may also have to be known. Some components may possess only very few rival explanations; some may possess many. These various factors and sequences, though difficult to fully specify in practice, are, I believe, what figure in causal explantions in medicine, science, and the law. Probability values, however, are often not presented in quantitative but are given largely in comparative terms, such as 'likely', 'very unlikely', etc.

What I am proposing then, when we are asked to provide a (causal) explanation – I believe the thesis urged here can be generalized to non-causal explanatory contexts – is a tacitly comparative causal sequence licensed by probabilistic generalizations. If the explanation is such that there is one primary candidate, little explicit reference will be made to the alternative rivals. If, for example, I am asked to explain, in Scriven's example [28], how the ink came to stain my rug, I may only refer to my knee knocking the desk. If, on the other hand, I was deep in thought and not so sure it was my knee, I may qualify the explanation and say probably it was my knee, possibly it was my unconsciously pushing a book across the desk which knocked over the ink bottle. *Very* unlikely, but still possible, is the explanation that a momentary earth tremor tipped the ink bottle off, and so on.

Similarly, *rival* explanations can be given for the bone-marrow transplant example, or for explanations of automobile accidents in which legal questions of responsibility would arise. In cases where the consequences are important, whether they be legal or practical ones (e.g., I want to avoid future ink spills) *utility* considerations may warrant further explanation of rival explanatory accounts in an attempt to modify the net probability of the rival explanations by further inquiry into the likelihood of initial or antecedent conditions, or even into the probabilities of the generalizations.

The schema advanced can be represented both quasiformally and in terms of an analogy. Quasiformally the model appears as:

$$\bigvee_{j=1}^{n}\ \bigwedge_{k=1}^{l}\left\{\left[\begin{array}{llll} \bigwedge_{i=1}^{m}\left[(x)(y)({}_kC_i^j \vdots\ldots(x) \overset{({}_kP^j)}{\Longrightarrow} {}_kE(y))\right] & & \bigwedge_{i=1}^{m+1}\left[(x)(y)({}_{k+1}C_i^j\vdots\ldots(x)\overset{({}_kP^j)}{\Longrightarrow}{}_{k+1}E\vdots\ldots(y))\right] & \\ \bigwedge_{i=1}^{m}\left[{}_kC_i^j\vdots\ldots(a_i)\right] & & \to\bigwedge_{i=1}^{m+1}\left[{}_{k+1}C_l^j\vdots\ldots(a_i)\right] & \\ \quad y=a_{m+1} & & \quad y=a_{m+2} & \\ \cline{1-1}\cline{3-3} \cline{1-1}\cline{3-3} & [{}_kP^j] & & [{}_kP^j] \\ {}_kE\vdots\ldots(a_{m+1})(={}_{k+1}C_i^j(a_{m+1})) & & {}_{k+1}E\vdots\ldots(a_{m+2}) & \end{array}\right]\right.$$

in which the symbols have the meaning given to them (see above). Here ${}_kE$ is one consequence; ${}_kE$ is equivalent to a succeeding cause ${}_{k+1}C$, which in turn probabilistically brings about ${}_{k+1}E$, and so on.

Analogically this schema can be represented as a complex network, with the explanandum as a node. Different strands (generalizations) lead to the same explanandum, the relative thickness of the strands representing comparative probabilities of the rival generalizations. Utility considerations may force increased attention to the 'thinner' explanatory accounts. 'Deeper' non-conflicting explanations could be introduced into such an analogy by adding a 'depth dimension'. 'Simpler' component explanations of generalizations could also be fitted into this schema, as when one explains the knocking over of a bottle of ink by appeals to simpler generalizations of object interaction, e.g., impenetrability, tipping, etc.

It might be useful to conclude by pointing out how this account of causal (and genetic) explanation relates to some of the problems which have occupied us, and also have stimulated Salmon to develop an alternative to Hempel's account of inductive statistical explanation.

Mackie's (and Anderson's) notion of a 'field' is, I believe, a useful addition to our causal inquiries. It can be added to the above account as a restriction of the inquiry into some finite list of plausible explanatory generalizations. Such restriction will of course depend on the present state of knowledge, historical considerations, legal contexts, and the like. Such a notion as a 'field' is a pragmatic one and it is quite coherent with the pragmatic spirit of the account of causal explanation presented here.

This account is also dependent on generalizations for explanatory and counterfactual force, though the generalizations are embedded in a multi-dimensional web of knowledge.

I believe that Salmon's examples, which led him away from the Hempelian schema, can be accounted for in the proposed explication. Salmon was concerned about explanations in which premises were true but irrelevant, and in which explanations met all the criteria for good D-N explanations. The explanation of a man's non-pregnancy premised on his taking birth control pills is such an example. In the analysis presented here such premises are *not* causal: their negation $\bar{C} \overset{P}{\Longrightarrow} E$ has the same probability; thus the presence of C does not make a difference, and the assertion is inadmissible.

Salmon's assertions, contra Hempel, about low weight explanations are I think assimilable within the present model. In general, one should prefer that explanation which offers the largest conjoint or net probability to its rivals. That probability could be low, but it would be the 'best' explanation.

In general, when there are viable competing explanations, the usual response is to 'hedge one's bets' and attempts to act so as to cover all contingencies. This is typical in medicine when, for example, the etiology of an infection is unclear and a broad spectrum antibiotic is prescribed to affect all likely infectious organisms.

In contrast to Salmon's recent views, the model defended here need not have a causal account superadded to it: the generalizations are themselves causal, though 'deeper' explanations are not excluded.

I close by noting what has not been pointed out in the present essay. Though I have been addressing the issue of causal explanation, I have not attempted to offer an explication of *causality*. This is a closely related issue but one which is best bracketed for the present. I also have not attended to motivational explanations and their relation(s) to causal explanations. Such an attempt would require an independent analysis of teleological and functional explanations.

I do think I have shown, however, how probabilistic generalizations which are so central to medicine, the biological sciences, and to law, function in an outline of causal explanation.[10]

University of Pittsburgh
Pittsburgh, Pennsylvania

NOTES

[1] In this essay the notion of interpersonal transactions and opportunities will not be further discussed except incidentally, both for reasons of space and also because I believe the main focus of my topic can be circumscribed within the debate about causality in the more restricted physical sense.

[2] Mackie's account is rich, and in a relatively short essay I will not be able to do full justice to its scope and complexity. I do want to point out that though I think that Mackie is fundamentally wrong on the issue of generalizations, I also believe that his account, taken together with the previously cited observations of Hart and Honoré, provide a useful framework for a current theory of causal explanation in law and medicine.

[3] The only point of emendation I would want to make of Mackie's "elliptical or gappy universal propositions" is to change 'universal' to 'general', so as to permit the use of *statistical* generalizations which may be excluded by connotations associated with the term 'universal'. I shall return to this point later.

[4] There are other conditions imposed on the model but they will not interest us here.

[5] It would take us beyond the scope of our topic to outline Salmon's proposals for explicating the nature of such a causal account in terms of production and propagation of modifications. See Salmon [26] for details.

[6] I will not have the opportunity in this brief summary of the theory to discuss these implications, tests, and will be able to cite only one application of the theory. I also can do no more than cite sources discussing the historical origins and elaboration of the theory.

[7] This point obviously cannot be developed in a short article but a review of Watson ([33], ch. 17), and Good [12] will support the thesis.

[8] It would be impossible to review here Gorovitz's and MacIntyre's arguments (or the critical responses their essay has stimulated by Martin [21] and Bayles and Caplan [2], [3] and Gorovitz's rejoinder [14]). It is to the point, however, to indicate in view of the theses concerning biomedical theory and causality which I suggest, that medical error and a correlated responsibility for medical injury, has several sources.

[9] I shall not explore various interpretations of probability here since I think the explication of probabilistic causal explanation can proceed reasonably far without an interpretation of probability as subjective, frequency, propensity, etc. In point of fact, the probability that enters into such generalizations may well not have a univocal interpretation.

[10] I want to thank H. Tristram Engelhardt Jr. and William C. Wimsatt for reading an earlier version of this paper and making valuable suggestions. I also want to acknowledge with gratitude support from the National Science Foundation and the Interdisciplinary Programs Branch of the Division of Associated Health Professions, DHEW.

BIBLIOGRAPHY

1. Arber, A.: 1954, *The Mind and The Eye*, Cambridge University Press, Cambridge.
2. Bayles, M. D. and Caplan, A.: 1978, 'Medical Fallibility and Malpractice', *Journal of Medicine and Philosophy* 3, 169–186.

3. Bayles, M. D. and Caplan, A.: 1978, 'A Response to Professor Gorovitz', *Journal of Medicine and Philosophy* 3, 192–195.
4. Beckner, M.: 1959, *The Biological Way of Thought*, Columbia University Press, New York.
5. Claman, H. N., Chaperòn, E. A., and Triplett, R. F.: 1966, 'Immunocompetence of Transferred Thymus-Marrow Cells Combinations', *Journal of Immunology* 97, 828–832.
6. Dray, W.: 1957, *Laws and Explanation in History*, Oxford University Press, Oxford.
7. Ducasse, C. J.: 1969, *Causation and the Types of Necessity*, Dover Publications, New York.
8. Fudenberg, H. H., Good, R. A., Witlitzig, *et al.*: 1970, 'Classification of the Primary Immune Deficiencies: WHO Recommendation', *New England Journal of Medicine* **283**, 656–657.
9. Gallie, W. D.: 1955, 'Explanations in History and the Genetic Sciences', *Mind* **LXIV**, 161–167.
10. Gardiner, P.: 1959, *The Nature of Historical Explanation*, Oxford University Press, Oxford.
11. Glick, B., Chang, T. S., and Japp, R. G.: 1956, 'The Bursa of Fabricius and Antibody Production', *Poultry Science* **35**, 224–234.
12. Good, R.: 1971, 'Disorders of the Immune System', in R. A. Good and D. W. Fischer (eds.), *Immunobiology*, Sinauer Association Incorporated, Stamford, Connecticut, pp. 3–16.
13. Good, R. A. and Bach, F. H.: 1974, 'Bone Marrow and Thymus Transplants: Cellular Engineering to Correct Primary Immunodeficiency', in F. H. Bach and R. A. Good (eds.), *Clinical Immunobiology*, Academic Press, New York, Vol. II, pp. 63–114.
14. Gorovitz, S.: 1978, 'Medical Fallibility: A Rejoinder', *Journal of Medicine and Philosophy* 3, 187–191.
15. Gorovitz, S. and MacIntyre, A.: 1976, 'Toward a Theory of Medical Fallibility', *Journal of Medicine and Philosophy* 1, 51–71.
16. Hart, H. L. A. and Honoré, A. M.: 1959, *Causation in the Law*, Clarendon Press, Oxford.
17. Hempel, C. G.: 1965, *Aspects of Scientific Explanation*, Free Press, New York.
18. Hempel, C. G. and Oppenheim, P.: 1948, 'Studies in the Logic of Explanation', *Philosophy of Science* **15**, 135–175.
19. Lewontin, R. C.: 1969, 'The Bases of Conflict in Biological Explanation', *Journal of the History of Biology* **2**, 35–45.
20. Mackie, J.: 1974, *The Cement of the Universe*, Oxford University Press, Oxford.
21. Martin, M.: 1977, 'On a New Theory of Medical Fallibility: A Rejoinder', *Journal of Medicine and Philosophy* 2, 84–88.
22. Merton, R. K.: 1968, 'On Sociological Theories of the Middle Range', in R. K. Merton, *Social Theory and Social Structure*, Free Press, New York, pp. 39–72.
23. Miller, J. F. A. P.: 1961, 'Immunological Function of the Thymus', *Lancet* **2**, 748–749.
24. Peterson, R. D. A., Cooper, M. D., and Good, R. A.: 1965, 'The Pathogenesis of Immunological Deficiency Diseases', *The American Journal of Medicine* **38**, 579–604.

25. Salmon, W. C.: 1971, *Statistical Explanation and Statistical Relevance*, University of Pittsburgh Press, Pittsburgh.
26. Salmon, W. C.: 1978, 'Why Ask "Why?"?', *American Philosophical Association* 51, 683–705.
27. Schaffner, K. F.: 1980, 'Theory Structure in the Biomedical Sciences', *Journal of Medicine and Philosophy* 5, 57–97.
28. Scriven, M.: 1959, 'Truisms as the Grounds for Historical Explanations', in P. Gardiner (ed.), *Theories of History*, The Free Press, New York, 443–475.
29. Scriven, M.: 1959, 'Explanation and Prediction in Evolutionary Theory', *Science* 130, 477–482.
30. Toulmin, S.: 1961, *Foresight and Understanding*, Hutchinson, London.
31. Warner, N. and Szenberg, A.: 1962, 'Effect of Neonatal Thymectomy on the Immune Response in the Chicken', *Nature* 196, 784–785.
32. Warner, N. and Szenberg, A.: 1964, 'The Immunological Function of the Bursa of Fabricius in the Chicken', *Annual Review of Microbiology* 18, 253–268.
33. Watson, J.: 1970, *Molecular Biology of the Gene* (2nd ed.), Benjamin, New York.

H. TRISTRAM ENGELHARDT, JR.

RELEVANT CAUSES: THEIR DESIGNATION IN MEDICINE AND LAW

Kenneth Schaffner has given an important and useful treatment of the meaning of causality and the extent to which it is best understood through an inductive statistical or a statistical relevance view of causality. Etiological accounts in biomedicine do indeed refer back to gappy universals and employ both deductive and statistical reasonings. However, there is an important point made by Hart and Honoré, and acknowledged by Professor Schaffner, which must be underscored in order to understand the role of causal language in law and medicine. Schaffner acknowledges the dependence upon practical interests in Hart and Honoré's concept of cause. *Causes* are abnormal conditions which are contrasted with *conditions*, which are the expected or proper state of affairs. As Schaffner notes, following Hart and Honoré,

> A special laboratory from which oxygen is normally excluded suggests that the presence of oxygen will be construed as a cause of fire rather than a condition. Practical interests including controllability may also dictate which element is identified as the cause, i.e., what 'makes the difference' in a series of conditions ([2], pp. 2–3).

It is this dependence upon *practical* interests that makes the law's understanding of causality in medicine an enterprise of policy as much as one of description or explanation. That is, the law looks to medicine not in order to identify all the causal elements of an event, all the insufficient but non-redundant elements of the unnecessary but sufficient condition of events, or the necessary conditions, or the necessary and sufficient conditions of an event, but those that are *useful* in assigning responsibility in human conduct. In this sense the lawyer's use of causality is similar to that of the clinician, not the biomedical scientist. The clinician is likely to speak of *mycobacterium tuberculosis* as the cause of tuberculosis, although it is only a necessary not a sufficient condition. However, the biomedical scientist will indicate all non-necessary conditions which in conjunction with the necessary conditions constitute sufficient conditions: genetic susceptibility, nutrition. Again, in contrast, a public health physician may speak of poor economic conditions as the cause of widespread tuberculosis. In the case of the clinician and in the case of the public health physician particular causal conditions have been

S. F. Spicker, J. M. Healey, and H. T. Engelhardt (eds.), The Law–Medicine Relation: A Philosophical Exploration, 123–127.

highlighted. This I take as well to be the goal of the law: to select and highlight particular causes for practical reasons.

Schaffner recognizes this when he signals the dependence of Hart and Honoré's identifications of causes upon appeals to 'human habit, custom or convention'. Law and medicine require thus not only an account of causality, but a rubric for selecting relevant causes. Again, relevant causes for clinical medicine are those conditions likely to be influenced through therapy or prevented through prophylaxis. As a consequence, the causes of interest to a clinician can be identified only by reference to the interests of particular groups of clinicians. Thus one may attend to the *genetics of phenylketonuria* as the cause of the disease and not our phenylalanine rich diets – that is, one will usually view phenylketonuria as a genetic not a dietary disease. The same holds as well for hypertension, which may be considered to be a disease due to various factors such as stress and genetic background, though sodium intake may be a necessary condition. In fact such studies might suggest that one could treat it as a dietary disease, just as one treats tuberculosis as an infectious disease, though genetic background and stress can affect the chances of developing the disease. My point is again that *one underscores or isolates certain of many causal conditions because they are the easiest or most useful conditions to address*.

The law similarly selects causal relations with a view toward supporting various practices of assigning responsibilities, which practices are supplemented by various non-causal modes of assigning responsibility. This view is supported by Hart and Honoré, as is shown by an examination of their account of omissions as causes. Hart and Honoré elaborate their account of omissions through developing such common sense notions as, e.g., a person's failure to take an umbrella with him is the cause of his getting wet if it rains [2]. Implicit in such an assertion is some notion of what it would have been *prudent* or normal to do. The fact that one has failed to build numerous shelters into which to seek protection should rain start will not be advanced as the cause of one's being wet. Such discrimination of causes depends upon distinguishing causes from conditions, where causes are circumstances that are not normal, and conditions are circumstances which are deemed normal.

The selection of some conditions as normal (and thus conditions in this special sense) and other conditions as abnormal (and thus as causes in the practice of assigning responsibility) will turn on particular ways in which we structure the world. Thus Hart and Honoré give the example of the gardener's failure to water the flowers as the cause of the flowers dying. One identifies the gardener's *omission as the cause* because of 'the special interests in the particular case'. Hart and Honoré indicate that one does not signal the physical conditions because such would show only

> what *always* happens when flowers die, *why* flowers die: whereas an explanation is wanted not of that, but of the death of *these* flowers when normally *they* would have lived: what made *this* difference was the gardener's omission – an abnormal failure of a normal condition ([2], p. 37).

However, to signal some conditions as *normal* and others as *abnormal* requires reference, as the example of the gardener shows, to a complex web of human obligations, duties and expectations. A cause of the flowers' dying was not the failure of passersby to water them. Such an account succeeds only given a particular set of views concerning usual obligations or duties, which set of views signals that passersby are not expected to stop. Such views specify the causal field of background conditions that allows one to focus on the relevant causes for the context under consideration.

It is here, I take it, that the need of the law to isolate causal conditions relevant for assigning responsibility engenders many of the conflicts between physicians' and lawyers' views of causality. These conflicts arise because physicians and lawyers have at times different views of what the normal state of affairs is, or should be. They differ because their views of what physician-patient duties should be, or reasonably can be, differ. Consider, for example, a recent finding of the Wisconsin Supreme Court to the effect that surgical nurses are not responsible for not having noted that a hemostat was missing, and thus had probably been left in the patient during surgery. The court decision turned, in part, upon the lack of an established duty of care on the part of nurses to perform a post-surgical instrument count [3]. In addition to presupposing certain special, perhaps non-causal senses of responsibility, the question at issue was the extent to which the nurses' omission was a normal condition or an abnormal condition, i.e., a cause of the hemostat being left in the patient. As in the case of the gardener and the unwatered flowers, the cause of the untoward effects is to be isolated only by reference to a duty, here a *convention* concerning the duties of nurses.

One should note as well how many of the controversies that arise in medical malpractice suits turn on who can competently distinguish causes and conditions. For example, consider the special role of the invocation of *res ipsa loquitur* in order to move to establish negligence without employing expert witnesses. Such an invocation presupposes that in a case at hand it is clear that an injury would not have occurred in the absence of negligence and that, therefore, laymen can recognize the differences between normal and abnormal conditions. Such issues raise the question of who has the expertise to distinguish conditions from causes. Often making such discriminations requires not only an expertise sufficient to grasp the scientific issues involved, but also an expertise regarding the standards of care and, therefore, the established duties which define the legal issues. To determine the line between conditions and causes requires determining, for example, the duties of gardeners to water flowers; of nurses and physicians to their patients.

Again, such selections of certain causes in the practice of assigning responsibility does not presuppose a notion of causality other than that generally used in medicine and the sciences. However, there are other non-causal or not-fully causally grounded ways of assigning responsibility, which I note here but shall not explore. One might think here, for example, of the practice of holding masters accountable for the actions of their servants, the vicarious responsibility of the captain of the ship for the actions of those under his command [1]. One might also think here of the assignment of responsibility for the consequences of the influence on the voluntary actions of others in procuring their illicit actions. Again. One might think of the responsibilities one incurs in joining a conspiracy [4]. With respect to conflicts between physicians' and lawyers' views of accountability, it is probably the case that the assignment of vicarious responsibility to physicians as 'captains of the ship' evokes a great deal of consternation because such assignments of responsibility to physicians can occur in the absence of an obvious, direct causal link. Insofar as there are practices that do not depend upon identifying a causal basis for responsibility, Schaffner does not deal with them, nor shall I, except in recognition that they often strengthen the notion, which Schaffner has shown is unfounded, that the concept of causality employed in the law differs from that employed in medicine and the sciences.

This last point is the one I wish to stress: namely, that *the basic meaning of causality does not vary among law, medicine and the sciences, though law and medicine select some and ignore other causes within particular practices of attributing responsibility for actions and omissions, or of characterizing circumstances with a view towards treatment and prevention.*

It is the varying views of how to structure such social practices of identifying relevant causes which probably underlie much of the disagreement between lawyers and physicians. One is here reminded of the different view of the proper standards of care one should require of physicians: the standards of the local community of physicians, the standards of a particular medical specialty, or the standards of care of the most competent physicians, etc. Such choices are, in the end, choices between calling certain circumstances 'conditions' and other conditions 'causes', that is, abnormal conditions. Causal language is thus enlisted in particular social practices which serve to highlight particular causes for particular social purposes. However, the significance of causal language, as causal language, need not be essentially different in the law from similar language employed elsewhere. Rather, *all that is required is that law and medicine select different causes and causal patterns for attention because they are different social institutions with different goals.* By selecting some conditions as normal, background conditions, and other conditions as the cause at issue, one gives direction to a practical undertaking. Professor Schaffner's defense of a unitary theory of causation can, as a result, hold. One must, however, be careful to notice that different social institutions attend to some causes, not others, in structuring certain endeavors. Each has special concerns that highlight some, not other, causal conditions as most relevant. Social institutions, it turns out, often reflect particular causal variables for particular practical purposes without employing different notions of causality.

Georgetown University
Washington, D.C.

BIBLIOGRAPHY

1. *Aktieselskabet Cuzco v. The Sucarseco*; 294 U.S. 394, 55 S.ct. 467.
2. Hart, H. L. and Honoré, A. M.: 1959, *Causation in the Law*, Oxford University Press, Oxford.
3. *Mossey v. Mueller*, 218 N. W. 2nd 514 (Wisconsin Supreme Court, June 4, 1974).
4. *U.S. v. Rabinowich*, 238 U.S. 78, 35 S.ct. 682.

THOMAS HALPER

TIME, LAW AND RESPONSIBILITY: ADDITIONAL THOUGHTS ON CAUSALITY

Let me confess at the outset that the subject of causality invariably puts me in mind of Augustine's famous complaint about the subject of time: "Quid est tempus? Si nemo a me quaeret, scio, si quaerenti explicare velin, nescio!" ([2], Bk. XI, Chap. XV). 'What is causality?' I inquire, warily and wearily. "If no one asks of me, I know; if I wish to explain to him who asks, I know not". I hope that I may be excused, therefore, if in my remarks I focus less on causality narrowly conceived than on three themes sutured to the concept by the thread of everyday life.

I. TIME

'Causality' – and such related terms as 'influence', 'consequence', and 'create' – is a notion we employ reflexively in everyday speech. In this, we rarely experience difficulties, perhaps because ordinarily we are more interested in prediction than in explanation.[1] We have noticed, for instance, that when a baseball hits a window, it shatters. Our concern is not whether the ball 'caused' the break. It is enough for our purposes that the break normally follows the ball's contact with the window – that the shattering of glass is predictable – for us to feel the need to chase young ballplayers away from our house.[2] Anyone seeking to explain the event in terms of masses and forces would be hard put, I believe, to find an audience.

It is the obvious utility of prediction and its widely perceived connection with causality, I suppose, that have helped reinforce the common assumption that causes must always precede effects. Yet even in this post-Age of Aquarius, it is not difficult to conceive of a clairvoyant, who, foreseeing a future event, acts to take advantage of what he sees. Nor is it easy to understand how the temporal assumption accommodates 'chicken and egg' problems, like those associated with such closed loop systems as the thermostat, once the process has begun. Does the heat cause the thermostat to start or stop the furnace? Or does the thermostat cause the heat to rise or fall? The well-worn aphorism that "a hen is an egg's way of making another egg" hardly settles the matter. Nor does the traditional family complaint, "insanity is hereditary: you get it from your children".

S. F. Spicker, J. M. Healey, and H. T. Engelhardt (eds.), The Law–Medicine Relation: A Philosophical Exploration, 129–136.

Professors Schaffner [32] and Mackie [25] avoid these problems by attending to causal rather than to temporal priority. A cause is prior to an event, that is, if and only if there is a time when the cause is fixed but the event is unfixed. (An event is fixed, if, given the world as it is at some point in time and given the operation of natural laws, the event could not but take place.) Implicit in this approach, however, is an apparent paradox that may be worth mentioning: if one posits a deterministic universe, there never existed a time at which an event was unfixed, and so in such a setting, there can be no causal priority, and, therefore, no causality. Thus, causality is incompatible with determinism, although determinism is ordinarily said to mean that 'all events are caused' ([7], p. 19).

II. LAW

Given the pervasive importance of causality, it is certainly not surprising that it plays a vital role in that effort to regulate human behavior known as the law. Whatever the metaphysical imponderables, however, causality has always been treated by lawyers along "broad common-sense lines rather than by any scientific analysis that is too subtle" ([41], p. 472). "A cause", says William Prosser, for example, "is a necessary antecedent ... the term embraces all things which have so far contributed to the result that without them it would not have occurred" ([31], p. 241). Law suits, therefore, normally allege some causal connection between the defendant's act or failure to act and the plaintiff's damages.[3] Specifically, the plaintiff must show that the defendant's wrongdoing both was a cause in fact of the harm and was the proximate cause of the harm. The search for the cause in fact "is not a quest for a sole cause" ([19], II, p. 1109), but instead is a down-to-earth inquiry into the alleged presence of a causal relation. This relation is most often determined by the 'but for' test. That is, the defendant's negligence is a cause in fact of a harm, where the harm would not have occurred *but for* the defendant's negligence ([35], pp. 103, 106, 109).

This ostensibly sound and practical approach, however, is fraught with difficulties. First, every event necessarily has a multitude of causes – not all of them known or perhaps even knowable – each of which in some sense produced the harm. Absent one or more of these causes, would the event have occurred? Since the events can rarely be reproduced like laboratory experiments, some irreducible doubt is apt to persist, like an ice patch on a March lawn. Thus, in recognition of this doubt and imprecision, judges are not permitted to instruct juries that they must find the defendant's conduct to be even the 'dominant' cause of the injury ([5], [37]). Second, if two causes contrive to bring about an event, but either could have brought it about alone, the test breaks down.[4]

If 'cause in fact' is merely a descriptive term, it remains for the inappropriately titled ([31], p. 282) 'proximate cause' to turn our attention to the matter of responsibility. Proximate cause suggests the notion of immediacy or nearness, and, indeed, was born in Lord Chancellor Bacon's maxim, 'In jure non remota causa, sed proxima, spectatur'.[5] But as it has evolved, the term concerns not the closeness of time and space, but simply whether the defendant was legally obligated to protect the plaintiff against the event which in fact took place ([18], pp. 11–43; [9], p. 402). The answer to this question, therefore, springs not from causal analysis but rather from public policy. "At bottom", write Whitecross and Paton, "the problem is one of balancing interests – how far is the protection of the plaintiff to be carried?" ([41], p. 473). There is no point in rehearsing old battles between would-be reformulators of proximate cause – those defining it as the responsibility of the last culpable actor ([40] p. 134; [35]) or as "a substantial factor in producing the damage complained of" ([34], pp. 103, 223, 229; [26]) or as harm 'justly attachable' to the defendant's conduct ([11], pp. 211, 343) – except to note that a leading commentator has aptly dismissed them all as 'fruitless' ([31], p. 288).

What is worth discussing, however, is the appositeness of the balancing approach itself. According to this approach, so highly regarded by lawyers for its practicality and workability, competing claims are balanced on a case-by-case basis, the weightier claim prevailing over the lighter one. Building upon a metaphor of the scales of justice – a metaphor spackled onto common speech and given tangible form in a thousand court house statues – the balancing approach rests upon a foundation legitimized by familiarity.

And yet as comfortable as the image is, there is something fundamentally disingenuous and misleading about it. For, in truth, the balancing test begs two central questions and thereby serves to camouflage the workings of unspoken assumptions that too often predetermine conclusions later so laboriously defended. First of all, the balancing test assumes that the claims to be weighed are as 'given' as weights on a scale. In fact, however, the claims are not really 'given' at all. The mode of their formulation can have a profound impact upon their power and relevance. And the selection of which two claims to weigh may entail ignoring other claims of arguably major significance.[6] Second, the balancing test assumes that the 'heavier' claim can be chosen in an objective fashion, requiring only that an observer be honest and careful in reporting what he sees. But claims are not tangible weights, subject to the impartial pull of gravity; they are melanges of data and contentions, molded for partisan purposes. As such, they call not for the simple skills of a passive observer, but for the highly developed skills of an active evaluator. Yet the balancing test, by pretending that choosing the better argument is truly analogous to choosing the heavier weight, hides this evaluation process – together with its necessarily subjective elements – from public view. Ordinarily, this would raise no cause for concern. After all, it is this same balancing approach – though in far less explicit and sophisticated form – that you and I use in making the innumerable unquantified selections that help to answer the cosmic and mundane questions that dominate our daily lives. Shall we choose this career or that one? this residential locale or that one? this salad dressing or that one? We 'weight' the competing perceived benefits and costs, reach our decision, and hope for the best. Perhaps, it is unrealistic to expect much more from public decision makers, since the din from their power and glory can scarcely exempt them from the limitations of the species. Yet the formalized balancing test and its rhetorical mumbo-jumbo, by shielding the messy and value laden process from rigorous scrutiny, interferes with popular understanding of the rationale of official action. In this way, the test complicates the implementation of the principle of accountability that must remain critical to the maintenance of a free society.

III. RESPONSIBILITY

After years of dowdy unfashionability, responsibility appears to be making a comeback?[7] It is hard to trace the origins of this rally – to a moralistic reaction to Vietnam and Watergate, perhaps, or to a belated recognition of the limits of the narcissism legitimated by the ubiquitous counter-culture – but, for the present at least, responsibility seems to be 'in'. Yet, used both to describe relationships and prescribe obligations, 'responsibility' has acquired a vagueness that sometimes seems indistinguishable from unintelligibility.

In the descriptive sense, of course, 'responsibility' is intimately intertwined with the notions of causality and explanation. But it is my purpose to stress the judgmental sense, in which 'responsibility' expresses approval or disapproval of individual actions. In these instances, it is necessary to consider not merely the effect of particular actions, but also such matters as voluntariness, knowledge of fact, and law and short and long-run intentions. Normally, judgmental responsibility involves the ascription of moral fault, and one need only recall the intense debate provoked by Hannah Arendt's *Eichmann in*

Jerusalem to understand how widely and deeply held is the belief in the necessity of this legal-ethical connection.

Yet this connection is not invariable. The common law in its earliest days held "men answerable for all the ills of an obvious kind that their deeds bring upon their fellows" ([30], II, p. 470; cf. [24], p. 589), regardless of intent. Emphasizing "the loss and damage of the party suffering" [23], the law sought to preserve peace by offering an alternative to private vengeance ([21], pp. 2, 3). As the task of keeping order shifted to other governmental agencies (mainly, the police), however, the moral anomaly of liability without fault came under increasing attack ([21], pp. 144–63; [35], pp. 241, 319, 409).

Nonetheless, the doctrine of strict liability – liability, that is, without fault – remains very much alive. Prosecution under certain laws not requiring *mens rea* has been held valid under the due process clause ([33], [38], [39], [27]), though the courts have insisted on strong evidence of legislative intent to dispense with *mens rea* and the crimes have usually been minor offenses with minimal punishments. In addition, in tort law, ultrahazardous activities entailing an inherent risk of injury often impose liability upon those engaging in them, regardless of the absence of negligence. Aiming at discouraging but not prohibiting dangerous activities while compensating the unfortunate victims, these laws seek a rough, practical justice.

As recourse to strict liability has grown in recent years – in order to reduce expense, delay, and inconvenience – 'responsibility' and 'causation' more and more have seemed to converge. But if "the notion of 'strict liability' in morals comes as near to being a contradiction in terms as anything in this sphere" ([20], p. 169), as Hart has so cogently argued, perhaps it is time to reconsider the claims to expediency and societal utility in the light of their increasing conceptual threat to one of society's most properly cherished values.

IV. A FINAL WORD

Our interest in causality, despite its triumphantly elusive character, is not hard to understand. For one thing, causality, as philosophers well appreciate, is a key operating notion of everyday life, and however structured in cognition, 'organizes' our experience so that we can come to know the world. What Nagel said of modern theoretical science, then, can surely be expanded to fill the countless interstices of all mental behavior: "it is difficult to understand how it would be possible . . . to surrender the general ideal expressed by the principle [of causality] without becoming thereby transformed into something incomparably different from what that enterprise actually is" ([28], p. 324). Secondly, as I have tried to show, causality is tied to a variety of fundamental philosophical and practical concerns, like time, law, and responsibility. Differences in analyzing causality, therefore, may be more a function of differing perspectives than of anything more profound and complex. For just as a butcher and a veterinarian may see different things when gazing at the same cow, so a physician and an attorney may choose to isolate and emphasize different causal factors when viewing (say) a victim of food poisoning. The former may think in terms of physiology and pathology, the latter in terms of rights, duties, and obligations, but their argument concerning what caused the problem reflects not a clash over the meaning of causality but simply over the implications of their specialized competencies and habits of thought.

But while it may be wise to leave the notion of causality undefined or poorly developed ([15], p. 127), it is impossible to discard it as a working assumption underpinning our systematic investigations of the world ([16], ch. I). Causality, as a consequence, may be no less valuable heuristically merely because it can never be demonstrated empirically. Maybe the problem of causality, as one astute social scientist has suggested, is simply another manifestation of the "inherent gap between the languages of theory and research which can never be bridged in a completely satisfactory way" ([6], p. 5). But though the gap cannot be bridged, it may still not be too much to hope that those of us who remain drawn to the abyss by its dangers and fascinations can be taught enough care and respect to prevent the tumbling destruction of our work.

Baruch College, City University of New York
New York, New York

NOTES

[1] Friedman seems to argue that, indeed, there is no difference between predictions and cause-and-effect statements ([17], pp. 7–13). Wold contends that causal relationships, instead, should be considered a subclass of predictions [42]. Arguably, however, causal statements are actually a subclass of associational statements, though everyone is familiar with the old saw that correlation does not mean causality. Few have expressed this trite point as vividly as Cohen, who observed that the International Association of Machinists' membership from 1912 to 1920 showed an impressive eighty-six percent correlation with the death rate in the Indian state of Hyderabad from 1911 to 1919 ([10], p. 92).

[2] But, of course, as Hume long ago pointed out, prediction is mere induction from a 'constant conjunction' in the past; and this conjunction can never be shown to be the 'necessary connexion' required in a causal relationship. Hume did not deny causality and claim that it was merely a subjective artifact of the mind of the observer, but he did hold that we could not isolate it or demonstrate its existence (See [22], p. 379).

[3] Thus, Epstein argues that cause is central to the ascription of legal responsibility. If you have done something, in other words, you should be held responsibile for it unless you can overcome that presumption with some exculpatory excuse ([12], p. 151; [13], p. 165; [14], p. 391).

[4] The defendant's action must be a material element and a substantial factor in causing the injury [1].

[5] "In law the near cause is looked to, not the remote one" ([3], Reg. I).

[6] Thus, in a number of free speech cases, courts have professed to balance the individual's interest in expression against such societal interests as national security or crime control, neglecting claims for the societal interest in free speech ([4], [8]).

[7] Thus, that ultimate arbiter of contemporary chic, the Cosmopolitan Girl, gurgled, "What is the very best thing a man can be if he really loves a woman? Responsible! That may sound a little unsexy but believe me it can be quite a turn-on!" [29].

BIBLIOGRAPHY

1. *Anderson v. Minneapolis*: 1920: St. P. & S. S. M. R. Co., 146 Minn. 430, 179 N.W. 45.
2. Augustine: 1912, *Confessions of St. Augustine*, Robinson and Reese, London.
3. Bacon, F.: 1914, *Maxims of the Law*, Robinson and Reese, London.
4. *Barenblatt v. United States*: 1959, 360 U.S. 109.
5. *Barrington v. Arnold*: 1960, 356 Mich. 594, 101 N. W. 2d 365.
6. Blalock, H. M., Jr.: 1964, *Causal Inference in Nonexperimental Research*, Norton, New York.
7. Blanshard, B.: 1961, 'The Case for Determinism', in S. Hook (ed.), *Determinism and Freedom in the Age of Modern Science*, Collier Books, New York, pp. 19–30.
8. *Branzburg v. Hayes*: 1972, 408 U.S. 665.
9. Campbell, R. V.: 1943, 'Duty, Fault and Legal Cause', *Wisconsin Law Review*, 402–28.
10. Cohen, M. R.: 1964, *Reason and Nature: An Essay on the Meaning of Scientific Method*, 2d ed., Free Press, New York.
11. Edgerton, H. W.: 1924, 'Legal Cause', *Univ. of Pennsylvania Law Review* 72, 211–50; 343–82.
12. Epstein, R. A.: 1973, 'A Theory of Strict Liability', *Journal of Legal Studies* 2, 151–86.
13. Epstein, R. A.: 1974, 'Defenses and Subsequent Pleas in a System of Strict Liability', *Journal of Legal Studies* 3, 165–91.
14. Epstein, R. A.: 1975, 'Intentional Harms', *Journal of Legal Studies* 4, 391–424.
15. Francis, R. G.: 1961, *The Rhetoric of Science*, Univ. of Minnesota Press, Minneapolis, Mn.
16. Frank, P.: 1961, *Modern Science and Its Philosophy*, Collier Books, New York.

17. Friedman, M.: 1953, *Essays in Political Economy*, Univ. of Chicago Press, Chicago, Ill.
18. Green, L.: 1927, *Rationale of Proximate Cause*, Longman Green, London.
19. Harper, F. V. and James, F., Jr.: 1956, *The Law of Torts*, Little, Brown, Boston.
20. Hart, H. L. A.: 1961, *The Concept of Law*, Clarendon Press, Oxford.
21. Holmes, O. W.: 1881, *The Common Law*, Little, Brown, Boston.
22. Hume, D.: 1878, *A Treatise on Human Nature*, Longman Green, London.
23. *Lambert v. Bessey*: 1681, 88 Eng. Rep. 220.
24. Levitt, A.: 'The Extent and Function of the Doctrine of Mens Rea', *Illinois Law Review* 17, 589–620.
25. Mackie, J. L.: 1974, *The Cement of the Universe: A Study of Causation*, Oxford Univ. Press, Oxford.
26. *Mahoney v. Beatman*: 1929, 110 Conn. 184, 147 A. 762.
27. *Morissette v. United States*: 1952, 342 U.S. 246.
28. Nagel, E.: 1961, *The Structure of Science: Problems in the Logic of Scientific Method*, Harcourt, Brace, and World, New York.
29. *New York Times*, January 15, 1976, p. 68, col. 1.
30. Pollock, F. and Maitland, F. W.: 1899, *The History of English Law before the Time of Edward I*, 2d ed., Cambridge Univ. Press, Cambridge.
31. Prosser, W. L.: 1964, *Law of Torts*, 3d ed., West, St. Paul, Mn.
32. Schaffner, K. F.: 1980, 'Causal Explanation in Biomedicine and the Law', in this volume, pp. 95–122.
33. *Shevlin-Carpenter Co. v. Minnesota*: 1910, 218 U.S. 57.
34. Smith J.: 1911, 'Legal Cause in Actions of Tort', *Harvard Law Review* **25**, 103–53; 223–64.
35. Smith, J.: 1917, 'Tort and Absolute Liability', *Harvard Law Review* **30**, 241–281; 319–64; 409–53.
36. *Stone v. Philadelphia*: 1931, 302 Pa. 340, 153 A. 550.
37. *Strobel v. Chicago R. I. & P. R. Co.*: 1959, 255 Minn. 201, 96 N. W. 2d 195.
38. *United States v. Balint*: 1922, 258 U.S. 250.
39. *United States v. Dollerweich*: 1943, 320 U.S. 277.
40. Wharton, J. F.: 1974, *Negligence*, Cox and Hodges, London.
41. Whitecross, G. and Paton, G.: 1972, *A Text-book on Jurisprudence*, 4th ed., Oxford Univ. Press, Oxford.
42. Wold, H. O. A.: 1966, 'On the Definition and Meaning of Causal Concepts', *Model Building in the Human Sciences*, Centre Internationale d'Etude des Problèmes Humains, Paris, France.

SECTION III

THE PSYCHIATRIST'S DILEMMA: DUTY TO PATIENT OR DUTY TO SOCIETY?

WILLIAM J. WINSLADE

PSYCHOTHERAPEUTIC DISCRETION AND JUDICIAL DECISION: A CASE OF ENIGMATIC JUSTICE

I. INTRODUCTION

On October 27, 1969, Prosenjit Poddar, a 25-year old graduate student from India, fatally shot and stabbed Tatiana Tarasoff, a young junior college student. One might suppose that this was a crime of passion with a familiar pattern: a spurned suitor's desire for revenge erupts into an uncontrollable (or perhaps only uncontrolled) impulse to destroy the rejecting woman. Not unexpectedly, the jury convicted Poddar of second-degree murder, despite a plea of insanity and diminished capacity that was considerably buttressed by psychiatric and lay testimony as to Poddar's bizarre behavior. Poddar's criminal trial might have ended with his conviction and sentencing, followed by his serving about five years (the average time served for second-degree murder [1]) and, if his prison behavior was acceptable, his release on parole.

However, Poddar's case was somewhat unusual. A closer look at the facts – both of the circumstances preceding the killing and the subsequent legal procedures that resulted in not only a *Poddar* case [8] but also a *Tarasoff* case [12] – will reveal some ways in which judges try to articulate general principles that must be applied to irreducible and stubborn facts that defy legal categorization, and psychotherapists try to cope with perplexing features of the human condition that cannot be effectively controlled by psychotherapeutic intervention.

After Poddar's conviction for second degree murder, his attorneys filed an appeal. The principal claim was that the trial judge had given inadequate instructions on diminished capacity to the jury. The California Supreme Court reversed the conviction on this ground [8]. Although this technical issue is of interest to legal scholars and criminal lawyers, our present interest in the *Poddar* case is in what it reveals about the administration of the criminal justice system. Despite the formalities of the legal procedures and the circuitous routes that one must sometimes take as a result of them, the cumulative effect of judicial review, the discretion of the prosecutor, and clever legal representation can contribute to an outcome that is partially understandable but also inconclusive, ambiguous and perplexing.

When Tatiana Tarasoff's parents learned that Poddar had been treated by

S. F. Spicker, J. M. Healey, and H. T. Engelhardt (eds.), The Law–Medicine Relation: A Philosophical Exploration, 139–157.

psychotherapists at the University of California Student Health Service at Berkeley and that he had been interviewed by the campus police at the request of Poddar's therapist, who thought Poddar was dangerous, the parents brought a civil lawsuit against the therapists (and their employers) and the police on the grounds that their negligence caused Tatiana's wrongful death. Tatiana's parents claimed that the therapists or the police had a duty to confine Poddar or at least to warn Tatiana or her parents of the danger to her.[2]

This lawsuit – the *Tarasoff* case – appeared to end very quickly. The trial court in which the complaint was filed upheld the claim by the defendants that Tatiana's parents had failed to state a cause of action – i.e., a legal basis for liability – in their complaint. When the trial court dismissed the complaint and gave no opportunity for the plaintiffs to amend it, the dismissal was appealed. The California Court of Appeal upheld the trial court decision. When the case was then appealed to the California Supreme Court, most interested observers, including the psychotherapeutic community and the law enforcement agencies, expected the California Supreme Court to agree with the lower courts. But much to everyone's surprise, the California Supreme Court reversed the lower court's opinion, holding that a cause of action for negligence did exist against the therapists and the police for failing to warn [11]. They remanded the case for trial.

The defendants immediately petitioned the Supreme Court for a rehearing, a request that is rarely granted. However, after an alarmed outcry from both the psychotherapeutic community and law enforcement agencies, the Court granted the petition. The first opinion delivered by the Court in the *Tarasoff* case on December 24, 1974, was legally placed in limbo until after the rehearing and the issuance of the second opinion. It was one and one-half years later – on July 1, 1976 – that the Surpreme Court finally rendered its final and official decision in *Tarasoff* [12]. By this time the first, but no longer official, opinion had already generated considerable national controversy. The second opinion, though anticlimactic, modified the first in certain important respects. The most significant revision was that, unlike the psychotherapists, the police were exempted from any potential liability on the grounds that they did not stand in a special relationship to Tatiana or her parents that gave rise to any legal duty to them ([8] p. 29). In addition, the language of the second opinion stated the legal duty of psychotherapists in broader terms than the first opinion. Therapists are said to have more than a specific duty to warn threatened victims; they have a general duty to use reasonable care to protect threatened victims from harm [12].[3] As we shall see later, this expanded ruling has potentially far-reaching consequences for the psychotherapist-patient relationship.

It will not be possible to explore all the implications of *Tarasoff* in this essay. For example, the case raises questions concerning informed consent to psychotherapy, the scope of confidentiality, the proper uses of involuntary civil commitment, the role of psychotherapists as agents of social control and a cluster of related issues.[4] What shall be explored here is a more limited set of problems. It will be argued that despite the initial alarm created in the psychotherapeutic community about the destructive implications of *Tarasoff*, its actual legal impact has been minimal. However, the *Tarasoff* rule does give rise to justified concern by psychotherapists that the ambiguity of the rule (1) creates confusion about their professional roles and responsibilities, (2) exposes them to serious threats of litigation even if liability is unlikely and (3) undermines judicious exercise of psychotherapeutic discretion.

II. PEOPLE *V.* PODDAR

A. *Factual Background*

When Prosenjit Poddar was tried for the murder of Tatiana Tarasoff, the fact that Poddar had killed Tatiana was not disputed; the trial turned rather on whether the defendant was capable of harboring the requisite intent to sustain a conviction for murder. Key facts of the case revealed during the criminal proceedings are as follows.[5]

Prosenjit Poddar was born into the lowest of 'untouchable' castes in rural India and had worked his way to the top of the Indian University System. He was "considered by some to be a genius". In September of 1967, his university had sent him to the University of California, Berkeley, to study naval architecture, and in the fall of 1968, he had met Tatiana Tarasoff, a college student of Russian descent who had come to the United States in 1963. Through weekly contact at folk dances at Berkeley's International House, a friendship had developed between them, and on New Year's Eve she had kissed him. To Poddar, who had had no previous experience with women and in whose culture pre-arranged marriage was preceded by no prior physical contact between the parties, her interest in him apparently signaled betrothal.

When she thereafter alternately encouraged and rejected him (at least in Poddar's eyes), he became confused and withdrawn, going through long periods during which he failed to appear for either his classes or his job, in both of which he had previously been highly motivated to succeed. During these periods he remained in bed, eating and sleeping little, brooding over his relationship with Tatiana and attempting to analyze it by playing over some 15 000 feet of tape recordings he had surreptitiously made of his conversations with her. He came ultimately to perceive her as a temptress and a tease, bent on his destruction. His obsession turned to thoughts of revenge.[6]

In June, 1969, Tatiana left the country for Brazil. In the same month a close Indian friend of Poddar's who had become alarmed at Poddar's condition arranged for him to see Dr. Stuart Gold, a psychiatrist at the university's student health service. Dr. Gold in turn referred the patient to a clinical psychologist on the university staff, Dr. Lawrence Moore. Both doctors diagnosed the patient as an acute paranoid schizophrenic. During the summer of 1969, Poddar received a total of nine therapy sessions, seven of which were with Dr. Moore. In one of the sessions, Poddar alluded to his intention to kill Tatiana. In addition, Poddar's friend who had arranged for the psychotherapy reported to Dr. Moore that Poddar intended to purchase a gun in San Francisco. Dr. Moore sought to evoke Poddar's assurance that he would not carry out his intention to kill Tatiana. When Poddar refused, Dr. Moore implied that he would have to take steps to prevent the threatened harm. On August 18th, Poddar left angrily and did not return for treatment.[7]

Dr. Moore then filed a report with the campus police [8] for the purpose of instituting involuntary commitment proceedings [2].[9] On August 21st the campus police investigated the threat to the extent of searching Poddar's room and taking him into custody for questioning. However, having failed to detect in him abnormal tendencies sufficient in their view to justify his commitment and having evoked his promise to stay away from Tatiana, they had subsequently released him. At the time of the investigation, Tatiana's brother Alex, with whom Poddar shared an apartment during the months prior to the killing in the fall of 1969, learned that Poddar had threatened to kill his sister; but because he believed that Poddar did not intend to carry out the threat, he took no action on the knowledge.[10]

In early September, Tatiana returned from Brazil. In Poddar's presence at a party she talked of her summer exploits with a Brazilian 'bootlegger'; Poddar thereafter accused her – to an acquaintance but within hearing distance of her – of 'whoring around'. He called daily at her home and attempted to see her, but she refused to have anything more to do with him. Her mother later testified that his persistence in calling Tatiana and following her around had made Tatiana fearful of him, and that the mother too was afraid and had threatened to call the police.

On Friday, October 24, Poddar again sought the help of Alex to intercede on Poddar's behalf with Tatiana. Again, Alex told Poddar to forget about his sister. Poddar and Alex subsequently fought; Alex overpowered Poddar who broke into tears. Poddar was warned by Alex that his father was prone to violence and might attack Poddar if he learned of Poddar's persistent attempts to see Tatiana. Nevertheless, at 8:00 a.m. on the morning of October 27, Poddar went to Tatiana's home. Although Tatiana was at home, she told her mother to answer the door and tell Poddar she was not at home. The mother, with tragic prophecy, told Poddar: "Why don't you go back to India where you belong?"

At 5:00 p.m., Poddar returned and found Tatiana home alone. She opened the door and let him in. She tried to make him leave but could not; when she screamed, he shot her with a pellet gun and, while following her into the yard, repeatedly stabbed her with a kitchen knife. Then he walked back into the house to call the police, stating he had just stabbed someone and wished to be taken into custody.

B. *The Criminal Trial*

At the ensuing criminal trial, which lasted 17 days, the central question was whether Poddar had the requisite intent for murder, was insane, or had diminished capacity at the time of the killing. Considerable anecdotal testimony from persons who knew or had contact with Poddar was presented. Poddar's extreme depression, confusion, anger and withdrawal from contact with friends, his work and his studies were well-documented. Not only to his therapists, but also to his friends and co-workers had Poddar expressed violent fantasies and described himself as feeling like an animal. He warned his closest friend to stay away from him at night because he feared that he might kill him. In addition, testimony of several psychiatrists was introduced concerning Poddar's 'paranoid schizophrenia' and his lack of ability to understand and control his feelings and behavior. However, it was also revealed at the trial that Poddar was capable of appearing rational to the police; Alex Tarasoff, who, it should be recalled, was Poddar's roommate for the months just prior to the killing, did not take Poddar's threats to Tatiana seriously. Even after the police investigated Dr. Moore's report and informed Alex of the threat, he did not believe that Poddar intended to kill Tatiana. After the killing, Poddar had enough composure to walk back into the house to call the police. We are also informed that while Poddar was in the Oakland jail and later imprisoned at Vacaville, he was competent to aid in his defense and was not suffering from any apparent mental disability.

In short, the evidence concerning Poddar's mental and emotional status prior to, at the time of and immediately after the killing was quite mixed. It would be possible to conclude that Poddar should be held fully accountable or to conclude that he suffered a significant loss of his capacity for rational control of his conduct due to his severe emotional conflict. The fact that the jury found him sane and not suffering from diminished capacity might well have ended the matter. But it is also understandable why the California Supreme Court, when it reviewed the record on appeal, may have felt ambivalent toward the case.

C. *California Supreme Court Review*

The technical issue before the court was whether the jury was properly instructed as to whether diminished capacity could negate implied malice as an element of second-degree murder. If the jury had determined that diminished capacity did preclude implied malice, then Poddar could have been convicted of manslaughter only. As the court unequivocally pointed out, "[t]he record discloses in the instant case that there was significant evidence of defendant's diminished capacity", ([8], p. 758). The Court added at another point that "[e]vidence was introduced which was almost overwhelming that by reason of diminished capacity defendant lacked malice aforethought", ([8], p. 761). Although most of the Court's opinion discusses the case's technical arguments germane to jury instructions concerning diminished capacity, it is clear from the above statements that the Court was persuaded of Poddar's diminished responsibility for his conduct. The reversal on technical grounds (subject to the possibility of a new trial) allowed the Court to give legal effect to their appraisal of the record. And a petition by the Attorney General for a rehearing was denied.

D. *The Results of Reversal*

The attorney who represented Poddar on the appeal maintained that the California Attorney General's office was quite upset by the reversal of Poddar's conviction on technical grounds, and the denial of the petition for a rehearing. Of course the case could have been retried – more than five years after the killing. But the clear message of the Supreme Court opinion was that Poddar's plea of diminished responsibility was likely to prevail on retrial. After the opinion was issued, Poddar's attorney made an *informal* proposal to the Attorney General's office that capitalized both on the Attorney General's discontent about the technical reversal and on the discretion of the prosecutor. It was proposed that Poddar be released from jail and not be subjected to a new trial on the condition that immediately upon release he would leave the United States and return to India. Poddar returned to India and is reported to be happily married – to a lawyer.

I relate this little known aspect of the *Poddar* case because it illustrates the ambiguous outcome of the case from a legal point of view. Poddar was convicted of murder and spent five years in custody but won a reversal of his conviction. Because he was not retried, the issue of his alleged diminished capacity was not put to another legal test. Thus, from a strictly legal point of view, Poddar's legal responsibility was not resolved. Nevertheless, his incarceration for five years gave practical effect to the original jury verdict. (Five years, you will recall, is the average time served by convicted second-degree murderers.)

The California Supreme Court, with an opportunity to review the criminal trial record from a perspective that provides sufficient psychological distance from the confusing human drama disclosed at the trial, felt that it, like the psychiatrists who testified, could discern substantial evidence of Poddar's diminished mental capacity. The impact of this evidence on the trial jury was undoubtedly less powerful than the fact of the tragic death of a young girl. Thus the role of the trial judge in giving jury instructions was especially important as a preliminary shaping of the issues. Within the limitations of legal procedures, the California Supreme Court responded both to a jury verdict that was not arbitrary, but was perhaps excessive, and to jury instructions that were not irresponsible, but were perhaps insensitive. Even so the reversal of Poddar's conviction did not automatically set him free; it only required that the case be reconsidered.

The anger of the Attorney General's office at the reversal of Poddar's conviction and the denial of a rehearing is also understandable. To add to the frustration of losing a criminal case on technical grounds, there was the reality, as a plausible dissenting opinion pointed out, of the substantial burdens that a retrial would impose on the criminal justice system in such a complex and controversial case.

When Poddar's attorney proposed an alternative that not only avoided a retrial but also provided for protection of society by means of a symbolic act of unofficial exile, it was an unusual but not an unwarranted exercise of the prosecutor's discretion to agree to release Poddar. Although the legal issues remain in limbo, and Poddar is free but not excused, there is a sense in which justice – as much as is humanly possible within the limitations of legal procedures – may have been done.

However, even if the results reached in the *Poddar* case conform to a rough sense of justice, it is what I call enigmatic justice – enigmatic because of multiple layers of permanent ambiguity that make it, like a riddle, obscure and perplexing. First, there are so many things about the facts that are and will remain unclear and unknown; we might call this *epistemological incompleteness*. These include uncertainties about Poddar's mental state and his intentions when he went to the Tarasoff home; the lapses on the part of Tatiana, her family, Poddar's therapists, and the police; the possibly prejudicial jury instructions; the jury's apparent disregard of the evidence of Poddar's diminished capacity – or did they take it into consideration in finding Poddar guilty of only second-degree rather than first-degree murder? Second, we have discussed what we might call legal inconclusiveness: no final adjudication of Poddar's legal responsibility for his conduct is made; Poddar is released from jail but not truly set free; the criminal process results in a technical legal limbo, but a practical problem is solved by informal negotiations. It is the particular combination of epistemological incompleteness and legal inconclusiveness that makes the Poddar case enigmatic.

III. TARASOFF *V.* THE REGENTS OF THE UNIVERSITY OF CALIFORNIA

A. *The Tarasoff Rule*

An inordinate amount of misunderstanding, especially in the psychotherapeutic community, still exists about the legal significance of the *Tarasoff* case. Thus, it is desirable to begin with a clarification of some of the legal issues. As I pointed out earlier, *Tarasoff* was appealed to the California Supreme Court prior to a trial on the facts. The specific issue before the Court was whether, assuming that the factual allegations in the complaint could be established, a cause of action could be stated against the psychotherapists, their employers or the police. The plaintiffs, Tatiana's parents, claimed that both the psychotherapists and the police should be held liable for failing to *confine* Poddar under California's law permitting the involuntary commitment for psychiatric evaluation and treatment of persons dangerous to others, and for failing to *warn* Tatiana or her parents of the danger that Poddar posed for her.

The Court made it quite clear that California law grants statutory immunity from liability to the publicly employed psychotherapists and police for failing to confine Poddar ([12], p. 31, 32). The Court also ruled in the second *Tarasoff* opinion that the police are not liable for failing to warn Tatiana or her parents of her peril ([12], p. 29). However, the Court held that the psychotherapists are not granted immunity for failing to warn Tatiana or her parents ([12], p. 29). Instead, the Court articulated a common law rule that in certain circumstances psychotherapists have a duty to a third party arising out of the psychotherapist's special relationship to a patient. The rule was expressed as follows:

> When a therapist determines, or pursuant to the standards of his profession should determine, that his patient presents a serious danger of violence to another, he incurs an obligation to use reasonable care to protect the intended victim against such danger ([12], p. 20).

The therapist's duty might be discharged by "warn[ing] the intended victim or others likely to apprise the victim of the danger, notify[ing] the police, or tak[ing] whatever other steps are reasonably necessary under the circumstances" ([12], p. 20).

B. *Approaches to Analysis of the Tarasoff Case*

The *Tarasoff* case can be analyzed from several different perspectives. One might examine the soundness of the technical legal reasoning that the Court displayed in reaching its conclusion. The 'special relationship' between the psychotherapist and the patient is said by the Court to give rise to duties to protect certain threatened third parties. However, a close look at the cases upon which the Court relies for finding duties to third parties will reveal dubious and uncertain analogies ([9], [13]). Furthermore, the case raises important questions about the analysis of the concept of legal duties in general and duties to third parties in particular. Although a detailed examination of these legal issues is desirable, it is beyond the scope of this essay.

Not only legal scholars but also social scientists might raise important questions about some of the assumptions and assertions made in the *Tarasoff* opinions. For example, each of the three opinions filed in the case – the majority opinion written by Justice Tobriner, the separate concurring and dissenting opinion by Justice Mosk, and the dissenting opinion by Justice Clark – makes some empirical claims about the predictability of violence, about the significance of confidentiality in psychotherapy, and about the (likely) impact of *Tarasoff* on the practice of psychotherapy.[11] For example, will psychotherapists be more inclined to use involuntary commitment with patients suspected of being dangerous? Will therapists refuse to treat potentially dangerous patients? Will therapists be disposed to give premature warnings to third parties or otherwise unnecessarily breach their patients' confidential communications?

Although the ideas expressed on these issues in the Court opinions rely to some extent upon empirical data, the disputed issues are not adequately resolved by any of the studies or other data cited in the opinions.[12] The *Tarasoff* opinions exemplify but do not satisfy the need for more systematic study of empirical issues germane to legal doctrines. The adversary process typically brings such problems to light, but judicial opinions rarely are grounded on sufficiently reliable empirical data to provide a sound empirical base for the decisions reached. The *Tarasoff* case is no exception to this general rule.

My concern is to explore neither the Court's legal reasoning nor the empirical issues still in need of social-scientific research. Rather I shall now focus attention on another aspect of the *Tarasoff* case: its implications for the exercise of professional discretion by psychotherapists. By examining this aspect of the case we shall clarify some important issues concerning professional responsibility as well as gain some appreciation of both the scope and limits of legal interventions in professional-client relationships in psychotherapy.

C. *Implications of the Tarasoff Rule*

(1) *Legal impact*. Dire predictions have come from the psychotherapeutic community about the disastrous legal consequences likely to flow from the *Tarasoff* rule. For example, Alan Stone has written that "the tragedy of Miss Tarasoff's death has set off a legal imbroglio in the civil courts that may long be with us" ([10], p. 358). However, the legal impact of *Tarasoff* in subsequent case law to date has been minimal. To my knowledge no similar cases have arisen in California or elsewhere in which the *Tarasoff* rule (or something similar) has been the basis for a ruling of tort liability.

One might argue that since the *Tarasoff* rule was not finally formulated until 1976, not enough time has elapsed for the rule to have an impact in case law. However, two considerations pull in the other direction. First, the notoriety of *Tarasoff* dates from late 1974 when the first opinion appeared. Second, the *Tarasoff* rule has not been extended to suicide cases. In *Bellah v. Greenson* [1], the parents of a young adult patient who committed suicide claimed that in virtue of *Tarasoff* their daughter's therapist had a duty to warn them that she was a suicidal risk. The California Court of Appeal restricted the *Tarasoff* rule to third parties endangered by a patient's threatened violence. Thus, we can at least conclude that the *Tarasoff* rule has had no immediate significant legal impact. We shall argue, however, that the potential legal impact does create serious problems.

(2) *Impact on attitudes of psychotherapists.* Perhaps the greatest impact of the *Tarasoff* rule has been on attitudes, and especially fears, in the psychotherapeutic community. In the absence of reliable attitudinal studies, one must at this time rely on anecdotal information and impressions formed from contact with psychotherapists. My own experience, in numerous situations where I have been asked to discuss the *Tarasoff* case in general or in connection with particular cases, has been that psychotherapists are quite alarmed about its implications. This was understandable in 1974 when the first *Tarasoff* opinion was rendered because it appeared near the peak of the so-called medical malpractice crisis. There also exists a generalized anxiety among professionals about the growing trend toward professional accountability and increased governmental regulation of professional practice. Futhermore, the *Tarasoff* rule may evoke fears of litigation even if one is sanguine about the possibility of liability. And it cannot be denied that litigation, apart from liability, is an unpleasant – time consuming, aggravating and costly – prospect.

An important concern is the belief held by many psychotherapists that the *Tarasoff* rule will undermine patient trust, especially if the therapist is viewed as a 'double agent' with loyalties divided between the patient's desire for confidentiality and the public need for protection.[13] For example, Poddar apparently believed that Dr. Moore could not be trusted to keep his secrets. After his first few therapeutic sessions with Dr. Moore, Poddar consulted Dr. Gold to express his doubts and to request a different therapist. Dr. Gold testified that he attributed this concern to Poddar's paranoia and sent him back to Dr. Moore. In view of Dr. Moore's subsequent conduct, Poddar's anxieties were not entirely irrational. Those patients who are most fully aware of their potentially violent proclivities are the patients most likely to have increased distrust. And psychotherapists, in turn, are more likely to shy away from treating such patients or exploring those aspects of a patient's character that may lead to a discovery of violent fantasies or that may trigger violent conduct.

(3) *Impact on psychotherapeutic practice*. As with the impact of the *Tarasoff* rule on attitudes, we lack reliable empirical information about how the rule has actually influenced patient care. It is reasonable to infer that the fear of litigation or liability has prompted psychotherapists to notify police more readily, to warn potential victims, to encourage voluntary hospitalization or to invoke involuntary commitment procedures. But only careful empirical study of psychotherapeutic practice can provide reliable data about the extent of the impact of the *Tarasoff* rule.[14] It is possible, however, to take a closer look at precisely what the *Tarasoff* rule does require of psychotherapists. The analysis will reveal that the vagueness of the *Tarasoff* rule understandably triggers the alarm in the psychotherapeutic community. Although the potential breadth of the rule is modified by language in the *Tarasoff* opinion which appears to limit its scope, the rule does impose serious restrictions on psychotherapeutic discretion.

(a) *Liability for Failing to Predict Dangerousness*

The *Tarasoff* rule states two possible bases of tort liability. The first is that if a therapist "pursuant to the standards of his profession should determine that his patient presents a serious danger of violence to another" ([12], p. 20), then a therapist can be held liable for failing to so determine. In other words, the therapist now has a duty to 'diagnose' or predict dangerousness and is potentially liable for failing to do so. On this issue the Court put forth a very qualified position. In the words of Justice Tobriner,

> We recognize the difficulty that a therapist encounters in attempting to forecast whether a patient presents a serious danger of violence. Obviously we do not require that the therapist, in making that determination, render a perfect performance; the therapist need only exercise "that reasonable degree of skill, knowledge and care ordinarily possessed and exercised by members of that professional specialty under similar circumstances" [citations omitted]. Within the broad range of reasonable practice and treatment in which professional opinion and judgment may differ, the therapist is free to exercise his or her own best judgment without liability; proof, aided by hindsight, that he or she judged wrongly is insufficient to establish negligence ([12], p. 25).

What this passage asserts is that therapists are required to exercise only responsible professional judgment. The legal rule invites the psychotherapeutic community to reflect on its standards of conduct, but it does not dictate to them what the standards should be. Because there is a wide range of opinion and disagreement in the professional community about the predictability of violence,[15] the potential liability for failing to predict violence, except in the most blatant cases of inept professional judgment, might at first glance appear to be very limited.

Nevertheless, significant dangers lurk behind the reassuring language of the Court. First, questions of liability for failing to predict dangerousness are likely to arise in a case, like *Tarasoff*, when someone has been killed or seriously injured by a dangerous patient. It is well-known that juries are sympathetic to plaintiffs in such cases. Second, because no clear standards do exist in the psychotherapeutic community concerning predictability of dangerousness, it will be difficult to avoid the temptation of proof aided by hindsight to establish negligence. Third, a battle of experts about predictability of dangerousness is likely to emerge in a jury trial.[16] Such controversy may influence a jury, like the criminal jury in the *Poddar* case, to disregard expert testimony and assign liability in accordance with their sentiments. At the very least this possibility may encourage litigation and pretrial settlements even if ultimately liability is unlikely.

The potential basis for liability for failing to predict dangerousness is uncertain, not because of the vagueness of this aspect of the *Tarasoff* rule, but because the standards for prediction are so controversial and because of the nature of litigation. Thus the reassuring language of the *Tarasoff* opinion will provide little comfort to a defendant psychotherapist whose undiagnosed-as-dangerous patient has committed a serious act of violence against another person.

(b) *Liability for Failure to Use Reasonable Care to Protect Threatened Third Party*

The second potential basis for liability arises when a therapist does determine, as Dr. Moore did with regard to Poddar, that a patient presents a serious danger of violence to another. Even if the therapist would not confidently predict that the patient will in fact commit an act of violence against another, the therapist may believe that the patient – like Poddar – is potentially dangerous. The therapist undoubtedly has incomplete information and must form his or her belief in the face of the inevitable uncertainty about human conduct. However, if that belief is reached, then the therapist 'incurs an obligation to use reasonable care to protect the intended victim against such danger" ([12], p. 21).

Prior to *Tarasoff* it was well established both in the law and in the literature of professional ethics that a psychotherapist had the *discretion* to disclose otherwise confidential information about dangerous patients. Such a disclosure was not then and is not now classified as a breach of confidentiality. The policy decision to *permit* psychotherapists to take such action has, as a result of the *Tarasoff* rule, been elevated to a legal *duty*.

At first glance the reasonable care requirement of the *Tarasoff* rule might seem to be a natural extension of the psychotherapist's social responsibility. Not only is protection of threatened third parties against harm a significant social goal, but also it allows the psychotherapist to intervene paternalistically to protect a dangerous patient against himself or herself. In this way the psychotherapist serves the best interests of both society and his or her patients. Indeed, some psychotherapists believe that the *Tarasoff* rule will have very little impact on their psychotherapeutic practice because it merely makes a legal requirement out of what they do already.[17]

It is difficult to deny that in situations in which a patient presents a highly probable and imminent threat of serious violence to another person, it is desirable for psychotherapists standing in special relationships to such dangerous patients to attempt to prevent threatened harm. As Justice Tobriner puts it, "[i]n this risk-infested society we can hardly tolerate the further exposure to danger that would result from a concealed knowledge of the therapist that his patient was lethal" ([12], p. 27). However, the language of the *Tarasoff* rule is not restricted to narrowly circumscribed situations. Extremely vague language is used to articulate the legal rule. The duty to use reasonable care arises when a patient presents "a serious danger of violence to another" ([12], p. 20). The Court makes no effort to define 'serious' or to specify what counts as violence. As a result the standard provides little guidance to psychotherapists about the scope of their legal duty.

One might think that this vague rule is desirable because its flexibility protects the discretion of the psychotherapist to assess carefully each situation that occurs. However, the vagueness of the rule in fact tends to undermine psychotherapeutic discretion. It creates a potential conflict for the psychotherapist between his or her particular duty to provide care for the patient and a general duty to protect third parties from harm. The presence of the latter duty can adversely affect the performance of the former. For example, when Dr. Moore confronted Poddar about his intentions to harm Tatiana and told Poddar that he might have to notify proper authorities, Poddar became angry and broke off the therapy. Since Tatiana was out of the country at the time of the confrontation, one might wonder whether Dr. Moore acted precipitously in notifying the police. If Dr. Moore had pursued therapy with Poddar more aggressively and worried less about Poddar's danger to others, could the tragedy have been averted? Once again we are faced with epistemological incompleteness.

In addition to the conflicting duties' issue, the reasonable care aspect of the *Tarasoff* rule creates other, more serious, problems. The Court could have stipulated that when a patient is determined to present a serious danger of violence to another, the psychotherapist is required, analogous to a physician treating a child whom he suspects to be a victim of child abuse, to make a report to appropriate authorities. In the case of a dangerous patient, the report normally would be to the police. Of course the psychotherapist should be free, in the exercise of professional discretion, to do more, such as to warn the victim or others, or to take other reasonable steps depending upon the circumstances. However, the Court did not structure the standard in this way. Instead, it merely stated that

> the discharge of this duty may require the therapist to take one or more of various steps, depending upon the nature of the case. Thus it may call for him to warn the intended victim or others likely to apprise the victim of the danger, to notify the police, or to take whatever other steps are reasonably necessary under the circumstances ([12], p. 20).

The greatest difficulty with this elaboration of the reasonable care requirement is that, as a practical matter, it seems to impose extraordinary responsibilities on psychotherapists, responsibilities that they are normally neither trained for nor equipped to carry out. How far must a therapist go to protect third parties against harm in our "risk infested society" ([12], p. 27)? Once again the Court includes some language in the *Tarasoff* opinion designed to reassure psychotherapists:

> We emphasize that our conclusion does not raise the specter of therapists . . . indiscriminately being held liable for damage despite their exercise of sound professional judgment ([12], p. 31).

Although the Court may be correct in claiming that psychotherapists may not indiscriminately be held liable, it overlooks the additional specter of litigation. The burdens of litigation – whether as a plaintiff or a defendant – are considerable. To protect oneself against the threat of litigation, it would be tempting for psychotherapists to be scrupulous, if not excessive, in satisfying the reasonable care requirement. This may encourage premature notifications of police or potential victims. This may not only weaken the psychotherapist-patient relationship but also exacerbate the general level of anxiety in a society that already tends to be alarmist.

Such a reaction to the specter of litigation is not wholly irrational when one considers the consequences of the *Tarasoff* litigation itself. It will be recalled, as Justice Mosk observes, that "Dr. Moore *did* notify the police that Poddar was planning to kill a girl identifiable as Tatiana" ([12], p. 34). And Justice Mosk also remarks that "[w]hether plaintiff can ultimately prevail is problematical at best" ([12], p. 34). We also know, from the testimony in the record of the criminal trial, that the police interviewed Poddar as well as Tatiana's brother Alex, who discounted the threat. Justice Mosk was correct in his prediction if he meant by 'prevail' that the therapist would not be held liable. However, in the *Tarasoff* case, the final outcome, reached on July 1, 1977, exactly one year after the Supreme Court opinion, was that an out of court settlement was reached and the complaints against the therapists were dismissed with prejudice. It is interesting to note that the settlement amount was not disclosed, thus adding still another ambiguous result to the *Poddar-Tarasoff* story. But the fact that the litigation in this case did lead to a settlement illustrates the basis for the fear that the *Tarasoff* rule invites litigation that in turn may lead to unduly self-protective practices by psychotherapists. Psychotherapeutic discretion may give way to defenses against litigation – a result analogous to the defensive medicine syndrome already widely recognized as a by-product of malpractice litigation in other branches of medicine.

IV. PODDAR AND TARASOFF: CONCLUDING OBSERVATIONS

The California Supreme Court played a major role in shaping the outcome of the *Poddar* and *Tarasoff* cases. One is tempted to speculate that their knowledge of the facts in *Poddar* may have influenced their position in *Tarasoff*. Whether or not the California Supreme Court was so influenced, its opinions reflect some of the uncertainties as well as the frustrations of attempting to apply the artifices of the law to the enigmas of human conduct. Both *Poddar* and *Tarasoff* illustrate the limitations of law as a human instrument; the problems that give rise to the need for legal intervention are often inherently intractable, and legal interventions are limited to technical rulings or formulation of general rules rather than resolutions of the underlying problems. The legal maxim that 'hard cases make bad law' is particularly applicable to the *Tarasoff* case.

Behind the veil of legal procedures and technical arguments about jury instructions in the *Poddar* case, the Court was sensitive to the complexity of the cultural, interpersonal and intrapsychic conflict that is revealed in the criminal record in the *Poddar* case. The opportunity for detachment from the immediacy of the crime enabled the Court to appreciate the complexity of the human drama in this case. The criminal record reveals not only Poddar's problems but also the failures of many persons – Poddar, Poddar's friends, Tatiana's family, Tatiana herself, the psychotherapists, the police – to intervene effectively in a sequence of events which perhaps could have been interrupted at many different points in the sequence to prevent the killing of Tatiana. On one reading of the transcript of the criminal trial one may not be particularly sympathetic to Poddar, but rather one may be saddened by the ineptness and impotence of human beings to prevent senseless tragedies. Poddar's cultural alienation and emotional immaturity, despite a precocious intellectual development, enables one to understand though not excuse his behavior. The Court's emphatic statements about Poddar's diminished responsibility might also be applied by analogy to the diminished foresight and limited power of the other principal participants in this drama. It is as if the court believed that it was unfair to hold Poddar solely or fully responsible when so many others failed to intervene in an effective manner.

Whereas the *Poddar* case pulls one in the direction of diffusion of responsibility or perhaps collective responsibility, the *Tarasoff* case pulls one in another direction. Perhaps the Court felt, after reading the trial record in *Poddar*, that somebody could have and perhaps should have prevented the tragic murder. In their first opinion the Court potentially implicates the police and the therapists. But the second opinion implicates only the therapists. At least someone is identified as potentially responsible for failing to prevent Tatiana's death. But as Justice Mosk's dissenting opinion brings out, the abstract rule articulated in *Tarasoff* ought not apply to the facts of the *Tarasoff* case. Is it possible that the Court responded with the *Tarasoff* rule as a frustrated reaction to the insolubility of the human problems underlying the *Poddar* and *Tarasoff* cases?

Poddar and *Tarasoff* are troubling cases with respect to the facts, the technical legal issues and the broader issues of public policy with which they are concerned. What I have tried to show is that we must not only acknowledge but also take very seriously the limited effectiveness of legal interventions in the context of human conduct (in general) and in the context of psychotherapy (in particular). At the same time one can sympathize with the Court in its efforts to arrive at results and articulate rules that do justice to the vast array of competing interests. But some human problems subjected to the legal process produce at best only enigmatic justice, i.e., justice that, even if it is not blind, is ambiguous, obscure and perplexing.

University of California at Los Angeles
Los Angeles, California

NOTES

[1] According to the Management Information Sector of the California State Department of Corrections, the median time served for first degree murder, as of 1977, is 125 months; for second degree murder, 61 months; and for second degree murder with a firearm, 54 months.

[2] For background on the evolution of the concept of duty to warn, see [13], pp. 156–57 and 162–64; [14], pp. 234–37 for arguments that legal precedent would *not* support a duty to warn in the *Tarasoff* context, see [13], pp. 156–57, 162–64; [9], pp. 554–57. For contrary view see [6], pp. 1026–31.

[3] [11], The *Tarasoff* case will be cited generally unless specific quotes are utilized.

[4] For discussions of informed consent as applied to psychotherapy, see [15], p. 1021; [6], pp. 1056–60. For discussions on confidentiality and related problems arising under *Tarasoff*, see [13], pp. 157–58 and 164–67; [15], pp. 1017–1022; [6], pp. 1040–1043. For a discussion on the therapist's role as an agent of social control, see [7], pp. 15–19.

[5] The facts of the case have been developed from the criminal transcript of the *Poddar* case, from the Supreme Court opinion in *Poddar*, from discussions with Poddar's trial attorney and his appellate attorney. No specific references to these sources will be made in the text.

[6] Poddar had once given Tatiana a copy of Eric Berne's *Games People Play* and accused her of playing 'Rapo'.

[7] This action on Poddar's part reflects exactly one of the fears raised by opponents of this opinion, namely, that the duty of the therapist to warn and the accompanying need to breach patient-therapist confidentiality, may lead potentially dangerous patients to curtail therapy and 'act out' the very danger which continued therapy may be able to prevent.

[8] Had the *Tarasoff* opinion been decided on the facts, the fact that Dr. Moore had told the police of the threat may have released him from further liability under the duty to warn rule of Tarasoff.

[9] Dr. Moore's superior, Dr. Powelson, was away when the report to the police was issued. Upon his return and after reading its contents, Dr. Powelson ordered the report withdrawn and the copies of it destroyed, though the latter never occurred. His stated motive was to protect the police, who "had to be free to use their own judgment".

[10] Warning to Alex also may have been sufficient to release Dr. Moore from liability under the rule of Tarasoff.

[11] See generally [10] and [4], [6], [9], [13], [14], [15] for further discussions.

[12] For example, for articles outlining the lack of reliability see [3], [6], [9], [15].

[13] For some discussion on the "double role" of a therapist, see [7], pp. 15–19.

[14] For articles discussing potential problems of overprediction, overcommitment etc., arising from *Tarasoff*, see [9], pp. 557–59; [13], pp. 157–58, 164–67; [15], pp. 1017–1022, 1018; [4], pp. 297–301. For the argument that the duty to warn will not threaten effective psychotherapy, see [14], pp. 238–239.

[15] For articles on this subject, see [15], p. 1018; [6], [3].

[16] For articles discussing these issues see [9], pp. 557–59; [13], pp. 157–58, 164–167; [15], pp. 1017–1022; [14], pp. 240–43; [6] generally.

[17] For some discussion on this issue, see [14], pp. 240–43; [6].

BIBLIOGRAPHY

1. *Bellah v. Greenson*: 1977, 73 Cal. App. 3d 911, 141 Cal. Rptr. 92.
2. *Calif. Welfare and Institutions Code* § 5150 (*West Supp*. 1974).
3. Diamond, B.: 1975, 'The Psychiatric Prediction of Dangerousness', *U. Penn. Law Rev*. **123**, 439.
4. Note, 'The Duty to Warn', *University of Colorado Law Rev*. **48**, 295.
5. Ennis, B. & Litwack, T.: 1974, 'Psychiatry and the Presumption of Expertise: Flipping Coins in the Courtroom', *Cal. L. Rev*. **62**, 693.
6. Fleming, J. G. and Maximov, B.: 1974, 'The Patient or his Victim: The Therapist's Dilemma', *Cal. L. Rev*. **62**, 1025.
7. 'In the Service of the State: The Psychiatrist as Double Agent': 1978, *The Hastings Center Report*: **8**, Special Supplement, April.
8. *People v. Prosenjit Poddar*: 1974, 16 C. 3d 750, 111 Cal. Rptr. 910, 518 P. 2d 342.
9. Note, 'Psychiatry-Torts – A Psychiatrist Who Knows or Should Know His Patient Intends Violence to Another Incurs a Duty to Warn': 1977, *Cumberland Law Rev*. **7**, 551.
10. Stone, A.: 1976, 'The Tarasoff Decisions: Suing Psychotherapists to Safeguard Society', *Harvard L. Rev*. **90**, 358.
11. *Tarasoff v. Regents of Univ. of Calif.*: 1975, 118 Cal. Rptr. 129, 529 P. 2d 553.
12. *Tarasoff v. Regents of Univ. of Calif.*: 1976, 17 Cal. 3d 425, 131 Cal. Rptr. 14, 551 P. 2d 334.
13. Note, '*Tarasoff v. Regents of Univ. of California: The Psychotherapist's Peril*': 1975, *Univ. of Pittsburgh L. Rev*. **37**, 155.
14. '*Tarasoff v. Regents of the Univ. of Calif.*: Psychotherapists, Policemen and the Duty to Warn – an Unreasonable Extension of the Common Law?': 1975, *Golden Gate University L. Rev*. **6**, 229.
15. Note, 'Torts – Psychiatry and the Law – Duty to Warn Potential Victim of a Homicidal Patient' – *Tarasoff v. Regents of the Univ. of Calif.*', 1976, *N.Y. Law School L. Rev*. **22**, 1011.

CHARLES M. CULVER AND BERNARD GERT

THE MORALITY OF INVOLUNTARY HOSPITALIZATION

I. INTRODUCTION

There is a good deal of recent dispute both within and outside of psychiatry about the procedure of involuntary hospitalization. (We use 'involuntary hospitalization' to cover both 2–3 day 'emergency' detentions and longer civil commitments. We discuss mainly detention here but do refer to commitment when appropriate.) While writers such as Szasz [10] believe that involuntary hospitalization should be eliminated entirely, it is more common to find disagreement about how wide or narrow the grounds for detaining patients should be.

Those who advocate narrow grounds are currently in the ascendancy. They prefer that detention be limited to those patients who not only are mentally ill, but who also exhibit evidence of clear and immediate physical dangerousness to themselves and/or others. Some commentators have suggested adding further conditions, such as incompetence of the patient to make treatment decisions and evidence that the patient's condition is in fact treatable (see American Bar Association [1] for a well-documented presentation of a narrow-grounds position).

Those who urge wider grounds also include mental illness as a necessary condition, but wish to eliminate physical dangerousness as a necessary condition, substituting instead any severe disruption of personal functioning (see Chodoff [2] for a well-argued presentation of this point of view; Chodoff includes 'treatability' as a third necessary condition).

Those who advocate wider grounds often point out that physical dangerousness is but one of many possible manifestations of severe mental illness and that it seems cruel and inconsistent not to treat other severely disabled patients who seem urgently to require it. Narrow-grounds advocates, however, feel that any relaxation of criteria in the direction of a 'disruption of functioning' rule would give physicians such wide discretionary power that civil liberties would generally be threatened.

We want to offer here a conceptual and moral analysis of the detention procedure which we believe leads to some clarification of the issues under dispute.

II. PATERNALISTIC AND NON-PATERNALISTIC DETENTION

In the overwhelming majority of cases, detention is carried out by the psychiatrist with the belief that it is for the good of the patient and for this as well as other reasons it is almost always a paternalistic act. However, in some instances detention may be done not primarily for the good of the patient but primarily for the good of third parties (namely, to prevent harm to them by the patient); in these cases we regard the detention as non-paternalistic. And there are some mixed cases where both the good of the patient and of third parties are involved.

We want to begin by considering paternalistic detention. We believe that when one appreciates that most detention is paternalistic and then focuses on the general question of when paternalistic interventions are justified, one can see more clearly the sources of some of the current disputes in this area. Finally, we will consider the problems raised by non-paternalistic detentions as well as a number of other critical issues.

III. PATERNALISTIC DETENTION

In order to show that (most) detentions are best understood as paternalistic acts, it is necessary to offer a general definition of paternalistic behavior and then measure acts of detention against that definition.

We believe the following definition (discussed in detail by Gert and Culver [4] makes explicit the important features of paternalistic behavior:

A is acting paternalistically toward *S* if and only if *A*'s behavior (correctly) indicates that *A* *believes that*:

(1) his action is for *S*'s good
(2) he is qualified to act on *S*'s behalf
(3) his action involves violating a moral rule (or doing that which will require him to do so) with regard to *S*
(4) *S*'s good justifies him in acting on *S*'s behalf independently of *S*'s past, present or immediately forthcoming (free, informed) consent
(5) *S* believes (perhaps falsely) that he (*S*) generally knows what is for his own good.

Let us explain each of the five features of this definition and discuss the extent to which acts of detention satisfy them:

Feature (1) emphasizes that *A*'s (e.g., the psychiatrist's) action is paternalistic only insofar as *A* believes he or she is acting for *S*'s (e.g., the patient's) own good. If the psychiatrist believes that he is acting *only* for his own good (which would almost never be the case) or *only* for the good of a third party then the action is not paternalistic. Of course actions can be more than paternalistic: they can be intended for the good of the patient as well as others; but what makes the psychiatrist's action toward the patient paternalistic is never the good of anyone other than the patient himself.

Detention, as noted above, is nearly always done with the belief that it is for the patient's own good. Even in those cases where there is concern for the patient's potential harmfulness toward third parties, it is usually true that the psychiatrist believes it is also in the mentally ill patient's own interests to be prevented from inflicting harm on others.

Feature (2) seems a necessary aspect of paternalism; for example it explains why a small child usually cannot be said to be acting paternalistically toward his or her parents even when all of the other conditions are satisfied. It has little relevance in the present context since a psychiatrist who is detaining a patient for what he or she believes is the patient's good would almost always believe that he or she is qualified to act on the patient's behalf.

Feature (3) explains why people often regard paternalism unfavorably. While a full account of what constitutes a moral rule and its violation is found in Gert [3], we may more simply state here that we count the following kinds of actions as violations of the relevant moral rules: killing; causing pain (physical or psychological); disabling; depriving of freedom, opportunity or pleasure; deceiving; breaking a promise; and cheating. We hold that all paternalistic acts involve the belief that one is carrying out one (or more) of these kinds of actions. All of these kinds of actions are universally regarded as requiring moral justification and it is for this reason that all acts of paternalism require moral justification.

Detention always involves violating the moral rule against depriving a person of his or her freedom. It also almost always involves, secondarily, causing the patient some immediate suffering during the detention process and, often, some later suffering throughout life secondary to the enduring knowledge that he or she was once involuntarily hospitalized.[1]

Feature (4) makes clear what distinguishes paternalistic psychiatric behavior from the bulk of instances where psychiatrists justifiably violate moral rules with regard to their patients – that in paternalistic behavior they believe their patient's good justifies them in doing so *independently* of having the patient's past, present, or immediately forthcoming consent. Note that expectation of receiving future consent does not prevent an action from being paternalistic; in fact such an expectation is present in most instances of justified psychiatric paternalism. Only past, present, or immediately forthcoming consent (as in pushing someone from the path of an oncoming car he or she does not see) completely removes an act from the class of paternalistic acts. Detention is virtually always done without the patient's consent and thus this aspect of condition (4) of the detention is virtually always satisfied.

Condition (5) makes explicit that we can only act paternalistically toward those whom we regard as believing that they know what is for their own good. Thus we cannot act paternalistically toward infants. Note that we can act paternalistically toward those who, we believe, do not in fact know what is for their own good, but we cannot act paternalistically toward those whom we do not regard as even believing that they know what is for their good. In fact the vast majority of adolescent and adult psychiatric patients do have the sort of minimal self-consciousness this condition describes. Detained patients almost always do believe they know what is for their own good – if nothing else, they usually believe it is not for their own good to be hospitalized.

IV. THE JUSTIFICATION OF PATERNALISTIC DETENTION

A. *The Justification Procedure*

To recapitulate, paternalistic behavior requires justification because it involves doing that which requires one to violate a moral rule with regard to a patient. We believe that the following kind of justification procedure may be most usefully applied to paternalistic acts (detailed more fully in [5]):

One must show that the evils (harms) one is probably preventing or ameliorating for the patient are so much greater than the evils (if any) one is causing through violating a moral rule with respect to the patient, that one could *universally* allow the violation of the moral rule under similar circumstances, or in somewhat more technical terminology, that one could publicly advocate this *kind of violation*.

What is necessary in each specific case, then, is to determine what *kind of violation* (of a moral rule) is involved in a given paternalistic act (such as detention) and then see if one could publicly advocate this *kind of violation*: i.e., if one would allow the universal violation of the moral rule under these circumstances. There are only three elements that should be assessed in specifying a given *kind of violation*:

(a) determining the moral rule(s) which is (are) violated;
(b) judging the probable amounts of evil (harm) to be caused and to be prevented or ameliorated by the moral rule violation (amount of evil includes both the kind

and severity of the evil, the likelihood it will occur, and the probable length of time it will be suffered);

(c) determining the rational desires of the person (patient) affected by the violation.

Since detention always involves violating a moral rule with respect to a patient, it always requires moral justification. In order for paternalistic detention to be justified according to the procedure outlined above, it must be the case: (1) that the amount of evil probably prevented or ameliorated by detaining a patient is very great; (2) that the amount of evil perpetrated by detaining the patient is so much less than the evil probably prevented that it would be irrational for one to prefer the latter to the former; and (3) that the patient has no adequate reason for suffering the evil that detention is intended to prevent. It is only when these conditions hold that all rational persons could consider allowing this kind of moral rule violation to occur.

Before proceeding we need to give a brief account of what we mean by the term 'rational desire' in the third element (c).[2] Certain actions, or intentions to act, are regarded as irrational, not only by psychiatrists but by people in general. If someone wants to commit suicide, then unless he has an adequate reason for wanting to do this, his desire is considered irrational. This is in contrast to other desires that we might have, e.g., a desire to go for a walk, for which we do not require a reason in order for our action to be considered rational. Desires for those things which it would be irrational to act on without a reason we call irrational desires. We believe that the following would be universally regarded as irrational desires: the desire to die; to suffer pain, physical or mental; to be disabled; to be deprived of freedom or opportunity or pleasure. This does not mean that it is always irrational to desire these things, only that it is irrational to desire them without some *reason*. For example, it is not irrational to want to have your arm cut off if you believe that you have gangrene and amputation is necessary to save your life.[3]

We believe that these elements of the justification procedure do in fact represent those features of individual cases we take into account in making judgments about the morality of individual detentions. Further, we believe that when we consider the elements of the justification procedure in somewhat more detail (see below), we can better understand some of the currently disputed issues.

B. *The Likelihood of Preventing Harm*

How likely is it that psychiatric detention does prevent serious harm to a person? It seems unfortunately true that there are few data available to answer this important question.

If we knew that 90% of those who were detained would have killed or seriously injured themselves without detention and that these evils are prevented for an appreciable period of time with, say, 72 hours of detention, then one element of the justification process would be strongly satisfied, i.e., it would be irrational to prefer a 90% chance of death or serious injury to 72 hours of detention. By contrast if only 1 in 10 000 would kill or injure themselves without detention this element would not be satisfied, for then the probable amount of evil prevented is extremely slight and it would no longer be irrational to prefer this small probability of death over the evils of detention.

Unfortunately, the actual percentage is at present unknown. Available studies ([1], p. 87) suggest it is in the range of one out of six if detention is appropriately limited to persons who show evidence of certain high-risk attributes (marked depression; recent history of impulsive and/or suicidal behavior; etc.).

Assume for a moment that the actual figure for a defined subclass of suicidal persons is 16%. Suppose a man had just suffered a heart attack and it was known that his risk of death was essentially zero if he remained in bed for one to three days (whether he liked it or not) but was 16% if he insisted, without any adequate reason, on being up and about. We believe that nearly everyone would view it as irrational if he did insist on being up, even though we knew that by universally recommending bedrest we were needlessly confining five people for every one person for whom it would be appropriate.

Suppose the figure were 10%. We believe that the large majority of people would still view it as irrational not to choose to be confined for a few days. How low the percentage would have to go before a significant number of people would think it rational to get out of bed we do not know. However, it seems very likely that if our subclass of suicidal persons were defined stringently enough, then the percentage of them who would suffer serious evils without brief detention would be sufficiently high that most people would view it as irrational to prefer that risk to the evils associated with detention. For example, suppose we detained only those who were markedly depressed, had a history of impulsive behavior, and were apprehended when they were apparently about to kill themselves. (We will assume that detention does prevent harm with sufficient likelihood in some subgroups that it would be irrational not to prefer it. However, more empirical research on this question is badly needed.)

C. *Application of the Justification Procedure*

Let us illustrate this justification procedure by applying it to a case where detention intuitively seems to be clearly justified:

Case (*1*) Mr. K. is pacing back and forth on the roof of his five-story tenement and appears to be on the verge of jumping off. When questioned by the police he sounds confused. When interviewed by Dr. T. in the emergency room, Mr. K. admits to being afraid that he might jump off the roof and says that he fears he is losing his mind. However he adamantly refuses hospitalization. Dr. T. decides that for Mr. K.'s own protection, Mr. K. must be detained in the hospital for a period of seventy-two hours.

Dr. T. is violating a moral rule by depriving Mr. K. of his freedom and is, in addition, causing him both the immediate and the probable future psychological suffering associated with being (and having once been) a detained patient. However, Dr. T. is very possibly preventing the occurrence of a very great evil: Mr. K.'s death or serious injury. Finally, since Mr. K. apparently has no reason for killing himself, his potentially self-destructive behavior appears to be irrational. Although it is rational to desire not to be hospitalized, it is irrational to prefer serious risk of death to a short deprivation of freedom. Thus the *kind of violation* which is involved in this case consists of *A*'s temporarily (72 hours) depriving *S* of his freedom and thereby also causing *S* a mild to moderate degree of psychological suffering (some of it temporary) in order to possibly prevent a very great permanent evil (death or serious injury); all of this occurs in a setting where *S* apparently has no adequate reason for death and where for *S* to prefer the serious risk of death over the less serious evils associated with hospitalization seems irrational. (It is important to note that there is a high probability that much of the evil imposed through detention will be temporary because Dr. T. believes Mr. K.'s condition is treatable. If the evil had to be imposed indefinitely that would significantly alter the situation.) We believe that essentially all rational people would agree that this kind of violation should be universally allowed and thus that Dr. T.'s paternalistic action is (strongly) justified.

According to our justification procedure, detention of apparently suicidal patients is morally justified only in those instances (1) where failure to detain would, with sufficiently high likelihood, be followed by death or very serious injury, (2) for which the person has no adequate reason, and (3) where detention probably will, in a relatively short time, lead to a significant decrease in the likelihood of serious self-injury. It is only in these instances that a rational person could universally allow the imposition of less serious and mostly temporary evils.

This is a very stringent test. It would never allow involuntary hospitalization *just* because someone was 'mentally ill', since the test demands the specification of what evils of what magnitude are probably being prevented or ameliorated; the (mere) designation of someone as mentally ill is imprecise on this point, though the presence of mental illness does play a role in the justification of detention (see below). It may be, in fact, that most or all patients correctly labeled 'mentally ill' are suffering evils of one kind or another for which they have no rational desire. But for detention to be warranted it is necessary that the present or probable future evils be very great *and* that there be a reasonably high likelihood that hospitalization will ameliorate or prevent them. That is, it must be irrational to prefer the possible evil to be suffered without hospitalization to the certain evil of hospitalization.

V. ISSUES IN THE JUSTIFICATION OF DETENTION

A. *The Seriousness of the Evils Prevented and Their Probability of Occurrence*

How are we to judge which present or possible future evils are sufficiently serious to warrant detention? The seriousness of an evil is determined by several factors, among which is the impact it will make on the person's life at a given time. On this test death is clearly the most serious evil, for nothing has greater impact than death. Thus potential suicide (of sufficient likelihood) is almost universally taken as grounds for detention. On this life-impact test, serious bodily injury, great physical or psychological pain, and social or economic losses can come out as relatively equal. A second factor is how permanently the harm will affect the rest of the person's life. Here again nothing is more permanent than death. But of the harms considered more or less equal on the last test, bodily injury will usually have a much more permanent effect than any of the others; e.g., brain damage and blindness are permanent. On the other hand it is almost always possible to reverse social and economic losses and to recover from psychological or even physical pain.

We think that it is only evils with great initial impact and permanence that are great enough to make it irrational for one to prefer the possibility of experiencing these evils rather than experiencing the evil of detention. This point is made even more strongly when we recognize that the evils of detention are certain but the evils to be prevented are only possible. We know that by detaining we deprive a person of freedom but it is almost never *very* certain that the person will suffer an evil if he or she is not detained. The fallibility of psychiatrists (or anyone else) in predicting this kind of low base-rate behavior is well known ([8], [1]).

Given the inherently lesser probability of preventing evils compared with the certainty of causing evil by detention, it is not surprising that the evils to be prevented must be so great in order to justify paternalistic detention. On the other hand, concentration on particular cases, especially after the fact, that is, when failure to detain *has* been followed by suicide, etc., tends to lead one to advocate more lenient standards for detention. In this controversy we can clearly come down against using what happens after the fact in a *particular* case as a legitimate argument for more lenient standards for detention. It is only the information available at the time of possible detention which can count in determining whether it is justifiable or not to detain. For example, consider the following case described by Chodoff [2]:

Case (*2*) Passersby in a campus area observe two young women standing together, staring at each other, for over an hour. Their behavior attracts attention, and eventually the police take the pair to a nearby precinct station for questioning. They refuse to answer questions and sit mutely, staring into space. The police request some type of psychiatric examination but are informed by the city attorney's office that state law (Michigan) allows persons to be held for observation only if they appear obviously dangerous to themselves or others. In this case, since the women do not seem homicidal or suicidal, they do not qualify for observation and are released.

Less than 30 hours later the two women are found on the floor of their campus apartment, screaming and writhing in pain with their clothes ablaze from a self-made pyre. One woman recovers; the other dies. (There is no conclusive evidence that drugs were involved.)

We think it is clear, on the facts given, that detention would not have been justified. The correlation between the kind of behavior described and subsequent suicide would be too low. The case is a tragedy but there will always be tragic cases regardless of how broad one's criteria are for detention: there will inevitably be people who fall just outside the criteria, who subsequently kill themselves.

B. *The Rationality of Desiring the Evils Prevented*

We are justified in detaining someone to prevent an evil only when it appears to be irrational for the person to want that evil. If the person does have an adequate reason for suffering a serious evil then detention is unjustified. Thus we should not detain a pain-ridden, terminal cancer patient who has only weeks to live if we learn that the patient intends to take a fatal dose of barbiturates: for such a person to prefer death to the evils of weeks of agony followed by certain death seems a rational choice. If would also be rational, of course, to choose to live out one's life under these circumstances rather than end it prematurely. But to allow a physician to detain a patient making the former choice would be (universalizing according to our justification procedure) to allow physicians to forcibly substitute *their* rational rankings of evils for *their* patients' equally rational rankings and that would be a *kind of violation* of a moral rule that would be unacceptable to rational persons.

We have noted that while it sometimes seems relatively clear that there is no adequate reason for persons to desire an evil, in other cases it is harder to judge. It is usually easier to judge the rationality of desires involving physical harm: such desires are usually irrational and in those instances when they are not (e.g., the above terminal cancer patient) it is usually relatively easy to determine that they are not. However, the rationality of what appear to be desires for social, economic or psychological harm is more difficult to judge. It is often not clear that, say, a man's squandering his money or acting in a way to ruin his reputation is clearly irrational. This is another reason, in addition to lack of permanence, why we may be more reluctant to detain someone to prevent apparently irrational nonphysical harms: viz., the greater likelihood that we may be wrong. For example, one patient with a history of mania ushered in a further episode by spending large sums of money on what appeared and later proved to be worthless speculative investments, all to his wife's (and later his own) great distress. However, it seems unlikely that speculative investment would ever be so clearly irrational as to justify detention.

The following case is more difficult:

Case (3) Mr. D. is a thirty-year-old single author who suffered an episode of mania two years ago. Since then he has been taking lithium and apparently doing well. He has just used up the small savings which had enabled him to continue writing, when he sells the novel he has been working on for the past several years. After the sale he abruptly stops taking lithium and within two months develops signs of mild to moderate hyperactivity, pressured speech, anorexia and insomnia. Soon thereafter a good friend of his becomes aware that Mr. D. has accumulated in his apartment, in cash, the proceeds from the sale of his book as well as the small amount of money remaining in his savings account. These funds constitute Mr. D.'s sole means of support for the foreseeable future; the friend is astounded to learn that Mr. D., normally a careful and frugal man, has begun burning and destroying the money. Mr. D. gives his friend no coherent explanation for doing so but tells him a rambling and jumbled story which involves not trusting the bank and also fearing that his home may be robbed. He wishes to destroy the money rather than let it fall into someone's hands. Mr. D.'s friend is alarmed by Mr. D.'s behavior; with

some effort he persuades Mr. D. to accompany him to see Mr. D.'s psychiatrist, Dr. L. After Dr. L. interviews Mr. D. and becomes familiar with the situation he informs Mr. D. that he ought to enter the hospital or at least begin taking his lithium again; in the meantime he should let someone else safeguard his money.

Suppose Mr. D. will accept neither hospitalization nor outpatient treatment of any kind. Should he be hospitalized involuntarily?

We think not, though this is a difficult case. However, we believe the evils Mr. D. is experiencing are not sufficiently intense or permanent in their effects to justify imposing the evils of detention. Also, while Mr. D.'s reasons for burning his money do not seem adequate, it is also true that socially aberrant actions like money-burning are sometimes carried out for quite adequate, if unusual, reasons; thus we hesitate to allow physicians to detain patients for such actions because of the definite possibility that physicians may incorrectly assess the rationality of the act. Even if one were convinced, after knowing the many facts in this case, that Mr. D. should be detained, it seems impossible to write a statute which would be sufficiently detailed to pick out just this kind of case. Any statute of the ordinary level of detail which would include Mr. D. would also include other cases for which detention would be inappropriate.

Of course Mr. D.'s mania may progress to a point where his hyperactivity, anorexia and insomnia do become life-threatening; then detention might be justified. But it might not progress to that point. It is his mania, in fact, which makes this a difficult case – a point to which we will soon return.

C. *The Evils Imposed and the Role of Mental Illness*

For detention to be justified it is necessary that the evils imposed by detention have a high likelihood of being transient: that after a limited time of detention the risk of the greater evil (e.g., serious injury) occurring be so much lower that detention is no longer necessary.

This is where the role of mental illness becomes important. For we know as a matter of empirical fact that those irrational desires which accompany recognizable conditions of mental illness (e.g. mania, depression, and schizophrenia) usually disappear when the mental illness is treated; thus there is a high probability that the evils we impose need be only transient, thus less in total amount, thus more justifiable.[4]

For how long should detention be allowed? If the evils associated with an episode of mental illness prove not to be readily reversible with a brief detention (2–3 days) what should be done next? It would be of practical utility to have available an additional two to three week extension of detention if there were compelling evidence that the patient would probably suffer severe evils if released. Because such an extension would greatly increase the amount of evil imposed on the patient it should not be allowed without the patient's having recourse to due process in the setting of a court or some impartial body; this would then be a civil commitment. An additional issue which could be considered at the time would be whether treatment should, if necessary, be given involuntarily. One necessary justification for involuntary treatment would be that the patient, even though in hospital, would likely die or suffer serious injury without it. If involuntary treatment were mandated it would usually be pharmacologic and two to three weeks would usually be sufficient time for these agents to have a therapeutic effect.

Only in extremely rare cases would commitment for a longer period of time be morally justified. It would be necessary (but not sufficient) to show that the evils associated with prolonged confinement were significantly less than the evils associated with freedom and that there was a significantly high probability that the patient could be successfully treated with prolonged hospitalization. Usually the patient should not be committed because the total amount of evil imposed by a long commitment is too great to be justified (see [2], p. 499; [8], p. 177, 180).

We agree with Stone [9] that in many cases it might be critical whether treatment were available in the hospital to which detention is made: as noted above it is unjustifiable to impose the evils of detention when there is little likelihood of reducing the evils experienced by the patient. We are unclear, however, how much force this point has, since in most cases temporary confinement alone eliminates the risk of immediate self-harm and substantially reduces the risk of future self-harm (see [1], p. 87). Of course if a longer commitment were necessary, then treatment availability might be critical.

D. *The Problem of Recurrent Manic Episodes*

The decision not to intervene in Case (3) is not an easy one. Many manic patients like Mr. D. manifest recurrent cyclical behavior which (1) can be financially or psychologically (but not physically) very harmful, (2) seems, by its conjunction with other known symptoms, to be almost certainly part of a manic episode, and (3) would almost certainly be treatable (reversible) in a short period of time, followed by the patient's gratitude that treatment had been carried out. It appears that manic patients are responsible for a large number of the troublesome instances where physicians feel some urge to detain but are unable to do so when narrow guidelines prevail. The situation is made more poignant by the fact that some patients subject to recurrent manic attacks are themselves concerned and apprehensive about the harm they may do if and when future episodes develop. Would it be possible to allow such patients to appoint a proxy or 'guardianship committee' (perhaps composed of spouse or parent plus patient-designated attorney plus psychiatrist?) which, if in unanimous agreement, could sanction future detention and treatment decisions, using broader criteria than immediate physical harmfulness? This might be called an Odysseus Pact or Odysseus Transfer and be thought of as a psychiatric analogue of the 'living will'. Such a committee might, in particular cases, choose to temporarily confiscate a person's funds rather than deprive him or her of freedom. We can see some difficulties with such a procedure but believe it merits discussion. Suppose a patient were insistent that he be allowed to appoint such a committee, and preferred to take what he believed to be the very slim chance of unjustified detention (or confiscation of funds) against the greater likelihood of future psychological and/or economic harm. Are there moral grounds on which one could refuse his request?

E. *Harmfulness Toward Others*

It seems clear that detaining a man to prevent him from inflicting harm on himself (absent an adequate reason) may be for his own good and is sometimes justifiable; what about detaining a man to prevent him from harming others? If a man is detained *primarily* because of potential harm to others, then clearly we are not dealing with paternalistic detention. Can detention of the mentally ill sometimes be justified on non-paternalistic grounds? We believe it can. But it should be emphasized that an intervention to prevent someone from harming himself and an intervention to prevent someone from harming others are, from the standpoint of moral justification, two entirely different kinds of actions. They are commonly compounded in discussions on this subject by the phrase 'danger to self or others', but this breeds confusion.

The kind of moral rule which is violated when one detains individuals who are potentially harmful to others is one where the physician inflicts certain evils on *S* in order to prevent *S* from inflicting evil on *T*. Several features of this situation distinguish it from the situation where *S* is potentially harmful to him or herself. We cannot use the degree of irrationality of *S*'s potential act as a test for justifying detention: one person's desire to harm another is never in and of itself irrational. Its irrationality depends upon the evil consequences that *S* might experience subsequent to his or her harming others (e.g., punishment); these consequences are usually much less certain than in acts of self harm. Often it would not be irrational to prefer the risk of these consequences to the evils of detention. Thus the kinds of tests we believe useful in assessing the justification of paternalistic interventions do not serve us here.

Should we then conclude that those individuals who are potentially harmful to others are to be left solely to the police? This would be a practical and simple solution to the problem, yet it runs counter to our intuition in many cases. For example, consider two men who are brought to the emergency room by the police. In each instance the police have been called because the man's wife has just reported that her husband has threatened her life. Each man admits to the emergency room psychiatrist that this is true.

In *Case* (4) the man has a history of paranoid schizophrenic episodes and as a part of a developing delusional system has recently heard voices instructing him to kill his wife. The psychiatrist feels there is a significantly high probability of the man's harming his wife if he returns home.

In *Case* (5) there are no symptoms of any major mental illness. There is a background of chronic marital discord and the psychiatrist feels there is a significantly high probability of the man's harming his wife if he returns home.

Most seem to believe that we are justified in detaining the man in *Case* (4) but not in *Case* (5). Of course a psychiatrist might be *motivated* to detain both men simply out of a desire to protect their wives but potential harmfulness to others does not provide a sufficient *justification* for psychiatric detention.

In general it seems to be held that psychiatrists should intervene in those cases in which, did they not intervene and the patients did harm someone, such patients might successfully escape punishment through use of an insanity defense. What seems to be critical in these cases is that we view the patient as having less responsibility for the carrying out of his or her harmful action. Were the man in *Case* (5) to harm his wife he would be seen as fully responsible (from the information given) while the man in *Case* (4) would not. To use another terminology, the man in *Case* (5) appears to have the ability to will to harm his wife or not to harm her while the man in *Case* (4), because of his mental illness, may not have the ability to will not to harm her. We will not develop this matter further here but simply summarize by saying that it seems to be the *irrationality* of the potential act which justified intervention with respect to self-harm and *involuntariness* which justifies intervention with respect to harm to others.

It is true that psychiatrists are often under pressure (sometimes from the police themselves) to detain persons in cases like (5), because the man *does* appear harmful and there is a feeling that something should be done. However, we believe that if the psychiatrist determines that there is no condition of mental illness present, then the person should be managed through police procedures: e.g., the use of assault laws if the person has threatened others, and/or the issuance of court orders temporarily prohibiting the individual from the presence of a party he has been threatening.

VI. CONCLUSION

We have tried to show that psychiatric detention is almost always a paternalistic action, and that although it always requires moral justification, in some cases justification can clearly be provided.

Our own position is one of advocating relatively narrow grounds for psychiatric detention. We believe that one necessary condition for the justification of paternalistic detention is that the evils likely to be prevented by detaining a person be of such great life-impact and permanence that it would be irrational to prefer them to the evils associated with being temporarily detained. A second necessary condition is that the person have no adequate reason for suffering the evils that detention is intended to prevent. We think that these are the important features of individual cases that account for the moral judgments we make about particular acts of paternalistic detention. When both of these conditions are present it seems not only justified for the physician to detain the person but that he would be failing in his or her duty as a doctor not to do so.

The dispute about what grounds are adequate grounds for paternalistic detention seems to us not only inevitable but welcome. In every act of paternalism there is a judgement on the part of *A* that *S*'s good justifies the harm accompanying the paternalistic act; that judgement is, of course, fallible. We are sensitive to evil intentions masquerading as good; we should be equally aware that purely beneficent paternalism can be distinctly immoral. In a fine essay Ira Glasser has recently written:

> The assumption of benevolence must be seen as an insufficient reason to grant unlimited discretionary power to service professionals. We must begin, at least legally, to mistrust service professionals as well as depend on them, much as we do the police [6].

By being as clear as we can be about what criteria justify detention we can hope to reduce the unnecessary evil committed by beneficent but fallible psychiatrists. But some acts of commitment seem to be not only morally justified but morally required. Thus we should also mistrust those civil libertarians who, out of their own benevolent intentions, urge us to regard temporary deprivation of freedom as a harm outranking even a significant possibility of death or serious injury. That policy too could lead to unnecessary evil. The dispute is welcome because each side tends to overlook the fact that it can commit excesses out of sincerely benevolent motives. One can only hope that what *is* best for patients will finally emerge.

Dartmouth College
Hanover, New Hampshire

NOTES

[1] Data obtained by Gove and Fain [7] suggest that, after discharge, detained patients do not retrospectively view their hospitalization particularly negatively; in fact a substantial majority of their patients (75.3%, as compared with 81.4% of a group of voluntary patients) felt that hospitalization had helped them. It is of course still the case that moral rules were violated with regard to their patients at the time of detention.

[2] A fuller account of rationality may be found in Gert ([3], pp. 20–43).

[3] Reasons are conscious beliefs that one's actions will help oneself or someone else to avoid or relieve some evil, or, alternatively, to gain some greater good (e.g., more ability, freedom, opportunity or pleasure). It is sometimes difficult to decide on the adequacy of a person's reason for acting on what would otherwise be an irrational desire. Saving your life is an adequate reason for cutting off your arm but getting rid of an ugly wart is not. But some cases are inevitably less clear.

[4] It is not necessary for our analysis that one accord any particular ontological status to the term 'mental illness'. All that is necessary is that one accept that there are recognizable conditions characterized by, say, marked depression, anorexia, insomnia, the desire to die, etc. and that these conditions and their associated evils are reversible when certain 'treatments' are carried out.

BIBLIOGRAPHY

1. American Bar Association: 1977, *Mental Disability Law Reporter* **2**, 73–159.
2. Chodoff, P.: 1976, 'The Case for Involuntary Hospitalization of the Mentally Ill', *American Journal of Psychiatry* **133**, 496–501.
3. Gert, B.: 1970, *The Moral Rules*, Harper and Row, New York.
4. Gert, B. and Culver, C. M.: 1976, 'Paternalistic Behavior', *Philosophy and Public Affairs* **6**, 45–57.

5. Gert, B. and Culver, C. M.: 1979, 'The Justification of Paternalism', *Ethics* **89**, 199–210.
6. Glasser, I.: 1978, 'Prisoners of Benevolence: Power versus Liberty in the Welfare State', in Gaylin, W., Glasser, I., Marcus, S. and Rothman, D. (eds.), *Doing Good. The Limits of Benevolence*, Pantheon, New York, pp. 97–168.
7. Gove, W. R. and Fain, T.: 1977, 'A Comparison of Voluntary and Committed Psychiatric Patients', *Archives of General Psychiatry* **34**, 669–676.
8. Livermore, J. M., Malmquist, C. P. and Meehl, P. E.: 1968, 'On the Justification for Civil Commitment', *University of Pennsylvania Law Review* **117**, 75–96.
9. Stone, A. A.: 1975, 'Comment on M. A. Peszke: Is Dangerousness an Issue for Physicians in Emergency Commitment?', *American Journal of Psychiatry* **132**, 825–828.
10. Szasz, T. S.: 1978, 'Involuntary Mental Hospitalization: A Crime Against Humanity', in Beauchamp, T. L. and Walters, L. (eds.), *Contemporary Issues in Bioethics*, Dickenson, Encino, California, pp. 551–557.

MICHAEL A. PESZKE

DUTY TO THE PATIENT OR SOCIETY: REFLECTIONS ON THE PSYCHIATRIST'S DILEMMA

My discussion of the essays by Professor Winslade and Professors Culver and Gert will obviously be influenced by my background as a clinical psychiatrist and a teacher of clinical psychiatry. Undoubtedly it will also be influenced by my European background and awareness of cross-cultural studies in the area of legal psychiatry. Finally, in the last three or four years, having served on a number of committees, I have been directly involved in the formulation of legislation in the area of civil commitment, competency to stand trial, and the insanity defense. This involvement in public policy issues clearly has afforded me the opportunity to learn how lawmakers perceive society's needs and psychiatrists' expertise. This does not necessarily run true to either our professional goals or our self-image. In a federal union, with fifty different jurisdictions writing statutes, fifty different state supreme courts interpreting the constitutionality thereof, and a federal judiciary often -overriding on appeal to state decisions, it is clear that policy is far from monolithic. Given the heterogeneity of American society, its different ethnic and religious mixtures, the issue of morality in public life and policy transcends philosophical debate and becomes quite often political instead. In turn many political problems become invested with ideological slogans. While the debate on civil commitment falls short of the heat generated by discussions of right to life versus right to abortion, it has caused sufficient acrimony and has led to many polemical articles. Only recently have two Supreme Court decisions in *Addington* [1], and *Parham* [3], hinted at a developing public policy in this area.[1]

Before entering the thickets of the imponderables of a philosophical discussion of the duty of a psychiatrist, it is my opinion that there is no absolute or clear cut way to differentiate the interest of a group from the good of its constituent members. This applies to the medical specialty of psychiatry since it recruits its membership from society at large and is itself already influenced and shaped by the values and mores of that society. Furthermore, in its practices psychiatry is regulated through licensing, and further controlled by legislation and court decisions which are clear expressions of the society it serves. In turn the practices and articulated goals of this medical specialty affect and influence society and its expectations of psychiatry. One could

S. F. Spicker, J. M. Healey, and H. T. Engelhardt (eds.), The Law–Medicine Relation: A Philosophical Exploration, 177–186.

therefore argue that the hypothetical patient and the hypothetical psychiatrist by their very membership in the same society benefit from each other's enhancement and welfare, and profit from the good of the society at large. The psychiatrist, by owing a duty to society which licenses and protects his professional interest, serves the individuals and is also protecting the interest of the patient; by treating the constituent member the psychiatrist, in turn, advances the general health of the group.

Clearly, many of the arguments on behalf of the rights of the mentally ill or the rights of the psychiatric specialty have lost sight of the fact that rights and obligations often coexist. If society has certain fundamental obligations and grants certain rights to its constituent membership, then there may well be an argument for reciprocal rights and obligations. The extent of the rights and obligations of both the mentally ill and of psychiatrists are still far from settled in the United States and are in the process of evolution, some would say devolution by court decisions. It is this lack of clarity and closure that has caused considerable concern *both* for patients and for the psychiatric profession in the United States. This ambiguity is not as obvious in Europe where the mentally ill have a specified right to treatment but very few rights to legal due process procedures.[2] The same obtains for the specialty of psychiatry which, as part of the various national health care systems, is invested with certain obligations and responsibilities both to the patients and to society. These obligations are legislated or are expressed as ministerial instructions.

The extent and flexibility of intervention would be limited by administrative regulations which would emanate from the appropriate governmental authorities. The freedom, and some would say looseness, with which psychiatry (as well as other medical specialties) is practiced in the United States, reflects a significant difference between Europe and the United States. But this freedom in turn begets a challenge, at times in the form of third party scrutiny, at times legal, in this series of essays, philosophical. In the United States, societal emphasis is placed on individual freedom. However, this freedom is usually held to have a legal parameter, it is a freedom from unreasonable incarceration.[3] The decisions and the problems being discussed are also clearly reflections that everything we do or abstain from doing touches on the lives of others and that complete and absolute freedom, however cherished in theory, may in fact have to be eschewed in practice.

These are extremely troubling times which tax the very character and commitment of a profession that is expected to do more than it can in practice achieve, while being denied expertise in the very areas where it stands paramount.[4] The previous essays illustrate some of the conflicts which translate into everyday problems faced in the clinical setting, which make the psychiatrist's professional life an Odyssean endeavor.[5]

The very fact that the practice of civil commitment is questioned in terms of morality or that the responsibility of psychiatry is so ambiguously defined should stimulate reflection. In 1975 I argued that the social standard of dangerousness was completely irrelevant to the concept of civil commitment [4], for the only viable medical ethical standard for involuntary commitment should limit such action to those who are psychiatrically incapacitated *and* unable to recognize their incapacity or reflect on the therapeutic alternatives. I stated that this incapacity, whether or not it resulted in dangerous behavior, should be the only standard by which a person could be coerced into treatment. I argued then and still maintain that society has a legitimate reason for ensuring that each constituent member be given every possible opportunity for achieving adequate education and health care. Those members in our community, who as a result of their psychiatric illness lose their ability to function effectively, may need to receive compulsory treatment *if* treatment is available and if there is a chance that they will profit from it.[6] The rights of the mentally ill include the right to appropriate treatment, not, as has often been argued by civil libertarian attorneys, as merely the right of legal due process. Such difficulties which arise, when strict standards of dangerousness are legislated, lead to what has often been called the 'criminalization' of mental illness. Civil commitment procedures become based on criminal court models, surely an abhorrent development; but those mentally ill who are not socially dangerous are neglected, become a public nuisance and are eventually arrested for minor offenses. Incarcerated in jails, they are not only deprived of freedom, of legal due process, but also of humane and competent treatment. It is pertinent, when discussing both the morality of civil commitment and the strict standards for such confinement, to be aware that there are many ways that society can deal with the socially deviant and the mentally ill.[7]

The comments by Professors Gert and Culver are in line with a standard of civil commitment which would restrict such treatment only to those individuals whose behavior jeopardizes their physical health or life; but where others use constitutional arguments these authors invoke a philosophical doubt in the process of helping the disabled. Arguments for such strict standards have often been expounded on the basis of either the denial of the existence of the entity of mental illness or on the denial of a long accepted tenet that mental illness in its severe forms indeed precludes the exercise of the person's free will. The most reasonable argument for strict standards of due process in the commitment of the mentally ill has been made by those civil libertarians who, while accepting the existence of mental illness and also the severe psychological disabling aspect of such disease, argue that mere psychiatric opinion without advocacy for the patient places too much power in the hands of psychiatrists.[8] From a theoretical point of view this argument is sound, though in practice more difficult to implement than might be supposed; in *Parham*, the United States Supreme Court expressed the following opinion:

> Common human experience and scholarly opinions suggest that the supposed protections of an adversary proceeding to determine the appropriateness of medical decisions for the commitment and treatment of mental and emotional illness may well be more illusory than real.

Most moral philosophers take one fundamental premise for granted and argue their philosophical positions on the keystone of free will and self determination. That is, each of the subjects of their moral debates is in principle capable of complete autonomy.

This, in my view, makes fundamental the question whether, or to what extent, free will is impaired by mental illness and whether most philosophical arguments about the morality or immorality of civil commitment or the ethics of paternalism are appropriately applied to the mentally ill. Our historical tradition dictates that for centuries, even before psychiatrists were trained, society's religious and legal institutions recognized the psychologically disabling effects of mental illness by whatever name they were given – lunacy, insanity, or idiocy. Issues of competency to stand trial or testamentary capacity have been adjudicated for centuries with or without the input of psychiatrists and certainly without an emphasis on such issues as social dangerousness.[9] If this issue of the impairment of free will is ignored, then clearly it is impossible to proffer any sound argument for civil commitment. Indeed, the best that can be argued is that it is a paternalistic act, a protective custody to prevent impulsive life-threatening behavior to self or others.

Somewhat paradoxically, one of the leading exponents of utilitarianism, John Stuart Mill, is also the most frequently quoted authority by those who oppose civil commitment on philosophical grounds. In his famous essay *On Liberty* ([2], p. 9) Mill writes:

> That the only purpose for which power can be rightfully exercised over any member of a civilized community, against his will, is to prevent harm to others. His own good, either physical or moral, is not a sufficient warrant.

What is inevitably omitted by those who cite Mill is the following statement:

It is, perhaps, hardly necessary to say that this doctrine is meant to apply only to human beings in the maturity of their faculties.

It would seem that the exception that Mill makes is critical to our discussion. Most of those who advocate banning civil commitment probably ground their position on both utilitarian as well as deontological principles derived from their personal political-social philosophy and understanding of or adherence to the Constitution of the United States. One of the utilitarian arguments derives in part from the analogy to the criminal system. Since it is better that one hundred guilty people go free than one innocent person suffer, so better that one hundred people possibly in need of hospital treatment remain untreated rather than one be hospitalized unnecessarily.[10] The deontological argument is based on the keystone of an ideological commitment to absolute freedom which at times may extract a price, in this case the mentally ill being abandoned and untreated.

I find the cases, particularly of the gentleman who burned his money, or the two women who stared into space, examples of the extent to which some in our society appear willing to sacrifice those who are mentally ill for the sake of their and our alleged freedoms.[11] During the *laissez-faire* period of our history, cripples and children were allowed to starve and to beg on the streets in the name of economic enlightenment.

It is worthwhile to emphasize the difference between the involuntary hospitalization of the non-protesting person and the involuntary hospitalization of the protesting patient. Most of the patients who are involuntarily committed are so disabled by their mental illness that they do not protest because they do not fully appreciate what is happening. This does not mean that the greatest degree of psychiatric professional care as well as attention to civil liberties should not be given such patients. However, the analogy is close to the patient brought to the emergency room in an unconscious or amnestic state. To expect every patient to fully participate in his treatment decisions and to give what can be regarded as his fully informed consent is a worthy goal but is unattainable in practice. Not to treat such patients is however unconscionable.

We thus face a very peculiar paradox in that the United States has gone some way in a social and legal standard for the involuntary hospitalization of the mentally ill. There are troubling parallels between what is currently argued as legal and moral in the United States, and what is being held up to public scorn and indignation as the abuse of psychiatry in the Soviet Union.

The Soviets have developed and adopted a nosology where politically unacceptable behavior is considered a variety of schizophrenia – sluggish schizophrenia. Hence the Soviets believe that when they diagnose their political opponents to be suffering from mental illness, they are fit subjects, by their standards, for confinement and involuntary treatment. In the United States psychiatrists are being asked to diagnose and predict *dangerousness*. The United States treasures life; the Soviets value political orthodoxy.[12]

It is a paradox today that there is thus a movement to minimize the medical aspect of civil commitment and to maximize the responsibility of the psychiatrist to society. The *Tarasoff* decision, discussed by Professor Winslade, is a good example. The California Court has in fact argued for the social responsibility of the psychiatrist but not of the assailant. It found the mental health profession theoretically liable for negligence to a third party, but not negligent for refraining from civil commitment. The ensuing public policy is in line with my argument.

It should be emphasized that the court did not make a judgement that the mental health professionals were in fact negligent to Tatiana Tarasoff, but only offered its opinion, binding in California, persuasive in other states, that there may be cause for action. This would be based on malpractice standards of negligence to a third party if damages were proved. Tatiana's death was the damage alleged; failure to warn her was the implied negligence. The lower trial court was left to determine whether this negligence met the standards of malpractice. What would have happened had the situation been adjudicated is for us a moot issue, since it was settled out of court. The court argued that the psychiatrist had immunity from alleged negligence for failure to commit, even if there was reason to assume presence of serious illness. One may in fact stand passively by, or so the court would have us believe, and allow a patient to commit an act which will not only be dangerous to others, but which will ruin his/her own life, reputation, and professional career. In Poddar's case it led to his deportation from the United States. The individual has a right to freedom; the police and psychiatrist have immunity for failure to act to detain; but the psychiatrist may owe a duty to a member of society.[13]

How can such a policy hinted at by the court be developed? Should a special administrative telephone line be established, presumably as part of the local police department, or some newly-funded hot line or Division of Victim Information? Would the agency have to evaluate and ascertain proof which would enable such communication to be taken seriously? Would that standard need to be 'beyond a reasonable doubt'? Would it have to be 'sure and certain'? Would that mean the psychiatrist would be subpoenaed to testify?

What weight could be placed on his/her testimony which would be hearsay and generated by patients' remarks, which certainly could then be seen as potentially self-incriminating and thus probably not subject to any further investigation? Would the psychiatrist need to do his own investigative work to track down the potential, threatened victim? In the course of discussion, it was also suggested that the analogy of the mandatory child abuse reporting could be entertained here. The analogy is really quite poor, since we report when there is evidence of child abuse, not when we have reason to think there *may be* child abuse.[14]

The psychiatrist embarks on the Odyssean journey in his quest for the faithful Penelope. He is confronted by the Scylla and Charybdis of malpractice for acts committed or omitted, by the one-eyed Cyclops of the California Supreme Court, and by the Singing Maidens of constitutional purism and due process. Then of course there are the faithful suitors, the other professionals, who claim that they can do as well without infringing on human and civil rights.

I believe that the only way we can fulfill our obligations to society is by devoting ourselves to the proper application of those professional skills that we have acquired, namely, the diagnosis and treatment of mental illness. Our duty may compel us to civilly commit persons for short periods of time until the adjudicating process can take over and enable us to make more permanent decisions.

But to serve society it is best that we fulfill our duty to our patients. It does society and the patient a disservice if psychiatry undertakes tasks which jeopardize our mandate as healers.

University of Connecticut, School of Medicine
Farmington, Connecticut

NOTES

[1] The United States Supreme Court is regarded as the final arbiter of the constitutionality of laws and statutes and has often led, though not without criticism, in legal constructions which are viewed as expressions of social conscience and thus societal morality. In *Addington v. Texas* (1979) the court wrote: "The State has a legitimate interest under its *parens patriae* powers in providing care to its citizens who are unable because of emotional disorders to care for themselves" [1].

[2] In *Parham v. J. R.* the United States Supreme Court, in 1979, wrote what may turn out to be a most revolutionary decision as regards *due process* in medical problems. "Due process has never been thought to require that the neutral and detached trier of

fact be law-trained or a judicial or administrative officer". This statement was shortly followed by "... due process is not violated by use of informal, traditional medical investigative techniques". Finally, Chief Justice Burger writing for the majority stated: "What due process is constitutionally due cannot be divorced from the nature of the ultimate decision that is being made" [3].

3 In *Addington*, the United States Supreme Court recognized legally what has been argued by many psychiatrists: "One who is suffering from debilitating mental illness and in need of treatment is neither wholly at liberty nor free from stigma".

4 It is somewhat perplexing and paradoxical that while Psychiatry is being denied expertise in the area of reliability and validity in the diagnosis of mental illness, it is also more frequently being asked to participate in social issues such as the adjudication of child custody problems. The specialty of Psychiatry is in a position to make psychiatric diagnoses with a reliability no less than other medical specialties, but is not in a position to make professional judgement on such issues as 'fitness to bring up children'.

5 There is a serious shortage of qualified individuals going into Psychiatry. According to a report prepared in 1978 by the American Association of Chairman of Departments of Psychiatry, the percentage of United States' medical graduates entering the specialty of Psychiatry dropped from approximately 12% in 1970 to 8% in 1974 and it is estimated that this percentage had dropped to less than 4% by 1978. There are many reasons for this significant decline in interest. It would be irresponsible to attribute this trend to some of the legal issues that have confronted the practice of Psychiatry. However, it is not at all unreasonable to speculate that the proliferation of law suits against institutional psychiatry, which are being perceived as legal harassment, will have a significant and deleterious effect on the small number of individuals training in Psychiatry who are considering public service as their career choice.

6 It is imperative that the precept of *primum non nocere* be reaffirmed in all aspects of clinical judgment, including the initiation of involuntary treatment. This is one of the most difficult and fundamental differences between clinical judgment and legal philosophy. One precept of legal philosophy is to seek to standardize and give equal treatment to all who are in the same class, so that equity be achieved. In clinical judgments one attempts to tailor treatment to the needs of the individual, taking into consideration all the social and medical options as well as the prognosis. Too often in the field of medicine, heroic treatments and fiscally ruinous procedures are undertaken which have little chance for a positive outcome, and may in fact do considerable harm. I do not subscribe to the popular notion that institutions engender the institutionalization syndrome of the schizophrenic. Anyone who has seen process schizophrenics treated or untreated over a period of time may observe the development of social regressive traits. But medical judgement has to consider the possibility and likelihood of positive outcomes. In the cases of the first break, acute schizophrenias and the manic or the mid-life psychotic depression, the prognosis is excellent. This is obviously not the case for socially and educationally handicapped individuals who manifest *process schizophrenia* or suffer from a second or third break. In fact it seems cruel to treat someone against his will who has made a marginal adjustment to his schizophrenic process when there is nothing to offer by way of improved social ties, status, or life style after discharge.

7 As a member of the Courts Diagnostic Clinic, I participate in evaluations of defendants for competency to stand trial. On one occasion, two out of four defendants were found competent and two incompetent to stand trial. Of the four, three were in the local

correctional center and one on bond in the community. One of the four defendants was accused of murder, one of disorderly conduct, one of possession of burglar tools in a parking lot, and one of cruelty to an animal. The person accused of murder was on the street; the others were in jail. Society begins to sequester such people via a different route when the standards of civil commitment become non-medical and governed by legal due process and proof which is outside the expertise of a psychiatrist.

[8] Many of the attorneys who specialize in problems of the poor, the handicapped, and the disadvantaged, and those who work in the area of *pro bono publico*, who were at one time quite ardent advocates of the Szaszian position, have recently discovered the benefits to be derived by their clients from claims for Social Security Disability on the grounds of mental illness. At times these disability payments are retroactive, and often the arrangement gives the attorney half of the allotment that the Federal Government owes the client.

[9] The United States Supreme Court has provided three rulings in the area of competency to stand trial. The decision which is most pertinent to my argument is *Dusky v. United States* [362 U.S. 405 1960]. The court ruled the legal criteria of competency as "whether there is sufficient present ability to consult with his lawyer with a reasonable degree of rational understanding, and whether he has a rational as well as factual understanding of the proceedings against him".

[10] In *Addington*, the United States Supreme Court wrote that the burden of proof may need to be different in criminal and civil cases. In the criminal case, "our society imposes almost the entire risk of error upon itself"; hence the beyond a doubt standard. Arguing for a lesser burden of proof – "clear, unequivocal and convincing" – the Court stated that a more stringent standard "may impose a burden the state cannot meet and thereby erect an unreasonable burden to needed medical treatment".

[11] An excellent example of this attitude is the conclusion of a letter to the *New York Times*, April 4, 1978, signed by Richard D. Emery and Chris Hansen (members of the New York Civil Liberties Union): "In a critical way, derelicts who resist psychiatric intrusion champion the individualism we all cherish. They are protecting all of us from the trend toward permitting the state to act as a parent by institutionalizing people in need. Compulsory institutionalization has for over a century restricted freedom, encouraged abuse, and has taken us further away, not closer, to the bright dream of helping people in need. Freedom should never be abbreviated on the say-so of self-appointed priests of normalcy who often respond to public and political considerations and not to their patients' true needs. No one should be trusted with that much power over other people".

[12] Generalizations are not only odious but unfair, but there appears to be a greater degree of extent of repugnance in the United States for crimes against people as opposed to crimes against property than is the case in Europe. At the same time social behavior, such as gun carrying and ownership, is tolerated to a much greater extent than is the case in Europe.

[13] I have often wondered whether the radical nature of the California Supreme Court decision in *Tarasoff* is not related in part to: (1) the idiosyncratic aspect of the California Civil Commitment Statutes (The Lanterman – Petris – Short Act) and (2) the fact that both psychologists and psychiatrists were involved in the treatment of the student, Poddar, who killed Tatiana Tarasoff. Society has learned what to expect from the medical profession, but the proliferation of various so-called 'psychotherapists', many

without professional training and most without a code or tradition of professional ethics, leaves many people with a sense of distrust.

[14] Everything has to be decided with some level of common sense. Confidentiality and the hallowed patient-doctor relationship can be violated as much by the physician as by the patient. If a patient, particularly in an institutional setting, threatens other people, threats which are heard by staff as well as the primary care physician, then it is unreasonable to expect confidentiality to prevail. Recently, while attending psychiatrist, I supported the decision of the staff to warn the girl friend of a patient who made threats against her life prior to his escape from the hospital. To have followed any other course would have been irresponsible, not only with respect to the safety of that individual, but also with regard to the long-term welfare of that very patient. Our decision and action would have been taken regardless of the decision in *Tarasoff*. It is my personal observation and experience that such judgments have often been made and such warning acts carried out prior to what has been viewed as a 'revolutionary' decision in *Tarasoff*.

BIBLIOGRAPHY

1. *Addington v. Texas*, 99 S.Ct. 1804, 47, U.S.L.W. 4473 (1979).
2. Mill, J. S.: 1974, *On Liberty*, Appleton-Century-Crofts, New York.
3. *Parham v. J. R.*, 99 S.Ct. 2493, 47. U.S.L.W. 4740 (1979).
4. Peszke, M. A.: 1975, 'Is Dangerousness an Issue for Physicians in Emergency Commitment?', *American Journal of Psychiatry* 132, 825–828.

SECTION IV

DECISION MAKING AT THE BEGINNING OF LIFE: MEDICINE, ETHICS AND THE LAW

STUART F. SPICKER[1] AND JOHN R. RAYE

THE BEARING OF PROGNOSIS ON THE ETHICS OF MEDICINE: CONGENITAL ANOMALIES, THE SOCIAL CONTEXT AND THE LAW

I. PROGNOSIS IN MEDICINE

In their retrospective evaluation of clinical rounds in medical ethics at Children's Hospital Medical Center in Boston, Melvin Levine, Lee Scott and William Curran surveyed the most frequently recurring issue which emerged in these sessions over a five-year period. Among some 17 issues and topics the question 'Who should decide?' emerged most frequently (37%). 'Acting on uncertain prognosis' involved only 6% of the cases and ranked in the 16th position ([24], p. 204). The point of interest here is the tendency of the researchers to qualify the topic of prognosis with the term 'uncertain'. The underlying assumption is clear: prognostications are typically uncertain since they are based on what Dr. Mark Siegler calls *'subjective appraisals'* ([43], p. 857). There is a tendency to assume that prognoses are *in principle* highly uncertain. This prevailing attitude perhaps accounts for the fact that many physicians consider prognoses as not really helpful and at times even harmful. This latter view is supported by arguments in Dr. Siegler's essay "Pascal's Wager and the Hanging of Crepe" [43]. The thesis of this essay is that physicians, in forecasting negative outcomes in serious cases, generate an intellectually dishonest, no-lose situation: when the physician encounters a case wherein the prospect of death is quite likely, for example, the outcome is either (1) the actual death of the patient and with it immediate testimony to the physician's knowledge and foresight, or (2) the patient's recovery after which the physician is imbued with supernatural healing powers. So the physician in such cases is either omniscient or omnipotent – predicates reminiscent of those ascribed to deity by medieval philosophers.

In *Clinical Judgment*, Dr. Alvan R. Feinstein discusses some additional inadequacies of prognoses, and points out that "Although contemporary diagnosis has become an act of extraordinary and often quantified biologic precision, prognosis remains a vague and often inaccurate generality" ([6], p. 116). Feinstein illustrates his point by citing the fact that "diagnosis and general statistics of *myocardial infarction* do not adequately specify the prognosis in different subgroups of patients" ([6], p. 116). Most importantly, "diagnostic names are inadequate both for indicating the nuances of current

S. F. Spicker, J. M. Healey, and H. T. Engelhardt (eds.), The Law–Medicine Relation: A Philosophical Exploration, 189–216.

clinical states and for predicting subsequent developments" ([6], p. 116). Yet in spite of these limitations, one should not be led to the mistaken conclusion that prognostications are useless or that physicians should desist from making prognoses in all medical situations. It may prove especially useful, in this regard, to return to the Hippocratic concept of prognosis; for in our time it is common to note the absence of adequate prognostic data when in fact they could be acquired and serve all concerned. That is, physicians have all too often abandoned the attempt to correlate specified clinical states with the morphologic categories of 'disease', which results in the condition that, as Feinstein points out, "the necessary clinical data were often lacking" ([6], p. 120). But this is nothing short of a nihilistic approach to medical prognosis accompanied by the false inference *that prognoses should not be made because perfectly precise prognoses cannot be made*. Feinstein is one of the few to observe that the real problem lies in the fact that "clinicians have not made the data respectable and available" ([6], p. 124). He reminds us, finally, that the clinician knows that clinical features "are his harbingers of prognosis and determinants of therapy. But he cannot express them specifically or consistently" ([6], p. 126).

The fact is, of course, that predictive thinking plays an essential role in clinical medicine. The ability to forecast future conditions is almost always on-going, albeit tacitly, and it does little good to the urgent search for specificity and precision to adopt an intellectual sulk and to simply claim that clinical predictions are never certain but are inherently probabilistic. We have in fact come a good way from Hippocrates' *Prognostic*, but even in this ancient text, in addition to the respect, creditability, and confidence in the physician which patients typically reveal, should prognoses prove accurate, Hippocrates foresaw the importance of prognoses in determining proper treatment.

> I hold that it is an excellent thing for a physician to practice forecasting. For if he discover and declare unaided by the side of his patients the present, the past and the future, and fill in the gaps in the account given by the sick, he will be the more believed to understand the cases, so that men will confidently entrust themselves to him for treatment. *Furthermore, he will carry out the treatment best if he know beforehand from the present symptoms what will take place later.*[2] Now to restore every patient to health is impossible. To do so indeed would have been better even than forecasting the future ([14], p. 7).

In illness, then, there are symptoms which point to certain consequences in either the near or the remote future. Accurate prognostications can provide a knowledge of the dangers ahead which might enable the physician to meet or even prevent them. We all know that the means of treatment available to Hippocrates were few in number, and hence prognoses by and large served to keep the patient's faith in his doctor. To this end Dr. Siegler's essay is well directed. But since today's doctors can do more, can *in fact* choose among numerous treatment options beyond those imagined by Hippocrates, the contemporary physician should be even more attentive to Hippocrates's suggestion that precise and adequate prognostic data can have great bearing on present treatment [31].[3] Furthermore, since questions arise regarding the selection of patients for non-treatment, withdrawal or discontinuance of treatment, medical prognoses take on ethical significance. For this reason there is an obligation to acquire accurate data in order to make more precise and clinically rigorous probabilistic predictions [37].

In what follows we intend to show that medical prognosis need not be a merely empty forecasting of future conditions likely to prevail given (1) that one is familiar with the natural history of the disorder or disease, (2) that certain conditions occurred in the past, (3) that other signs and symptoms exist in the present. That is, accurate prognostication often has (1) direct bearing on treatment/non-treatment decisions, (2) ethical significance, and (3) important implications for legislation and social policy, which is to say that prognosis is not merely a cognitive exercise expected by patients to periodically excite the muscle of the physician's mind.

The thrust, then, of what follows is *not primarily* directed to 'medical ethics', but is better appreciated as an exploration in the wider domain of the philosophy of medicine; for a closer look at the concept and import of medical prognosis is long overdue, the failing here being partly explained by the powerful tendency to focus on the *process* of medical diagnosis.[4] But, after all, it not infrequently happens that patients and their physicians are soon quite clear in the matter of the diagnosis; the chief problems then become (1) the accurate projection of the future course of the malady, based on the prognosis, however tacitly unstated, (2) the appropriate management and therapeutic plan, and (3) a projection of the broad social setting in which the surviving patient will function.

II. ETHICS, PROGNOSIS AND MENINGOMYELOCELE

Wherein, we may ask, lies the ethical significance of prognosis on treatment/non-treatment decisions in clinical medicine? The answer to this question may be found by turning our attention to a particular long-term analysis of the natural history of a major congenital malformation. Such long-term studies are rarely performed in academic centers and are notoriously lacking for most disorders and diseases. But there are elegant and systematic exceptions. One such exception can be found in the work of Dr. John Lorber, who has undertaken extensive studies of infants born with a congenital anomaly known in Britain as 'myelomeningocele', and labeled 'meningomyelocele' in the United States.

Meningomyelocele is a defect in early fetal life which results from the failure of the neural tube to close. This malformation produces a disorganization of local neural elements of the spinal cord and attendant muscular weaknesses.

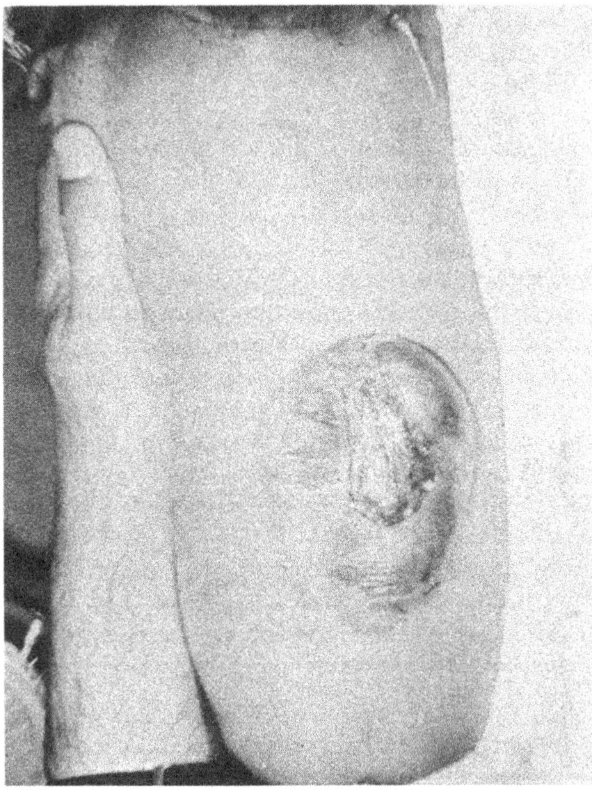

Fig. 1.

In a high percentage of cases associated with this spinal anomaly there is a structural alteration of the central nervous system which interferes with spinal fluid circulation and results in hydrocephalus.

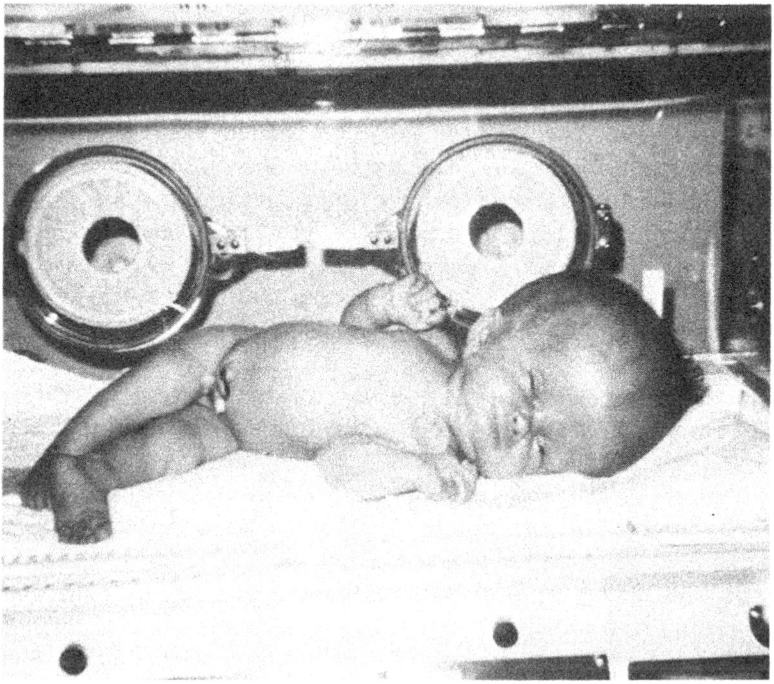

Fig. 2.

In 1966 K. M. Laurence reported that during the period 1956–1962 in the mining valleys of South Wales the average incidence of spina bifida cystica was 4.1 per thousand births; the national average for Britain being about 2 per thousand births ([22], p. 17) and 1 per thousand births in the United States. Myelomeningocele is the most common severe congenital malformation of the central nervous system.

Any long-term clinical, epidemiologic study must begin with a well-defined total population, and the utmost care must be taken in the selection of patients to be described. In 1971 Dr. Lorber reported on his twelve-year study of 524 infants [25]. In 1972 he published the results of his study of 270 additional infants [26]; and in 1973 he reported the results of 37 new cases [27].

In the first study, all 524 infants were treated vigorously with all that was available in the medical armamentarium. Not too many years prior to Lorber's work, infants born with myelomeningocele were 'treated' with an attitude of benign neglect. In cultures where outright infanticide was not practiced, these infants were given only the benefit of simple comfort until death ensued. After 1963 a policy of vigorous therapy was followed in Sheffield, England, and all newborn infants with this congenital anomaly were given a treatment regimen which included covering the spinal defect with skin and diverting the cerebrospinal fluid to other absorptive sites by ventriculo-cardiac or ventriculo-peritoneal shunts. These procedures markedly improved overall survival, and as these infants aged, they were classified into three groups – those with minimum, moderate and severe handicaps. Those in the most severe group, were they at all ambulatory, required braces and crutches. Confinement to the wheelchair was quite common since most of these children were not functionally ambulatory. Repeated urinary tract infections as a result of the inability to void spontaneously required surgery to establish alternate drainage pathways. In a relatively short time, technological developments enabled the shunt to operate more satisfactorily in the control of the hydrocephalus in many if not all such infants. These and other medical achievements have been viewed (and perhaps rightly so) as 'medical miracles', some of the prosthetic devices dubbed 'orthopedic magic'. Such technological achievements, then, enabled pediatric and neurological surgeons to approach infants with various forms of myelomeningocele as a new challenge rather than in despair. As a result this 'new patient' without a well-defined prognosis, 'replaced' the earlier but paradoxically accurately prognosed infant, whose early death was assured. The traditional medical ethic could now once again prevail: The physician has a duty to preserve, spare, and prolong human life wherever and whenever he or she can, and must fight against death in all circumstances! Given the present standpoint, controversy centered around the timing of surgical interventions, especially those procedures which would allow for the closure of the cystic lesion on the infant's back, lesions as high as thoracic (T-12) and as low as sacral (S-1).

The focal question was whether closure should be done in the first 24–48 hours of birth or conservatively delayed to some more efficacious point in time. In 1963 W. J. W. Sharrard and his colleague in Sheffield published the results of a controlled trial of immediate (under 48 hours) and delayed closure of spina bifida cystica [38]. "The main conclusion of this trial", they write, "was that operative closure of a myelomeningocele should be regarded as a surgical emergency" ([38], p. 22). This general conclusion was based on the fact that the immediately operated group fared significantly better in terms of morbidity with regard to local sepsis, meningitis and ventriculitis, muscle paralysis in the lower extremities, and duration of hospital stay[5] ([38] p. 22; [35]; [39]; [40]).

In addition to the normative considerations ingredient in scientific and clinical research, ethical dilemmas in medicine have emerged as the result of recent technological advances. The reason for this can be simply stated: morality and conduct come to the fore when persons have options among which they may and even must choose. Technological achievements expand the realm of human choice, and this is no more in evidence than in the case of infants born with congenital anomalies, e.g., myelomeningocele. When, not so many years ago, nothing could be done to enable such newborns to survive, virtually all died in the first few months of life. Even when surgical interventions were employed to assist in the control of hydrocephalus, the risks of dying from the complications of a severe cystic lesion were as great as the complications associated with the treatment of hydrocephalus. In this context, then, the surgeon might have as easily justified non-treatment, as treatment was not particularly efficacious.

As a result of early closure, the use of antibiotics to deal with ventriculitis, and other surgical procedures, a general policy of actively treating all infants with myelomeningocele came into being. This meant closing the back, shunting the hydrocephalus, and offering continuing orthopedic, urological, neurological, and psychological care.

III. THE PRINCIPLE OF SELECTION

John Lorber begins his comprehensive article of 1971 with the following observation:

> Intensive treatment of spina bifida cystica in recent years has resulted in a much increased survival rate. More and more infants are being surgically treated. It is felt by some that all affected infants should be operated upon even if it is certain that many survivors will *suffer*[6] from multiple handicaps ([25], p. 279; see [30]).

Before proceeding further it is important to note the way in which Lorber signals that the *suffering* of the survivors is an essential and inescapable outcome of decisions to vigorously treat all such disabled and/or deformed neonates: " . . . there are large numbers who are so severely handicapped at birth that those who survive are bound to suffer from a combination of major physical defects" ([25], p. 279). A few pages further on the reader is given the humanitarian basis for Lorber's approach to the neonate with a myelomeningocele:

> If we wish to spare children and their families prolonged suffering[7] and to give better

attention to those who are more likely to benefit from total care, we may have to select suitable cases for intensive treatment and others for no treatment ([25], p. 288).

In this third study Lorber announces a "second revolution in the management of myelomeningocele" ([27], p. 202). Through personal communications from "most paediatricians and paediatric surgeons in Britain", he records "an almost universal acceptance of selection", an acceptance, he notes, "which has been officially recognized as legitimate practice" by the Department of Health and Social Security. Lorber's 'triumph', then, having influenced Britain's national policy in the treatment and care of infants born with spina bifida cystica, is testimony to his own clearly humanitarian motives. He remarks, "There has been no difficulty with the nursing staff, who fully understand the humane purpose and the need for such practice, so long as they are taken into the confidence of the medical staff" ([27], p. 202). In 1971 he closed his first major study with the words, "Objective data are presented to suggest that selection for treatment can be made on a humanitarian basis" ([25], p. 301).

There is no reason to question Lorber's intention to minimize pain and suffering. In our day, when philosophers, theologians and others struggle with the limitations of a plethora of ethical theories, like the various forms of consequentialism (rule and act utilitarianism), and deontological theories, it is becoming more and more difficult to resist the appeal of traditional medical ethical principles or maxims – (1) save life, (2) above all do no harm, (3) do what is best for the patient and abstain from any harm or injustice ([55], 34). That is, humanitarian and equalitarian ethics might well replace the utilitarian formula – seek the greatest amount of happiness for the greatest number – with a principle that implores us to seek the least amount of avoidable suffering for all, that is, minimize pain and suffering. This principle may have important implications for equalitarian public policy. One advantage of this principle is that an urgency accompanies it which does not accompany the utilitarian principle. Providing help to others by way of minimizing suffering, and even preventing it, seems useful here. Another clear advantage is that "in most cases we can do most for our fellow men by trying to remove their miseries". Moreover, as J. J. C. Smart observes, "people will be less ready to agree on what goods they would like to see promoted than they will be to agree on what miseries should be avoided" ([46], p. 30). In short, a negative utilitarianism may be worth consideration as the possible foundation for ethics in medicine, since by 'suffering' in this context one understands misery involving actual pain, not just unhappiness. (There are, of course, dangers in this position, for on this view one might well be able to argue in favor of annihilating the human race.)

Given the end of minimizing pain and suffering, it is now easier to understand Lorber's position. In order to "decide our priorities to ensure that, with all the intensive effort and good will, we shall not do more harm than good" ([25], p. 300), "it would be of considerable value", he tells us, "if one could foretell from simple physical signs present on the first day of life the likely future of a baby if he were untreated, and compare this with his chances if he were given the total care as is known today" ([25], pp. 279–280).

In his study, published in 1971, Lorber provided an analysis of those important features which have a bearing on late prognosis. The project was designed "to correlate accurately observed data obtained on the first day of life with the subsequent progress of the children. Such a prospective analysis would give in any individual baby, with particular signs, probabilities of various severe handicaps and also relatively minor handicap or of none" ([25], p. 288).

The importance of Lorber's work, for our purposes, is to determine the bearing of prognosis on the ethics of medicine. He has been able to provide abundant data which permit the forecasting of outcomes from birth. His comprehensive study clearly allows the conclusion which he draws: "Those who are against selection often state that it is not possible to withhold treatment from any infant with myelomeningocele, as one can never tell what the outlook is for an individual case. The data presented here make such a position untenable." He concludes, "*It is possible to forecast* from a purely clinical assessment with accuracy *the minimal degree of future handicap* in an individual even if *it is impossible to forecast the maximum degree of disability* which he may suffer, if he survives" ([25], p. 299).

With Lorber's work, then, the pendulum has swung from treating all infants with myelomeningocele to selecting those for treatment who do not show adverse signs at birth signaling a so-called 'hopeless prognosis' [22]. In Lorber's original prospective study of infants, 116 of 201 (58%) which compose series two *would have been* excluded from treatment; in his study of 37 infants, published in 1973, 25 (68%) *were not* given treatment ([27], p. 201) and died by nine months of age. Of the 12 who were treated only one died; the remaining 11 were living "normal or moderately handicapped" lives. One should point out that for Lorber "selection for no treatment" means (1) no antibiotic therapy should infection like ventriculitis occur; (2) no provision for intensive care, oxygen or tube feeding; (3) infants would be fed on demand and no more. Lorber specifies his list of contraindications to active therapy:

At birth: Gross paralysis of the legs (paralysis below 3rd lumbar segmental level with at most hip flexors, adductors, and quadriceps being active). (2) Thoracolumbar or thoracolumbosacral lesions related to vertebral levels. (3) Kyphosis or scoliosis. (4) Grossly enlarged head, with maximal circumference of 2 cm or more above the 90th percentile related to birth weight. (5) Intracerebral birth injury. (6) Other gross congenital defects – for example, heart disease, ectopia of bladder, and mongolism ([27], [32], p. 44). After closure, in the newborn period: Meningitis or ventriculitis in an infant who already has serious neurological handicap and hydrocephalus. Later: in any life-threatening episode in a child who is severely handicapped by gross mental and neurological defects ([27], p. 204).

Those critical prognostic indicators and sequelae, e.g., gross congenital anomalies such as heart disease and severe birth injury are, for Lorber, "of the gravest prognostic significance" ([25], p. 295).[8]

It should be pointed out that Lorber's criteria have been supported by others, with minor deviations ([50], [47], [16]). These physicians agree that a careful neurological examination in the newborn period can delineate with a high degree of certainty the neurological deficit of the infant. This knowledge provides accurate prognostication for ambulation, the risks of hydrocephalus, bowel and bladder problems, and major orthopedic abnormalities.[9] In short, if any one of Lorber's initial adverse criteria is present, survival is not possible without severe multisystem physical defects often but not invariably associated with mental retardation ([28], p. 307). Those researchers who follow Lorber to the extent that they recommend a policy of selection all share in the following moral principle: 'minimize suffering'. Dr. Gillian M. Hunt writing in *The Lancet* in December, 1973, closes his "Occasional Survey" with the following remark: "To minimize the suffering caused by this condition [myelomeningocele] operation at birth should not be recommended for those cases for whom severe disability can be predicted" ([17], p. 1312).

IV. OBJECTIONS TO LORBER'S PRINCIPLE OF SELECTION

Notwithstanding the fact that a policy of selective treatment has been adopted in many medical centers, its acceptance is not in fact universal. The most frequent challenges are offered on both medical and ethical grounds. Sometimes physicians appeal to the norms of their profession, as when John M. Freeman, M.D., of The Johns Hopkins University remarks that "Major codes of ethics which cover our behavior can be reduced to a common denominator. Love thy neighbor: Do unto others as you would have them do unto you" ([8], pp. 145–146). The weakness of this view is notorious, of course, even when the ambiguities of such expressions are clarified. Yet in spite of the oversimplification of this ethical stance, Dr. Freeman does sharply formulate the ethical dilemma:

Since early surgery will improve both the quality and quantity of survivors, ethical problems now exist which were not present before. Is it moral to encourage the survival of a child who will be paraplegic, incontinent, and will require multiple surgical procedures for hydrocephalus, orthopedic deformity, and bladder dysfunction? If the back is closed, should the hydrocephalus be treated? Are we to treat these two acute problems and allow a child to die slowly of renal decompensation? If we elect *not* to treat a child, what becomes of him? Is he to be fed and watered while the physician waits for him to develop meningitis? Is he to be sedated and fed inadequately so that he dies slowly of starvation without making too much noise? Are we to kill him overtly? Or covertly? Actively rather than passively? Or are we to embark on the long, difficult, and costly total care of such a child? ([10], p. 14)

In point of fact, Dr. Freeman objects to Lorber's position, notwithstanding the fact that both physicians agree, in principle, with the principle of selection for no treatment, i.e., Lorber selects and gives comfort care; Freeman would select and terminate the life. Lorber's view is as follows: selection is a humanitarian principle in infants born with myelomeningocele; but the active killing of these selected for no treatment "could be an extremely dangerous weapon in the hands of unscrupulous individuals" ([28], p. 308).[10] In Lorber's view it should remain illegal, as it is in the United Kingdom and the United States. However, those selected for no treatment ought to be given comfort care until death naturally ensues. Dr. Freeman maintains that the withholding of treatment from a selected group (which may be as high as 60%) entails the intention not to appreciably lengthen their lives; in this case this intention is indistinguishable from the intention to shorten the life by killing the infant directly. But killing is illegal, therefore we should follow a policy of active treatment for all. No better illustration of a physician's ambivalent position can be found in the literature. Freeman summarizes it as follows:

Since the editor feels that a slow, natural death over weeks or months is not humane for the child, the family or the staff forced to care for the infant, he is left in the schizophrenic position of advocating either active euthanasia or vigorous treatment. Until active euthanasia for the most severely afflicted children becomes acceptable to society, we must opt for vigorous treatment, to make these children and their families as intact as we are able ([10], p. 21).[11]

A further consideration in rejecting Lorber's position is based on the projected fate of the untreated group. Freeman maintains that " . . . many untreated children do not die quickly, and some do not die at all" ([10], p. 15). That is, many will live longer with more handicap than if they had been treated, thus producing greater morbidity in this group than was necessary. Severely affected infants whose back has not been surgically repaired may survive with greater disability than they would have had with early surgical intervention. In "The Short-Sighted Treatment of Myelomeningocele: A Long-Term Case Report", Freeman presents a case in which only 'partial treatment' was provided. This is a case of 'routine care' advocated by Lorber for infants selected for no surgical treatment or other sophisticated medical interventions. The result for this surviving child was "the worst possible outcome" ([9], p. 312). Dr. Lorber, in the same number of *Pediatrics*, offered his comment on his selective policy:

> . . . such selective policy does not solve the problem and occasionally leads to the kind of total disaster as is reported here by Freeman . . . . This is a very real and well-founded fear, but experience in several large series indicates that only a very small minority of such untreated infants would survive long ([28], p. 308).

Lorber's 'solution' for such difficult cases is to re-evaluate the infant at six months and determine if the infant is likely to survive indefinitely; if so,

> such infants must be taken back into the 'fold' and all their problems treated as if they had been treated from birth. They must be kept under close observation by the 'team' and not left to their fate . . . . No doubt, one will still occasionally come across properly 'selected' untreated patients who will survive longer. Their handicaps will not necessarily be graver than the thousands who survive with all the operations. Occasional hard cases should not sway the discerning physician to do what he considers the best for his patient and his patient's family ([28], p. 308; [26], p. 871).

It should be clear that although he argues on consequentialist grounds for the justification of selection, Lorber is not arguing for the right to secure the infant's death at any time.

Another objection to Lorber's principle and policy of selection has been raised by Robert M. Veatch. In "The Technical Criteria Fallacy", Veatch proffers the following thesis in criticism of Lorber's principle of selection: "In principle it is a mistake . . . to assume that any set of technical criteria will be able to make a definitive separation between babies to be treated and those not to be treated". Veatch here challenges the "concept that *any* list of objectively measurable criteria can be translated into decisions about selection for treatment and nontreatment" ([56], p. 15). We think this criticism is inapplicable to Lorber's position although (as we shall see) there *are* grounds for rejecting his policy of selection. The key to the weakness of Veatch's criticism is given in his own words: "When Lorber uses the phrase 'contra-indications to active therapy' he is medicalizing what are really value choices"

([56], p. 15). Now the term 'medicalizing' need not be construed pejoratively. It is abundantly clear on a careful reading of Lorber's papers that the employment of his particular set of 'contraindications' is based on his conception (however much we may disagree with it) of personal and cultural values. That is, however much we may challenge Lorber's principle of selection (and we shall) it will not do to claim he commits the technical criteria fallacy, for Lorber is not only well aware of the value-laden basis of his position – what he construes as the extant parental, societal and humane values of his social context – but one might say that the entire drive of his newly-acquired and accurate prognoses is to show the *systematic connection* between these values – e.g., minimize pain and suffering, achievement of a functional quality of life – and their inherence in the six major signs which serve as contraindications for treatment. Indeed it seems that Veatch offers us a quite abstract view in granting no conceptual connection between a set of physical signs *and* treatment decision. It seems to us that Lorber is free of *this* criticism, since he never construed his contraindications (even if we call them 'physical signs') as a *mere* set of corporeal, technical criteria. However much we may criticize Lorber's position, he is on the mark in *seeing in* the severe hydrocephalus, kyphosis and scoliosis certain limitations to activity, function, and the realization of interests by these children. It should be clear, then, that Lorber *never claims* that prognosis with respect to future disabilities is the sole determiner of moral choice, a position apparently attributed to him by Veatch.[12] Prognosis of a rigorous sort which forecasts with great accuracy the minimal degree of future handicap in an individual is itself rooted in Lorber's conception of prognosis *which includes a minimally acceptable quality of life for each infant*. And it is here that one should focus one's criticism. That is, it is not the case that Lorber commits the informal fallacy of translating a set of mere physical signs into value-laden decisions by a slippery cognitive manoeuvre, but rather that he asks too much in urging us to share in decisions for nontreatment *primarily* on the basis of *his version of a minimally acceptable quality of life*. So though some may "run the risk of seriously misunderstanding the nature of the difficult decisions that must be made" ([56], p. 15) in such cases, as Veatch reminds us, it might be presumptuous to direct such a charge against Dr. Lorber and his associates in Britain. Indeed, as Freeman remarks, "Lorber's assessment of the effects of treatment represents a courageous attempt to evaluate what we are doing with our vigorous treatment" ([10], p. 219). Whatever may be said, then, Dr. Lorber as physician is not a scientist *manqué*.

V. PAIN, SUFFERING AND SOCIETAL REJECTION

Notwithstanding the humanitarian import of Lorber's work on the prognosis of infants born with myelomengocele, it is now appropriate to focus on the truly ethical significant of prognosis. What clarifies this issue are the continuous references to the pain and suffering which it is said these neonates undergo in the early months in which a policy of universal treatment is employed. Keep in mind that Lorber's initial study of 523 infants was prospective, that is, all infants were given vigorous treatment, which means that early surgery to close the back was performed. In his explication of the results of vigorous treatment, Lorber includes descriptions that suggest to the initiate Lorber's pre-judged position regarding selection. For example, he discusses "One normally intelligent girl of 9 years of age who has had 18 major operations, including 7 revisions of her shunt and two extensive spinal osteotomies in an attempt to correct her extreme kyphoscoliosis". He continues, "A long metal rod was passed through the bodies of her vertebrae along the length of the vertebral column: unfortunately she had such a compensatory lordosis that this rod emerges from the thoracic vertebrae and through the skin to bridge the lumbar lordosis and enter the lowest lumbar vertebrae and sacrum" ([25], p. 284). One infant with hydrocephalus developed ventriculitis some time after the revision of a ventriculo-cardiac shunt, and survived three separate episodes "but died later of shunt complications, having had 7 shunt operations in her 11 months of life" ([10], p. 298). With such reports, it seems obvious that pain and suffering are essential accompaniments of vigorous treatment. But is this in fact the case? After years of experience in the treatment of infants with myelomeningocele, R. B. Zachary of Children's Hospital, Sheffield, remarks: "I personally have seen little evidence that the babies have pain in the newborn period . . . " ([60], p. 1461). Even in the most critical study confirming Lorber's prognostic data, Gordon D. Stark and Margaret Drummond make no reference to early pain and suffering, although they point out that "the large majority of survivors have major physical defects and are often mentally retarded" ([50], p. 680). If, as Eliot Slater suggest, "prevention of suffering comes before preservation of life" ([5], p. 286), then we need be provided ample evidence of pain and suffering in these neonates in the first few months in order to justify Lorber's policy. In the 'Report of a Working-Party', which sustained Lorber's recommended policy of selection, the authors refer to "The suffering in question . . . born by the child who may have to face a long series of painful, and ultimately ineffective operations" ([34], p. 85).

These opinions notwithstanding, pediatric neurosurgeons deny the truth of this claim. Knowledge of the anatomical and physiological states of affairs indicates that since neurological function is absent in areas below the lesion, in the kinds of cases we have been discussing, no significant pain phenomena exist on which one may formulate a moral argument against operative interventions. Dr. Joan L. Venes notes that in these cases " . . . actually the amount of physical suffering is quite minimal" ([57], p. 1). Furthermore, the sophisticated techniques available today with respect to ventriculo-atrial shunt insertion, turn out to be an overnight procedure with minimal acute pain at the point of insertion of the shunt. It is important in this discussion to distinguish acute from chronic pain and to distinguish pain which is not a moral evil *simpliciter*, from pain which is clearly a moral evil, perhaps a greater evil than death [29].[13] In the vast majority of the cases we have been discussing, pain phenomena, which would serve to justify selection on the principle of 'minimize suffering', do not appear to be a significant factor.

From what has been said it is clear that Lorber's position in fact rests on a *quality of life* argument, not *life* in the first few months or first year, but beyond two years into early childhood and adolescence. This quality of life 'argument' in Lorber's view does not, we hasten to point out, center on the absence of *cognitive development*, but rather tends to focus on the fate of the *physically* handicapped child in its social context.

Lorber, in the closing discussion of his second study, published in 1972, concludes that

> The fate of infants born with myelomeningocele is of increasingly grave concern to doctors, . . . the general public, and most of all, to parents. Many, including parents, would prefer that such babies be allowed to die peacefully in early infancy, if their predictable quality of life would be beset with grave, multiple handicaps ([26], p. 871).

The final despairing note is added soon after:

> There is, however, no advance in sight which could make more than a marginal difference to the quality of the survivors with adverse criteria. No amount of orthopedic skill could create muscle power where the spinal cord has failed to develop; no medical or surgical treatment of extreme hydrocephalus could restore lost brain function; and no method of treatment could lead to an acceptable quality of life in infants with gross multiple malformations ([26], p. 872).

Thus Lorber advocates treating the problems of the less handicapped children in order to improve the quality of life of the long-term survivors. The weaknesses of the so-called 'quality of life argument' are well known and extant in the literature: Since babies cannot judge what shall be worthwhile life from their own standpoint, their views are of course unavailable. But substituting our preferences for those of the infant, i.e., asking the question whether "we ourselves would find such a life preferable to death" ([11], p. 161), is also unsatisfactory. People disagree in particular cases even when various thought-experiments are performed in phantasy; imagining ourselves in the place of such infants is inadequate for deriving what one *ought to do* or what is morally preferable and justifiable ([12], pp. 365–369). Most important of all, of course, is the fact that a quality of life argument rests on the future state of affairs, the full social context, the availability of support systems of all types, including the facilities for daily care, schooling and occupational programs. And here we come to the essential point mentioned only too briefly by Lorber:

> The worst-affected children are those who were illegitimate and others who were immediately abandoned by their families. They live in institutions, retarded and often permanently bedridden. Their chances in life are so unfavorable that the criteria for active treatment should be even stricter ([25], p. 296).

At this point one should at least mention the significance of various sociological factors. As Rosalyn Darling points out, Lorber "suggests, although he does not consider in detail, the possibility of 'social' criteria such as illegitimacy" ([1], p. 12) having significant bearing on the outcome for these infants. In addition, parental rejection of the newborn or, later on, parental overprotection ([2], p. 442) as well as inadequate care in state-operated institutions, inadequate special education programs, virtually nonexistent occupational programs [23] for the adolescent, harassing or extremely inconvenient transportation 'systems', psychosocial and sexual isolation, and social immobility, are among the most adverse factors affecting the lives of the survivors. One researcher in London remarks:

> At its most gloomy, the picture is one where the condition myelomeningocele is associated with severe social isolation, frequent misery and depression .... The picture is brightened to an extent by the apparently good relationships with parents and sibs that were usually reported and the ability to establish relationships at school.

But the gloomy picture is not as inevitable as Lorber might lead us to believe. David B. Shurtleff and others have made an extensive exploration of the potential for improving the transition from deformed infant to effective adult by setting realistic goals and socialization objectives for the patients and their families. Shurtleff is, of course, speaking of the severely, congenitally malformed infants, and reminds us that this is a "significantly increasing population" ([42], p. 22).[14]

Hence the suffering on which much ink is spilled needs to be relocated in the social arena in early childhood and adolescence. Given a horrendously inadequate care setting for infants with myelomeningocele, one might well conclude with Lorber, Stark, Drummond and others [3] that "The morality is doubtful . . . of recommending early operation on infants for whom a full range of medical, surgical, educational and social support cannot be promised" ([50], pp. 680–681; [51]). It may be that, at one extreme (e.g., third world countries) where medical, social, educational and occupational resources are severely limited, one might by *default* or by established social policy support Lorber's policy of selection, since one may do more harm than good in sustaining the lives of severely deformed infants; whereas in countries with an *embarras des richesses* such a policy calls for moral censure, and 'default' takes on moral significance. It is, in fact, still a decision if one elects to make no adequate provision for the least advantaged among us.

VI. LEGAL CONSIDERATIONS AND SOCIAL PERCEPTION

One question that arises immediately is whether legislation, which ought to be concerned with the achievement of long-term social goals, should be enacted to require that social and medical policies be aimed at maximizing the long-term expectations of these least advantaged myelomeningocele infants. For the demand here is not only (1) to minimize suffering and pain but (2) to improve the plight of the least advantaged, the latter principle requiring, no doubt, a form of redistributionism, since resources are not inexhaustible, either in the form of dollars or support personnel.

Is it not the case that a just society will *seek to compensate these least advantaged persons*? Is it not unjust to allow myelomeningocele infants to remain alive under a policy of vigorous treatment within a social setting which remains ill equipped to provide appropriate care to minimize what is essentially psychological suffering?

In any discussion of the importance of the social context for determining a morally appropriate approach to treatment of severely affected infants, one must introduce a few legal considerations. In addition to legislative action which could conceivably be designed to assist parents who find themselves unprepared for the burdens (and the joys) of caring for a severely disabled infant, one ought to mention the importance of the liability of parents, attending physicians, other health care professionals, including the potential for formal prosecution of such participants [36]. At the present time there does not seem to be a formally agreed upon policy which clearly defines the pediatric neurosurgeon's liability should he or she elect to follow Lorber's principle and policy of selection. In a pluralistic society it behooves us to make a formal argument to justify a policy of selection, a policy we believe should be rejected in a society such as ours. One of the difficulties that has emerged, of course, is the ambiguity of the very term 'selection', for one can *select* infants for nontreatment on at least two widely divergent bases: (1) following Lorber one could 'select' on the basis of a projected *quality of life* in a world already prejudged to be incapable of adequately sustaining and caring for such infants; (2) following others, like Dr. R. B. Zachary, one could 'select' on the basis of "sound medical and surgical principles" as well as a knowledge of the prospects with and without surgery ([60], p. 1461). These divergent views reflect an entirely different ethical standpoint. Lorber would have us prognose the *quality of life and the presumed suffering* of those neonates and thereby detemine what one *ought* to do by way of treating some and refusing to treat others. Dr. Zachary, on the other hand, does not rest his case on a quality of life argument; he is well aware of the rather limited force of the argument that rests on the premise that the neonate suffers intractable pain. In point of fact Dr. Zachary challenges the method of management of those infants who receive no treatment in clinics where such a policy has been adopted. He finds that these babies actually received very poor care and that some "received 60 mg/kg body weight of chloral hydrate not once but four times a day". "No wonder", he adds, "these babies are sleepy and demand no feed, and with this regimen most of them will die within a few weeks, many within the first week" ([60], p. 1461). In short, these babies did not fall but were pushed to death. The question arises, then, as to whether such 'treatment' is presently outside the law and should remain so. If such 'treatment' should remain illegal, as John Robertson and Norman Fost remind us, "hospitals could adopt rules prohibiting medical staff from not treating defective newborn infants, or, at least for following certain procedures when faced with those decisions" ([36], p. 886).

Such a legal approach could lead to a medico-legal policy which could well assuage the worry of physicians and other health care personnel that they will face litigation regarding infants selected for nontreatment. From the medical perspective, then, such a 'treat all' policy might seem advantageous. For there is little doubt that a policy like Lorber's which advocates selection for non-treatment for as high as 60% of infants with myelomeningocele raises serious worries for medical professionals; at the very least a policy of selection would of necessity entail additional decision makers. We have seen this approach applied elsewhere, ([33], p. 363) that is, in cases where neither the patient, nor the parents nor the physician are considered appropriate agents for decisions to discontinue treatment, or to inhibit its very employment ([36], p. 887).[15] Those physicians who opt for a policy of selection, e.g., Freeman and Lorber, advocate that the physician make that particular determination, but they do so in a context where the prognostication is based on the infant's quality of life. And that is to establish criteria on the basis of social utility, development potential, the "presence or absence of capacity", ([20], p. 32; [15], p. 123) and the financial burden to parents and society, the latter totaling as much as twenty thousand dollars annually as the cost of inpatient care alone ([26], p. 868).

A 'treat all' policy, of course, will enable significant numbers of infants to survive, but it should not go unnoticed that anomalies like anencephaly or extremely severe and unmanageable hydrocephalus will quite soon take the life of the neonate. In these clear cases, following Dr. Zachary, treatment is unwarranted, *not because a prognosis of the infant's quality of life demands it, but simply because sound medical judgment concludes that no immediate benefit from further interventions is possible*. The clear cases, infants with severe intracranial hemorrhage or other life-threatening anomalies, need not be treated through operative interventions; for to close the back will have no bearing at all on the impending death. Dr. Zachary also selects some neonates for nontreatment when "the chances of primary healing after surgery would be small: there would be a risk of wound breakdown, which would be far worse than no operation at all" ([69], p. 1461). Hence there are, of course, unsalvageable cases, that is, infants for whom no medical intervention would be beneficial even if the social context were ideal [59]. Once again, the results of Lorber's prognoses can be made applicable in resource allocation decisions, since such allocations are themselves future oriented. Precisely what will be needed in the way of support of infants, children, and adults with myelomeningocele can be determined from careful studies such as those of Dr. Lorber. But with the projection of resources required of an ever-increasing population of such handicapped persons, there is the inevitable problem of evaluating competing needs, since infants with myelomeningocele are not the only ones who require support. Such complex allocation questions in the face of limited resources and competing interests must not be treated with insouciance and indifference, and for this reason alone the law may one day have to reflect *our selection of priorities*.

A scheme worked out by our legal colleagues should, in effect, provide the necessary help to those least advantaged persons who are born with disability and thus alleviate as much as possible the distress caused by these disabilities.

Such a system, once again, would call upon all types of resources and will surely add to already existing burdens. Any other strategy only sustains Dr. Lorber's originally humanitarian proposal, notwithstanding the clearly compromising policy of selection. But the fault lies in the nature of the dialectic which is generated by societal values on the one hand and the desire to minimize suffering on the other. If we fail to provide for the least advantaged among us, we may be compelled to select the very severely infirm for nontreatment and early death. We trust there is little stock in the view that would sustain these lives in the early weeks at all costs, on the basis of a sanctity of life principle, yet fails to make provision for continuous support however demanding that may be. This would be nothing less than to permit persons, that is, children, to suffer in order to serve as living (or dying) sacrificial idols to our merely symbolic gesture to life.

VII. THE PUBLIC'S PERCEPTION AND ITS SOCIAL COMMITMENTS

Whether advanced life support and maximum therapeutic efforts are to be instituted in the case of neonates who are judged to be severely deformed and where the anticipated outcome is a rather early death, serious medical, legal, ethical, and economic questions arise in terms of justifying continued efforts and treatment. What we ought to do in the case of infants born with myelomeningocele is never an easy matter. Paradoxically, two eminent pediatric neurologists disagree on this too: Dr. Freeman remarks that with respect to the decisions involved in selection, the decision not to treat some infants is 'the easy path' ([10], p. 21). Dr. Lorber, across the Atlantic, takes the opposite view: "Whether a line should be drawn, or where it should be drawn, are matters of opinion. It is easier not to draw a line, that is, to treat" ([25], p. 300). The issue is not one of selecting easy paths, for the correct policy will never be easy. In fact it demands nothing less than a return to traditional norms which must now be preserved in a very complex and contemporary context.

We are not suggesting here, however, that government through legislation further assume the role of surrogate parent, because we have already learned that we cannot coerce parents into caring for their disabled and/or deformed infants. Precisely because such coercion is in the end inefficacious, a better tactic is to assist, by whatever supportive means, the parents whose burdens are excessive in the face of the most severe anomalies borne by their children. Nor are we calling for various forms of public charity usually accompanied by disastrous effects such as humiliation, degradation, intrusion, incarceration, punishment and stigmatization. Now stigmatization is generally taken to refer to the labeling process which the typically healthy members of the society impose on those less fortunate and especially those severely handicapped. The very interesting results obtained by psychological researchers make this point worthy of mention as we conclude.

In "Atypical Physique and the Appraisal of Persons" Beatrice A. Wright reports on the phenomenon of *spread* in rehabilitation psychology. This is a description of a psychological process which reveals that we tend to *perceive* other characteristics of such persons with equally negative valence, especially since there is an additional tendency to "weight negative aspects of something more heavily than positive aspects" ([58], p. 111). This perceptual set regarding the disabilities of affected infants, children and adults is usually rooted in a *context* such that the nature of this context determines to a large extent whether the disability assumes a central or a more peripheral role in forming the total impression of a person. The two chief contexts or orientations are what Wright calls the 'coping' and the 'succumbing'. She adds:

> The succumbing framework highlights the difficulties and tragedy of being handicapped in terms of its devastating impact, not in terms of its challenge for meaningful adaptations. Emphasis is on what the person can't do, what is denied the person, the problems that beat the person down. Such a state is experienced as pitiful. The coping framework, on the other hand, orients the evaluator, whether it be the insider or outsider, to scan problems in search of solutions and satisfactions. Persons with disabilities are seen as playing an active rôle in attempting to mold their lives constructively, not as being passively devastated by difficulties ([38], p. 112).

The results of such research should not, of course, lead one to assume that the coping context precludes attention to the suffering that accompanies handicapping conditions; but this suffering and pain are felt to be manageable, precisely because satisfactory aspects of this person's life are also recognized. Hence the lesson is one of preparing the public for a way of perceiving and establishing a context that will enable all of us to meet the challenge of disability, since "a person is not equivalent to an impairment" ([58], p. 113). Our current cognition and perception of the handicapped, especially the severely handicapped, is evidence of the most *abstract* attitude, through which we single out the handicapping impairment and unwittingly generalize or 'spread' it over our entire perception of that person. As a consequence of this research, it is clear that one line of attack is to present handicapping phenomena within a coping rather than a succumbing context. In our discussion, this comes to the need to assume *abilities* and *potentialities* for all afflicted persons, and this is nothing less than a call for societal change, which must begin at the perceptual level, that is, in the very way we *see* persons with handicaps; for we cannot simply claim to be willing to have our society support those on whom it imposes an unwelcome burden ([4], p. 492). We need not dwell, then, on the all too obvious fact that persons with more severe handicaps, disabilities, and deformities are systematically kept from our gaze and, even worse, are kept hidden from our children's vision.

So we conclude this exploration of the bearing of prognosis on the ethics of medicine in much the same fashion as one of us (S.F.S.) concluded his first tiptoe into medical ethics. In "The Execution of Euthanasia" he urged that we "foster the most humane care settings for the terminally ill" ([49], p. 91). Our societal commitment to the least advantaged among us requires that we expand our concept of medical prognosis and construe its use in a social-contextual fashion. It is no longer fruitful to view the notion of prognosis as a mere reference to forecasting the natural progression of disease and illness. Our exploration suggests that the work of Lorber and others signals the need for a wider understanding of future social conditions which bear on decisions to select patients for nontreatment. In short, decisions taken at birth ought to be intrinsically connected to the quality of *social* life in which medically assisted neonates will one day have to function. We can then assist health care professionals to live up to the spirit of the tradition which originated on the island of Cos. Our physician colleagues did take an oath. Rather than close with the obvious reference to Hippocrates, it might be more appropriate to restate the modern form of the Oath of Hippocrates so eloquently stated by Dr. Zachary:

> Under no circumstances would I administer drugs to cause the death of the child. There is no doubt that those who are severely affected at birth will continue to be severely handicapped. But I conceive it to be my duty to overcome that handicap as much as possible and to achieve the maximum development of their potential in as many aspects of life as possible – physical, emotional, recreational, and vocational – and I find them very nice people ([60], p. 1462).

The University of Connecticut, School of Medicine
Farmington, Connecticut

NOTES

[1] I am especially grateful to Drs. John Freeman and Joan L. Venes for their suggestions and comments during the initial formulation of this essay. I am also indebted to Professor Sally Gadow for her critical reading of an earlier draft and for the useful suggestions which she provided.

[2] Our emphasis.

[3] See ([31], p. 1196); Dr. Motulsky remarks: "Knowledge of the natural history of untreated disease becomes particularly important in decisions regarding initiation of treatment and assessing the effect of various modes of therapy on the course of a given disease. A bias in most published data regarding prognosis and natural history of chronic disease suggests worse outcomes than actually apply. Inappropriate therapeutic decisions may result".

[4] We call the reader's attention to the forthcoming appearance of the edited proceedings of a "Workshop on the Logic of Discovery and Diagnosis in Medicine". This excellent conference convened October 6–8, 1978, under the auspices of the University of Pittsburgh School of Medicine and was co-sponsored by the Center for the Philosophy of Science and the Program for Human Values in Health Care.

[5] It is interesting to note that these researchers – Sharrard, R. B. Zachary, J. Lorber and A. M. Bruce – were extremely sensitive to the ethical implications of their research design. For in this study, composed of two groups, the management of the groups was the same, apart from the early operations performed on the experimental group. After 40 infant patients had been included, 20 of whom received immediate operative interventions, the trial ended. The researchers remark that "Although statistical analysis does not allow firm conclusions to be drawn about any single aspect of the analysis, summation of the trends in various aspects was sufficiently conclusive to us to make it ethically unjustifiable to continue the experiment and investigation further" ([38], p. 22). Perhaps at this juncture it should not go unnoticed that scientific research with bearing on accurate prognoses reveals *internal* norms. For in addition to the dedication, persistence, discipline of the researchers, the fortitude to resist their own prejudices, and the commitment to share the evidence and results of their research with the scientific community and the public, these and the other investigators were aware of the ethical dimension of their work beyond the internal norms of the scientific activity itself [19].

[6] Our emphasis.

[7] See also ([4], p. 488). Drs. R. S. Duff and A. G. M. Campbell also discuss a case in which the parents felt that "much of the suffering of their baby, themselves, and their other children was senseless and destructive". This suffering, we should note, was due not to chronic pain in the care process, but by 'the hostility of the staff', and trying to cope at home with inadequate financial and personnel support when complications arose.

[8] See [52]. In 1974 Drs. S. C. Stein, L. Schut and M. D. Ames of Children's Center, Philadelphia, in their retrospective study of selection procedures for treatment of myelomeningocele, suggest that lacunar skull deformity (LSD) correlates significantly with mental retardation; this is a neonatal skull X-ray finding in newborns with myelomeningocele. This, in principle, follows Lorber's model; the difference being that LSD and any *two* of Lorber's major adverse criteria are viewed as sufficient contraindications for treatment. In this study myelomeningoceles presented in the following locations: thoracolumbar (39%), lumbar and lumbosacral (57%) and sacral (4%).

[9] See ([10], pp. 24–25). J. M. Freeman notes that "The higher the lesion, the greater the neurological deficit and the higher the risk of hydrocephalus".

[10] See ([34], p. 88). Report by a Working Party: "Infants not selected for treatment are likely to have a very short life-span. We believe that there is no occasion for actively shortening it still further".

[11] See ([10], p. 21). "Active euthanasia might be the most humane course for the *most severely* affected infants, but it is illegal. 'Passive euthanasia' is legal, but it is hardly humane. Therefore, in an ambivalent fashion we feel that *virtually* every child should be given optimal care." In their letter to the editor of *The Journal of Medical Ethics*, ([1], p. 153) entitled 'Active and Passive Euthanasia', A. G. N. Flew and R. G. Twycross complain about the current employment of the terms 'passive' or 'negative' euthanasia, since they rightly point out that good terminal care "is anything but passive or negative". They worry that those who are opposed to euthanasia will call for 'furor therapy' in cases where this view is productive of greater harm to some individuals.

[12] During the discussion which followed the presentation of this paper on November 10, 1978, Robert M. Veatch offered further clarification of his published position (see [56]). In his letter of November 21, 1978, Veatch further clarified his interesting concerns:

"I think we would agree that the values you identified are indeed those held by Lorber and that it is impossible to reach the conclusions he reaches without holding some set of values such as the ones you describe. Our disagreement is over whether he is fair in acknowledging that the values have to be combined with the empirical measures he identifies in order to reach his conclusions. It seems to me that on many occasions, he states the criteria as if they were medical indicators for nontreatment independent of any normative framework. Certainly he does not go out of his way to point out that the criteria should be used only by those who share his values or their equivalent.

In terms of deductive logic I accuse him of arguing from a minor premise to a conclusion without stating any major premise. The fact that you can find what his major premise must be by looking elsewhere in the Lorber literature, does not seem to let him off the hook. I think there is a very practical problem because many professionals use the criteria as if they were independent of evaluations and unsuspecting parents are not given an adequate opportunity to accept or reject the use of the criteria based on values other than those held by the professional".

We tend to agree that Lorber does not acknowledge in any detailed discussion the role personal values and norms play in the decision to select some infants for nontreatment, and that Lorber's empirical indicators may lead some to conclude that his view rests on nothing more than a biological check list devoid of normative considerations. However, it seems too strong to state that Lorber is in some sense illogical, simply because he has not formally stated the major premise of his argument, one which, we believe, is easily gleaned from his publications which reveal his general commitment to the principle to minimize suffering. That is, the major premise is that 'chronic suffering and pain for the infants ought not to be prolonged by means of additional medical (surgical) interventions'. Given this major premise, the minor premise (which he does offer) – 'Treating all myelomeningocele infants necessitates the perpetuation of inhumane suffering' – permits his conclusion: 'Do not treat (surgically) all myelomeningocele infants'. The obvious eliciting of the major premise does indeed let Lorber off the hook. But, as we shall argue, he is not entirely free of hooks. In this we agree with Veatch. Finally, the force of our extended argument is in accord with Veatch's final concern, namely, criteria for determining treatment/nontreatment decisions of these infants must include reference to the norms of social context, in which health care is generally provided to myelomeningocele infants. But the issue is wider than the values of parents and health professionals, since general social policy with respect to the care of myelomeningocele infants lies behind what we ought to do for each infant with myelomeningocele at the time of birth.

[13] Professor McCullough's interesting distinction between pain *simpliciter* (which is not a moral evil) and pain which is a moral evil, rests on the claim that only pain that overwhelms our independence and autonomy is a moral evil. But not only are pain claims notoriously incorrigible, the newborn infant could not possibly have an *autonomous* existence in any meaningful sense. One difficulty here for McCullough, then, is that on his view we cannot ascribe moral evil to the pain experienced by newborn infants, and that seems counterintuitive, irrespective of the empirical question of whether or not pain is experienced by neonates undergoing treatment for myelomeningocele.

[14] One would be overly optimistic to assume that preventive screening tests, e.g., amniocentesis, will make this discussion moot, since myelomeningocele could conceivably in time be eliminated. Notwithstanding the existence of a test for x-fetoprotein material in the amniotic fluid, the tests are (1) still unreliable for prenatal detection of myelomeningocele and (2) unfeasible for application in all pregnancies, especially since this congenital anomaly is not associated with a woman's age as is the chromosomal anomaly which is productive of Down's Syndrome.

[15] See ([10], p. 14) where Dr. Freeman writes: ". . . I feel the decision to treat, or not to treat must ultimately be made by a physician from the team which will be responsible for the long-term care of that child – a physician who is aware of his own prejudices toward the problem". Also see ([25], p. 290) where Dr. Lorber remarks: "All such decisions [for selection for nontreatment] should be made by consultants with special experience in this field of medical and surgical paediatrics. They must not be delegated to junior staff". Since these physicians suggest that physicians should decide in particular cases which infants would receive vigorous treatment, they are perhaps assuming that "an individual with scientific expertise in a particular area also has expertise in the value judgments necessary to make policy recommendations simply because he has scientific expertise" ([55], p. 29). Robert Veatch refers to this assumption as 'the generalization of expertise'. The argument advanced for rejecting this assumption is cogently made by Veatch, but one should also point out that some persons with medical expertise often *have expertise* in those evaluative considerations which are entailed in the formulation of policy. Veatch, regrettably, does not tell us what precisely constitutes "moral or policy expertise" ([55], p. 39). It is equally important, of course, to insist that the ethicist not assume to generalize his expertise when, simply because he is qualified to make evaluative analyses and policy recommendations, he assumes he has expertise in understanding the clinical and scientific aspects of medicine.

BIBLIOGRAPHY

1. Darling, R. B.: 1977, 'Parents, Physicians, and Spina Bifida: A Study of Values in Conflict', *The Hastings Center Report* 7(4) 10–14.
2. Dorner, S.: 1976, 'Adolescents with Spina Bifida: How They See Their Situation', *Archives of Disease in Childhood* 51, 439–444.
3. Duff, R. S. and Campbell, A. G. M.: 1973, 'Moral and Ethical Dilemmas in the Special Care Nursery', *The New England Journal of Medicine* 289(17), 890–894.
4. Duff, R. S. and Campbell, A. G. M.: 1976, 'On Deciding the Care of Severely

Handicapped or Dying Persons: With Particular Reference to Infants', *Pediatrics* 57(4), 487–493.

5. Eckstein, H. B., Hatcher, G. and Slater, E.: 1973, 'Severely Malformed Children', *British Medical Journal* 2, 284–289.
6. Feinstein, A. R.: 1967, *Clinical Judgment*, Robert Krieger Publishing Co., Huntington, New York.
7. Flew, A. G. N. and Twycross, R. G.: 1975, 'Correspondence: Active and Passive Euthanasia', *Journal of Medical Ethics* 1, 153.
8. Freeman, J. M.: 1973, 'To Treat or Not to Treat', in R. H. Wilkins (ed.) *Clinical Neurosurgery: Proceedings of the Congress of Neurological Surgeons, Denver, Colorado, 1972*, Williams and Wilkins, Baltimore, Maryland, pp. 134–146.
9. Freeman, J. M.: 1974, 'The Shortsighted Treatment of Myelomeningocele: A Long-Term Case Report', *Pediatrics* 53(3), 311–313.
10. Freeman, J. M. (ed.): 1974, *Practical Management of Meningomyelocele*, University Park Press, Baltimore.
11. Glover, J.: 1977, *Causing Death and Saving Lives*, Penguin Books, Middlesex, England, Chap. 12, 'Infanticide', pp. 150–169.
12. Hare, R. M.: 1976, 'Survival of the Weakest,' in S. Gorovitz *et al.* (eds.) *Moral Problems in Medicine* Prentice-Hall; New Jersey, pp. 364–369.
13. *Hartford Courant*, 1978, 'Children Save Deformed Cat'.
14. Hippocrates: 1959, *Prognostic* in *Hippocrates*, Vol. II, transl. W. H. S. Jones, Loeb Classical Library, Harvard University Press, Cambridge, Massachusetts.
15. Holder, A. R.: 1977, *Legal Issues in Pediatrics and Adolescent Medicine*, John Wiley and Sons, New York, Chap. IV pp. 107–133.
16. Hunt, G. *et al.*: 1973, 'Predictive Factors in Open Myelomeningocele with Special Reference to Sensory Level', *British Medical Journal* 4, 197–201.
17. Hunt, G. M.: 1973, 'Implications of the Treatment of Myelomeningocele for the Child and His Family', *The Lancet*, 1308–1310.
18. Husserl, E.: 1960, *Cartesian Meditations: An Introduction to Phenomenology*, Transl. D. Cairns, The Hague: Martinus Nijhoff. The original text, *Cartesianische Meditationen und Pariser Vorträge*, heraus. von S. Strasser, *Husserliana I*, Den Haag, Martinus Nijhoff, 1950.
19. Jonas, H.: 1976, 'Freedom of Scientific Inquiry and the Public Interest', *Hastings Center Report* 6(4) 15–20.
20. Jonsen, A. R. and Garland, M. J.: 1977, 'A Moral Policy: Life/Death Decisions in the Intensive Care Nursery', *Medical Dimensions* April, 28–35.
21. Kass, M., Shaw, M. W.: 1976–77, 'The Risk of Birth Defects: *Jacobs v. Theimer* and Parents' Right to Know', *American Journal of Law and Medicine* 2(2) 213–243.
22. Laurence, K. M.: 1966, 'The Survival of Untreated Spina Bifida Cystica', *Developmental Medicine and Child Neurology* 8 (Suppl. 11), 10–19.
23. Laurence, K. M. and Beresford, A.: 1976, 'Degree of Physical Handicap, Education, and Occupation of 51 Adults with Spina Bifida', *British Journal of Preventive and Social Medicine* 30, 197–202.
24. Levine, M. D., Scott, L. and Curran, W. J.: 1977, 'Ethics Rounds in a Children's Medical Center: Evaluation of a Hospital-Based Program for Continuing Education in Medical Ethics', *Pediatrics* 60(2), 202–208.

25. Lorber, J.: 1971, 'Results of Treatment of Myelomeningocele', *Developmental Medicine and Child Neurology* **13**, 279–303.
26. Lorber, J.: 1972, 'Spina Bifida Cystica: Results of Treatment of 270 Consecutive Cases with Criteria for Selection for the Future', *Archives of Disease in Childhood* **47**, 854–873.
27. Lorber J.: 1973, 'Early Results of Selective Treatment of Spina Bifida Cystica', *British Medical Journal* **4**, 201–204.
28. Lorber, J.: 1974, 'Selective Treatment of Myelomeningocele: To Treat or Not to Treat?', *Pediatrics* **53**(3), 307–308.
29. McCullough, L.: 1979, 'Pain, Suffering and Life-Extending Technologies', in R. Veatch (ed.) *Life Span*, Harper and Row, New York, pp. 118–141.
30. Merrill, R. E., McCutchen, T., Meacham, W. F., and Carter, T.: 1965, 'Myelomeningocele and Hydrocephalus', *Journal of the American Medical Association* **191**(1), 111–118.
31. Motulsky, A. G.: 1978, 'Biased Ascertainment and the Natural History of Disease', *The New England Journal of Medicine* **298**(21), 1196–1197.
32. Oppenheimer, S.: 1977, 'Comparative Statistics – Treatment Versus Non-Treatment', in R. L. McLaurin (ed.) *Myelomeningocele*, Grune & Stratton, New York, pp. 41–52.
33. Pontoppidan, H., *et al.*: 1976, 'Optimum Care for Hopelessly Ill Patients', (A Report of the Clinical Care Committee of the Massachusetts General Hospital) *New England Journal of Medicine* **295**(7), 362–364.
34. Report by a Working Party: 1975, 'Ethics of Selective Treatment of Spina Bifida', *The Lancet*, 85–88.
35. Rickham, P. P. and Mawdsley, T.: 1966, 'The Effect of Early Operation on the Survival of Spina Bifida Cystica', *Developmental Medicine and Child Neurology* Suppl. 11, 20–26.
36. Robertson, J. A. and Fost, N.: 1976, 'Passive Euthanasia of Defective Newborn Infants: Legal Considerations', *The Journal of Pediatrics*, **88**(5), 883–889.
37. Shapiro, A. R.: 1977, 'The Evaluation of Clinical Predictions', *The New England Journal of Medicine* **296**(26), 1509–1514.
38. Sharrard, W. J. W., Zachary, R. B., Lorber, J. and Bruce, A, M.: 1963, 'A Controlled Trial of Immediate and Delayed Closure of Spina Bifida Cystica', *Archives of Disease in Childhood* **38**, 18–22.
39. Sharrard, W. J. W., Zachary, R. B. and Lorber, J.: 1967, 'The Long-Term Evaluation of a Trial of Immediate and Delayed Closure of Spina Bifida Cystica', *Clinical Orthopaedics and Related Research* **59**, 197–201.
40. Sharrard, W. J. W., Zachary, R. B. and Lorber, J.: 1967, 'Survival and Paralysis in Open Myelomeningocele With Special Reference to the Time of Repair of the Spinal Lesion', *Developmental Medicine and Child Neurology*, Suppl. 13, 35–50.
41. Shaw, M. W.: 1977, 'Genetically Defective Children: Emerging Legal Considerations', *American Journal of Law and Medicine* **3**(3), 333–340.
42. Shurtleff, D. B.: 1977, 'Independence Achievement of Congenitally Physically Handicapped Children', *Pediatrics Digest*, 15–22.
43. Siegler, M.: 1975, 'Pascal's Wager and the Hanging of Crepe', *New England Journal of Medicine* **293**, 853–857.

44. Singer, P.: 1975, *Animal Liberation: A New Ethics for our Treatment of Animals*, Avon Books, New York.
45. Singer, P.: 1977, 'Can Ethics Be Taught in a Hospital?', *Pediatrics* 60(2), 253–255.
46. Smart, J. J. C. and Williams, B.: 1973, *Utilitarianism: For and Against*, Cambridge University Press, Cambridge, England.
47. Smith, G. K. and Smith, E. D.: 1973, 'Selection for Treatment in Spina Bifida Cystica', *British Medical Journal* 4, 189–197.
48. Snyder, R. D.: 1976, 'Doctor as Prognosticator', *New England Journal of Medicine* 294(5) 281.
49. Spicker, S. F.: 1978, 'The Execution of Euthanasia: The Right of the Dying to a Re-Formed Health Care Context', in S. Spicker (ed.) *Organism, Medicine, and Metaphysics: Essays in Honor of Hans Jonas on His 75th Birthday*, D. Reidel Publishing Co., Dordrecht, Holland and Boston, Mass. pp. 73–94.
50. Stark, G. D. and Drummond, M.: 1973, 'Results of Selective Early Operation in Myelomeningocele', *Archives of Disease in Childhood* 48, 676–683.
51. Stark, G. D.: 1974, *Spina Bifida: Problems and Management*, Blackwell, Oxford, England.
52. Stein, S. C., Schut, L. and Ames, M. D.: 1974, 'Selection for Early Treatment in Myelomeningocele: A Retrospective Analysis of Various Selection Procedures', *Pediatrics* 54, 553–557.
53. Tedeschi, G.: 1966, 'On Tort Liability for Wrongful Life', *Israel Law Review* 1(4), 513–538.
54. Tribe, L. H.: 1973, *Channeling Technology Through Law*, The Bracton Press, Chicago, Illinois.
55. Veatch, R. M.: 1973, 'Generalization of Expertise', *Hastings Center Studies* 1(2), 29–40.
56. Veatch, R. M.: 1977, 'The Technical Criteria Fallacy', *Hastings Center Report* 7(4), 15–16.
57. Venes, J. L., 'Personal Communication' Aug. 17, 1978, 1–9.
58. Wright, B. A.: 1978, 'Atypical Physique and the Appraisal of Persons', *Connecticut Medicine* 42(2), 109–114.
59. Zachary, R. B.: 1968, 'Ethical and Social Aspects of Treatment of Spina Bifida', *The Lancet*, ii, 274–276.
60. Zachary, R. B.: 1977, 'Life With Spina Bifida', *British Medical Journal* 2, 1460–1462.

JOHN A. ROBERTSON

SUBSTANTIVE CRITERIA AND PROCEDURES IN WITHHOLDING CARE FROM DEFECTIVE NEWBORNS[1]

I. INTRODUCTION

Passive euthanasia of defective newborns through selective non-treatment is now widely practiced in England and the United States. Many persons defend the practice as a morally and socially justified way to prevent suffering. However, a practice of withholding necessary medical care from defective infants to cause their death does not square easily with basic norms of liberal democratic society that accord equal respect to the life of all persons whatever their physical, mental or social characteristics.

By way of comment on Professors Spicker's and Raye's essays I would like to examine two assumptions upon which the justice of this practice depends. The first assumption is that there exists a class of persons from whom necessary medical care can be withheld on the basis of a prognosis about their mental and physical characteristics, consistently with basic legal and ethical norms. The second assumption is that present procedures for withholding care accurately select for non-treatment only those patients who fit into the putative class, and not others who justifiably should be treated.

II. IS THERE A CLASS OF PERSONS JUSTIFIABLY SELECTED FOR NON-TREATMENT?

There are two possible grounds for identifying a class of newborn infants for whom non-treatment may justifiably occur without their consent when such care is necessary to maintain their life.

A. *To Advance the Infant's Interests*

It is often asserted that passive euthanasia of defective newborns is justified to save the infant from the suffering inevitable in its handicapped state. The infant with severe congenital defects will not be able to participate in many ordinary activities of life, may be stigmatized, resented by families, or condemned to live under horrible institutional conditions. Thus it is said that humanitarian concern for the infant's own well-being requires that it be

S. F. Spicker, J. M. Healey, and H. T. Engelhardt (eds.), The Law–Medicine Relation: A Philosophical Exploration, 217–224.

allowed to die, through withholding necessary care, to avert the suffering it will face in life as a physically or mentally disabled person. On this view, withholding care violates no right of the infant, for it prevents rather than causes harm.

It is doubtful, however, whether this claim justifies the widespread practice of selecting defective infants for death through passive means. For there are few conditions so disabling that we could say with reasonable certainty from the infant's perspective that continued living is a fate worse than death. Such cases may of course arise. The clearest of them would involve incessant suffering, unrelievable pain, which would make it impossible to realize any of the experiences or states of being which make life, even for disabled persons, a good.

But short of such an extreme case, it is difficult to say that death is preferable to life for newborn infants who lack the physical and mental capacities of ordinary mortals. Most cases of Down's Syndrome, myelomeningocele and many other congenital anomalies, though they involve hydrocephalus, kyphosis, incontinence, non-ambulation, and mental retardation, do not fit this category. These infants may suffer, and of course do not know the diversity and richness of life of ordinary people. But the perspective of the healthy, normal individual is the wrong perspective to take here. The view of ordinary people who know ordinary capacities for experience and interaction, and who may view the infant's existence as a fate worse than death, does not tell us how the infant who has no other life experience would view it. For him life in a severely disabled form would seem better than no life at all, even if his life is lived in a custodial ward of a state institution.

Thus, attempts to justify non-selection for treatment on grounds of benefit to the child – presumably the humanitarian reasons that Dr. Lorber and others cite – should be suspect and a heavy burden placed on those advocating it to establish that such infants indeed fall into the category where, from their own narrow perspective alone, no life is better than some life. That claim is not impossible to make. However, in most cases it will not exist and may mask a decision to withhold treatment to advance interests other than those of the infant.

B. *To Advance the Interests of Others*

Although the interests of the defective infant is often asserted as justification for non-treatment, the absence in most cases of benefit to the child from non-treatment masks what may be the most prevalent reason for non-treatment:

to relieve parents, the family, doctors, and perhaps society of the burdens that care of such persons entails. The parents will face continued existence of a defective newborn who may or may not be cared for at home. The doctors and nurses may not want to treat an infant that may not be able to relate very well to them and who has a very poor prognosis. And society (taxpayers) may well have to endure very heavy financial burdens as a result. Persons who adopt this position are frankly utilitarian. They claim that the burden to parents, family, doctors and society from treatment are so great that it outweighs the benefits to infants who will end up in a retarded or physicially defective state, and therefore treatment may be withheld. This view ignores the fact that the infant's interest even from its diminished perspective is to live, by assuming that life to the infant cannot be a good which outweighs their own interest.

Before assessing the moral validity of such a position, it is important to be more precise about the burdens and benefits that a policy of full treatment entails. For I agree with Spicker and Raye the burdens may not be as great as imagined at the moment of diagnosis, and there may be benefits from treatment not easily appreciated by persons involved in such a decision.

Consider the matter of the suffering or cost to parents and family if treatment is required. Many persons view the parents as victims of a cosmic injustice, which medical treatment would only compound. On this view the parents should have the right to avoid further suffering by causing the child's death through selective non-treatment. But this argument ignores the fact that the major source of the parents' suffering is the birth itself and that additional burdens from the continued existence of the defective newborn depends on whether or not they retain custody and care for the child. Selection for non-treatment is usually seen as a way to relieve parents of the burdens of continued care. Yet there is no reason why they must continue to care for the child. If the child can be treated and cared for without their continued involvement, then the parents' suffering can be minimized consistent with the child's interests in life. It is true that they will know that the child exists in an institution and is being cared for by others at state expense. They may feel guilty and wish the child would die from natural causes. But this suffering seems a much less weighty interest than if they were required to keep the child at home at great expense to them and with the possible disruption of family and individual life-plans. Since there are legal procedures in nearly every state for parents to relinquish their obligations and responsibilities to a defective newborn and shift the burden of custody and care of the child to the state, the presumed suffering of the parents does not seem a sufficient condition to override the infant's right to a life that is otherwise in its interest to have.

Shifting custody and responsibility for the child from the parents to the state (and all taxpayers) does not eliminate the dilemma, though it does shift its focus in an important way. The utilitarian argument for passive euthanasia must then turn on the claim that perinatal and subsequent medical and institutional care for defective newborns will be too costly in light of the benefits of these expenditures. But what are the benefits? Two can be identified. One is the benefit to the treated infant, who now will be able to live. A second benefit is the respect for all human life that treatment of the most severely disabled necessarily entails. Protecting all human life, regardless of social worth and potential, reinforces the general societal commitment to equal respect for all lives, which ultimately benefits everyone.

The utilitarian argument for passive euthanasia through non-treatment ultimately depends on a rejection of the equivalency of all human life. It assumes that some lives are less worthy of protection than others, and that treatment can be justifiably distributed on the basis of the physical, mental, and social characteristics of the person in need. While treatment would clearly be justified and, indeed, obligatory regarding persons who would thereby enjoy ordinary capacities for social living, the benefits to individuals and to society in general from treating the severely defective are too slight to justify the enormous costs of treatment. In the final analysis, then, the existence of a class of infants from whom treatment may justifiably be withheld on the basis of the interests of others depends upon a willingness to make quality-of-life assessments when significant costs are involved. If we can justifiably make such assessments, then the utilitarian approach leads to identification of a class from whom care may be withheld. If such assessments conflict too strongly with the societal norm of equal respect for all lives, or seem too likely to lead to abuses, then defining a class on this basis fails.

A complete analysis of this issue is not possible here, for it is a central issue in medical ethics, philosophy, and law. However, it is worth noting that the courts are beginning to accept the idea that persons with extremely attenuated capacity for consciousness and relational ability might not enjoy the same right to have others (family, doctors, society) incur burdens to maintain their lives, as they would if they had greater capacities. Such a recognition has begun to appear in cases involving withholding necessary treatment from persons who are chronically "vegetative", or incompetent and terminally ill. For example, in the famous case of Ms. Karen Ann Quinlan, the New Jersey Supreme Court ruled that the guardian had no duty to provide essential medical care to a patient who was "chronically vegetative, with no reasonable possibility of recovering cognitive and sapient ability".[2] Although the court tried to justify this holding as reflecting the patient's inferred choice under the substituted judgment doctrine, it is difficult to view the case other than as an official recognition that quality life assessments, based on extremely diminished capacity for consciousness, are sometimes proper. Similarly, recent decisions in Massachusetts such as *Saikewicz*[3] and *Dinnerstein*[4] reflect the view that there is no obligation to treat terminally ill, incompetent patients even though treatment could result in additional weeks or months of life. These cases may also be understood as reflecting a judicial recognition of the view that the benefit to individuals with severe mental and physical incapacities of continued existence is not so great that substantial burdens ought to be incurred by others to provide it.

The case of the defective newborn is much harder than the precedents which have been set with regard to treatment of the comatose and incompetent terminally ill, because it usually involves patients who are conscious but not dying, and thus clashes more sharply with the norm of equal respect for the life of all. A societal judgment that non-terminally ill, conscious persons may be denied a right to life because their incompetent lives are not worth the costs, on some assessment of their physical and mental abilities, would be a major departure from the hardwon idea of equality that even strict utilitarians might wish to reconsider. However, we may expect the courts to carve out on a case-by-case basis additional exceptions to the general duty to treat all persons. If bright lines that do not encroach too much on the principle of equal respect for the lives of all persons can be drawn, we may expect the courts, when faced with such cases, to identify in effect a class of infants from whom necessary care may be withheld, on the ground that the resulting benefits to them do not justify the costs of treatment.

From the above analysis, I conclude that there exists a narrow class of infants who may justifiably be selected for non-treatment consistent with our notion of equal respect for the life of all persons. The class consists of those infants (1) whose suffering is so great that continued life is not in their interests or (2) whose conscious existence is so greatly diminished that investing in their care appears to reasonable people to yield no benefits that it need not be done, e.g., where the infants are irreversibly comatose or where death is imminent. Beyond these narrow categories, severely defective infants must be accorded the same rights as healthy infants and therefore must be treated.

III. ARE PRESENT PROCEDURES OF SELECTION FOR NON-TREATMENT SUFFICIENTLY ACCURATE?

The second assumption underlying the justice of passive euthanasia of defective newborns is that current procedures accurately select for non-treatment only those infants from whom care is justifiably withheld. Whether one defines the class for whom passive euthanasia is justified narrowly or broadly, many infants with congenital defects will not fit the category and must be treated. The fact that some defective infants are justifiably non-treated does not mean that care may be withheld from all defectives. Non-treatment can be justified only if certain criteria are met which all defectives do not meet. Otherwise some newborns with a right to be treated would die in order to benefit infants, parents and others in cases in which care may be justifiably withheld. A high rate of non-justified, passive euthanasia would increase the social costs, and alter the utilitarian calculus. The justice of a policy of passive euthanasia thus depends upon the accuracy of the selection procedures employed.

While firm empirical data on the extent of passive euthanasia is unavailable, several facts suggest that many more infants than would meet the criteria for justifiable selection for non-treatment are not being treated. First, most of these decisions are not made on the basis of articulated, clear criteria. They vary with the doctor, the hospital, and a mixture of factors that are not explicitly stated. Secondly, there are no legal or other checks on the discretion of doctors and parents. There is no required decision-making procedure, and though non-treatment currently would be illegal and criminal in nearly every jurisdiction, the law has not been enforced and is not much of a check. Thirdly, these decisions are often made in a highly emotionally-charged setting, soon after birth, when parents are still grieving the 'loss' of a normal child. They may not have considered all the alternatives, such as institutionalization, and may not be fully informed about the psychosocial potential of a retarded child. Indeed, a full medical work-up to determine the extent of neurological damage may not even be done. Fourth, pediatricians and pediatric neurosurgeons have reported that they would consider repair of duodenal atresia in a Down's Syndrome child to be 'extraordinary care' and therefore would not treat, even though this case is least justified for non-treatment. Finally, many anecdotal reports from doctors and nurses confirm that selection for non-treatment occurs on a large-scale, willy-nilly fashion, without careful attention to morally justifiable criteria for non-treatment.

In any event, the actual extent of the present over-inclusion of infants for non-treatment may be less important than the risk that it may occur under a revised social policy that openly permitted non-treatment. If non-treatment is to be socially acceptable and legally recognized, there is a need for a selection process that would minimize errors. Standards of substance and procedure are inextricably linked. If non-treatment is morally justified, it is morally justified only for those infants meeting the criteria and not for those who do not. It becomes much less tolerable if it can occur only by selecting many infants for non-treatment who did not fit this class. Policy-makers must pay as much attention to procedures adopted for applying the substantive criteria as they do to the substantive criteria itself. For the procedures used to apply the substantive criteria will, in effect, determine the limits of non-treatment, and may expand the practice beyond the justifiable limits of those not treated. A further reason for attention to the procedure is that it is constitutive of the respect that we show for those from whom care is withheld.

If selection for non-treatment is to be morally and socially acceptable, two conditions must be met. The first is that the decision be made according to criteria that are authoritatively articulated and publicly announced. The criteria cannot be whatever individual doctors and families decide, for the question is which of their decisions are morally and socially defensible. Rather, they should be developed by an authoritative body that is representative of the community as a whole, such as a legislature, a national commission or some other publicly constituted body that reflects a wide range of societal views. The norms articulated by this body should circumscribe the limits of non-treatment, for they would reflect the community's consensus as to which infants can be justifiably allowed to die through non-treatment.

The second condition is that doctors and parents making the decision according to these criteria should follow a specific process for assuring that a given infant falls within the category of those who may be justifiably selected for non-treatment. Since the cost of an error of under- or over-inclusion is very great to the patient, investment of time and resources is justified in order to reduce the frequency of errors. In the Quinlan case, for example, the court required that a hospital committee confirm the doctors' prognosis that the patient would not recover cognitive and sapient abilities, before necessary care could be withheld on the basis of the patient's mental state. Such a procedure was justified by the need to reduce the possibility of an error that would be very costly to a patient – premature termination of necessary care.

A variety of procedural arrangements could minimize the frequency of errors without incurring high costs to the participants and the medical care system. These could include confirmation by two consulting physicians, by a committee, or even in certain cases, by the courts. The most workable procedures would involve operationalizing or applying clearly articulated standards that could be easily translated into medical criteria. If the criteria for non-treatment are broader and involve application of more general principles to individual cases, such as whether or not treatment is in the best interests of the child, a more elaborate procedure, possibly including an adversary hearing before a judge, might be required.

IV. CONCLUSION

I have argued that only those infants should be selected for non-treatment and early death who satisfy publicly articulated criteria for withholding care, according to a procedure for applying criteria which minimizes errors of over-inclusion. One may object that publicly articulating criteria for non-treatment will do irreparable damage to societal norms of equal respect for life and that this entire matter is better kept out of the public realm and left to the privacy of the newborn nursery, trusting to the good judgment of doctors and parents. Such a solution might be attractive if the only problem here were rationalizing a gap between private practice and public norms. But the problem is greater, for it concerns the fate of those who suffer from such a gap – those infants who are erroneously and unjustifiably selected for non-treatment, even if non-treatment is in some cases justifiable. Those infants are persons with rights too, including the right to life. There is no reason why they should be sacrificed to assure non-treatment in cases where it may be justified, any more than they should be sacrificed to benefit future patients. As Justice Brandeis once said, there is no disinfectant like sunlight. Moral and public sunlight is sorely needed in the newborn nursery if societal norms of equal respect for life are to continue to constitute the essence of our social life.

University of Wisconsin
Madison, Wisconsin

NOTES

[1] Comments on Spicker and Raye's 'The Bearing of Prognosis on the Ethics of Medicine', in this volume, pp. 189–216.

[2] *In re Quinlan*, 70 N.J. 10, 355 A. 2d 647 (1975).

[3] *Superintendent of Belchertown State School v. Saikewicz*, 370 N.E. 2d 417 (1977).

[4] *Matter of Dinnerstein*, 380 N.E. 2d 134 (1978).

ANGELA R. HOLDER

IS EXISTENCE EVER AN INJURY?: THE WRONGFUL LIFE CASES

Although my topic is the wrongful life cases: Is existence ever an injury?, the basic question, however, is not whether or not one's life may be considered an injury, philosophically or physically, but whether or not being alive is ever, in law, something for which one should receive monetary compensation from another.

The confusion about what trends are developing in this area of law is primarily the result of the fact that cases of very different sorts have been collectively discussed as 'wrongful life' cases, when in fact very different legal principles are involved. Some involve suits by parents on their own behalf, either alleging negligence in performing sterilization operations, so that an unwanted child was later conceived and born, or alleging negligent obstetrical care in failing to discover that a fetus had a severe defect. Others involve suits brought on behalf of the infants themselves, in which they claim damage to themselves, either before their conception or by the physician's failing to appreciate their defects *in utero*. The infant plaintiffs claim their existences to be compensable events, on the theory that their positions would have been better off if they had never been alive. These infants argue that one has a fundamental right to be born healthy or not to be born at all. These cases brought by the children with deformities are the only ones that actually can be called 'wrongful life' cases, but this paper will discuss also those decisions in which the parents have brought their own causes of action.

The wrongful life cases are of very recent origin in the jurisprudence but have been based, for the most part, on well-known principles of American tort law. Thus, before discussing what the law seems to be now, it probably would be helpful if we go back and look at the beginning of this legal trend.

At common law, injuries sustained by a fetus were not compensable. The unborn child was considered to be a part of the mother and in an action arising from an accident that injured both of them, she was the sole plaintiff [14]. In 1946, however, the District of Columbia Appeals Court upheld a right of action on behalf of a child who was seriously handicapped as the result of injuries sustained in an automobile accident while his mother was pregnant ([3], [10]). Other states followed this precedent in numerous cases involving wrecks, medical malpractice involving pregnant women and a variety

S. F. Spicker, J. M. Healey, and H. T. Engelhardt (eds.), The Law–Medicine Relation: A Philosophical Exploration, 225–239.

of other personal injury cases. It is now clear that in all jurisdictions a live child, who was injured before birth, does have a cause of action against the person who negligently caused the damage to him.

The usual difficulty in this case is proof of causation – that the interference with the fetus more probably than not caused the handicap, and that the deformity was not the result of a congenital anomaly. Where that is established by medical evidence, however, the right to recovery is clear [17]. If the child can present medical evidence to show that he would have been normal if the accident had not occurred, the elements of damage are the same as those in any other personal injury suit: present and future pain and suffering, costs of medical care and loss of present and future income ([11], [33], [36]).

Some states, beginning with a Minnesota Supreme Court decision in 1949 [39], began to interpret their Wrongful Death statutes in such a way as to allow wrongful death actions to be brought by the families of unborn children who were killed prior to birth, but after they had become viable, usually during the last month or six weeks of pregnancy. About 20 states are believed by most commentators to indicate recognition of such a cause of action [1]. At least that many states, however, have refused, some in quite recent decisions, to allow a couple to bring a wrongful death action on behalf of a still-born child – on the theory that a fetus is not 'a person' under the applicable Wrongful Death statutes.

The majority of cases involving wrongful death actions on behalf of newborn infants allege medical negligence during labor or delivery. Most cases arising from the death of a child during delivery are, however, brought with the mother as sole plaintiff alleging medical malpractice by the obstetrician. The fact that the child died is argued as an element of damage to her and as factual proof of the medical negligence involved [25]. Although the majority of states still do not permit a wrongful death action to be brought for the death of a viable fetus, in all jurisdictions, obstetricians are liable for such lack of due skill, care and knowledge in their treatment of the pregnant woman that injury is caused to that part of her body known as the fetus ([27], [30]). For that matter, death of an entire pre-viable embryo, as the result of medical negligence, is actionable but the damaged patient is clearly the mother, not the embryo. No state allows an action for recovery of damages for the wrongful death of a pre-viable fetus, but negligence that causes an early miscarriage is certainly compensable in all jurisdictions.

In all these cases, the person who is sued is charged, as in any form of personal injury case, with having done something that actively interfered with fetal development. The driver of the car who injures the mother causes active damage to the fetus. The physician who inappropriately gives a mother a drug with a high risk of fetal damage, likewise, is an active participant in the harm that results.

Concurrent with these prenatal injury cases, courts began to consider the legal rights of parent and child when an unplanned infant is born as the result of a negligent sterilization operation, either a tubal ligation or a vasectomy [5]. Because it is still very difficult to prove negligence in the performance of either a vasectomy or a tubal ligation, most early cases involving unsuccessful sterilization operations were brought on the theory of breach of contract ([2], [21]). Most of those concluded that as long as the child born to the plaintiff was normal, although the mother could recover some damages for the pain and suffering of childbirth and pregnancy, damages would not, as a matter of policy, be awarded for the cost of raising the child.

Where a sterilization operation was undertaken because of the high probability that a child would be born deformed, however, and such deformity occurred, the courts were apparently willing to allow damages for the cost of child care if negligence was proved. In the case of *Doerr v. Villate* [16], for example, a man had a vasectomy after he and his wife had two retarded children. The operation was unsuccessful and the couple had a third child, who was also retarded. It was held that the couple had a cause of action for the cost of raising the child against the urologist who performed the vasectomy with an awareness of the couple's situation.

In most states, however, it has been held that the birth of a normal child is not a compensable event. Most courts that have considered the question hold that expenses of raising a normal child are offset by the pleasures he brings his parents [37]. This is known as the so-called 'benefit rule', that even if one is subject to a clearly tortious act, if the results accrue to one's advantage, the amount of damages awarded will be offset by the value of the advantage. There is, however, a trend toward allowing recovery in these cases. Although courts commonly refer to them as 'wrongful birth' cases, what is really involved is 'wrongful conception' and those courts hold in these cases that an element of damage in negligent failure to sterilize is the cost of raising a child to adulthood. The first decision to that effect was *Custodio v. Bauer* [13]. The plaintiff had a tubal ligation but subsequently became pregnant and gave birth to another child. She sued for negligent performance of the operation and negligent misrepresentation that she was sterile. The appellate court held that her allegations stated a cause of action and that she should have the right to a trial to prove that the operation had been performed negligently and upon such proof, she should at least be reimbursed for any outlay for the unsuccessful operation. The court also held that she could recover for all physical complications and mental and physical damage that she, the mother, suffered from the unwanted pregnancy.

In another recent case, *Coleman v. Garrison* [12], from Delaware, a woman had a tubal ligation at the time she delivered a baby but thereafter became pregnant and had another child. The court allowed a cause of action for expenses of the last child. It held that the Supreme Court decision in *Griswold v. Connecticut* [19], which declared that a state could not constitutionally forbid the use of contraceptives, created a constitutional right not to have children. The appellate court said that the jury, therefore, should have been allowed to weigh the benefits of parenthood against the economic burden of child-raising. The mother was clearly entitled to recover for her own pain and suffering, medical expenses and other reasonable consequences of the failure of the procedure. Further, the court held that the mother could recover for the cost of the change in the family life-style and economic consequences to her resulting from the birth of an additional child.

In *Troppi v. Scarf* [38], a woman whose prescription for contraceptive pills was improperly filled – she was given tranquilizers – became pregnant, sued the druggist and argued that she should be allowed to recover the cost of raising the child. The court held that the plaintiff had a right to recover those damages against the druggist.

In 1977 there were several cases in various states on the subject of failed sterilization operations. In almost all of them, the mothers who had had the unsuccessful tubal ligations were allowed to recover damages for their own medical expenses and loss of earnings, but in most states, courts ruled that they were not allowed to recover damages on behalf of a healthy child.

In one, however, *Sherlock v. Stillwater Clinic* [34], the father of the infant, the eighth in the family, had had a vasectomy at the time the seventh child was born; it was unsuccessful. The parents sued, alleging that they had the right to damages equal to the costs of raising the child and the court permitted them to do so, holding that

> Where the purpose of the physician's action is to prevent conception or birth, elementary justice requires that he be held legally responsible for the consequences which have, in fact, occurred.

The court did, however, point out in that case that this cause of action is exclusively that of the parents, since it is they and not the unplanned child who have sustained both physical and financial injury by the physician's negligence. The court further stated:

Compensatory damages for the cost of rearing the child to the age of majority would also, in our opinion, serve the useful purpose of an added deterrent to negligent performance of sterilization operations.

The same doctrines enunciated in the sterilization cases were then applied in two recent decisions where women's pregnancies were misdiagnosed and they could not, therefore, have early abortions. In both cases the women had decided against the risk of a late abortion and proceeded to have their babies, both of which were normal. In one jurisdiction the court allowed recovery and in the other, no cause of action was held to exist.

In the New York case, a woman consulted the defendant doctor in May, 1971 for the purpose of obtaining contraceptive pills. She then consulted the defendant on several occasions over the next few months because she thought she was pregnant and he repeatedly assured her that she was not. In December, 1971, she was advised by another physician that she was 4½ months pregnant. The husband and wife brought separate causes of action against the physician; the wife sought to recover damages for pain, suffering and mental anguish incident to the birth of her child, for the responsibility of the education and the medical expenses of the child and damages for her inability to work outside the home as a result of her obligation to raise the child. The husband sought to recover medical expenses, damages for the loss of consortium and damages arising from his responsibility for the cost of raising a child. The defendant appealed from denial of a motion to dismiss the actions and the appellate court held that the woman did have a cause of action [42]. The court found that the action was basically one for malpractice, which it defined as "recovery for damages sustained as the result of the physician's failure to use due care in diagnosis or treatment", and pointed out that in a malpractice action, which is one for personal injuries, the person responsible for the injury must be responsible for "all damages resulting directly from and occurring as a natural consequence of the wrongful act". This is the ordinary doctrine of 'foreseeability', applied throughout negligence law – that the reasonable man would expect that the actual consequences might have occurred as the result of the negligent act or negligent failure to act. Quite obviously, the forseeable consequence of negligent failure to diagnose a pregnancy is that the patient will, in due course, have a baby.

Almost at the same time, however, in an almost identical case, the Supreme Court of Wisconsin refused to allow a woman to recover damages [31]. The defendant physician made a diagnosis that she was not pregnant and she eventually consulted another obstetrician who discovered that she was seventeen weeks pregnant. The court found that the action was one for damages based on the birth of a normal, healthy child and that public policy may vitiate recovery, even when the chain of causation is complete and direct. The court held that to permit the parents to keep their child and enjoy him but shift the entire economic responsibility of his upbringing to a physician who failed to determine or inform them of the pregnancy would be to create a new category of 'surrogate parent'. The court found that such results would be wholly out of proportion to the culpability involved in making the misdiagnosis and that allowing recovery would place an unreasonable burden upon the physician under the facts alleged. Therefore, it held that even in view of proof of negligence, no cause of action for support of the child was stated.

The next developments in the progression of the law are the genuine 'wrongful life' cases brought by infant plaintiffs who claim that they would have been better off never having existed. This concept was first formulated by the Supreme Court of Illinois [41]. A plaintiff born to an unwed mother sued his natural father, who was married to someone else, for the social injustice and injuries he suffered because of his illegitimate birth. The court dismissed the case, on the theory that even though there may have been a tort, adverse social circumstances were not capable of recompense in the court because there was no applicable measure of damages. The second wrongful life case was a child whose mother had been a patient in a New York mental institution and was raped, thus resulting in the child's conception [40]. The child sued the state of New York for failing to provide adequate care to his mother during her hospitilization, thus resulting in his illegitimate birth. This case was also dismissed.

The first suit against a physician for the wrongful life of an infant was a decision of the New Jersey Supreme Court, in 1967 [18]. The plaintiff, Mrs. Gleitman, contracted German measles during the first trimester of her pregnancy. She consulted her obstetrician who told her, in effect, not to worry about it. The infant was born with very serious defects and both the parents and the baby sued the physician. The Court found that the parents might have a substantial case for recovery of damages for their own injuries; it denied recovery for the infant-plaintiff on the grounds that "the infant-plaintiff would have us measure the difference between his life with defects against the utter void of non-existence, but it is impossible to make such a determination". The court noted, moreover, that at the time that cases was decided, abortion for this woman would have been illegal under the law of the state of New Jersey and to advise her to have an abortion, the physician might well have been performing an illegal act.

About a year later, the New York lower courts decided the case of *Stewart v. Long Island College Hospital*. Mrs. Stewart also contracted rubella; her physician advised her of the risk that her infant would be deformed. A hospital review committee advised her, however, that she did not need an abortion and that she should not seek one elsewhere. Her child was born deformed and the infant and the parents sued the hospital. The jury awarded the child $100,000. The court allowed recovery solely on the grounds that the hospital had not informed the plaintiff's mother that two of the four doctors on the committee had recommended that she have an abortion, which was held to be a breach of the duty to disclose. This was, therefore, not actually a wrongful life action; it had much more in common with the more usual cases involving informed consent to treatment. The decision, was, however, eventually reversed on appeal and the infant recovered nothing [35].

In *Jacobs v. Theimer* ([4], [22]), the parents of a child born with numerous defects brought a malpractice suit against an obstetrician who had failed to diagnose German measles in the mother during her pregnancy. He had thus not informed her of the substantial risk that the infant could have resultant defects. The parents sued the physician for damages for medical expenses required to treat and care for the child and for their own emotional suffering. The Supreme Court of Texas held that the physician was under a duty to make reasonable disclosures about rubella and its dangers to the unborn child, and that simply to provide such information could not make the physician an accomplice to a criminal abortion even though abortion was illegal at the time. The court dismissed the action for the parents' emotional damage on grounds that it was too speculative, but permitted the cause of action for recovery of expenses reasonably necessary for care and treatment of the child, and remanded the suit for trial for determination of damages.

In this case the obstetrician did not realize that the infant's mother had had rubella; Mrs. Jacobs had contracted it on vacation. When she returned home she was hospitalized and while there, Dr. Theimer discovered that she was pregnant. She asked him if she might have had measles and he said no. This was not a situation in which the physician knew that a woman had rubella but knowingly failed to tell her about the possible consequences to the child. Unlike the preceding cases involving negligent intervention into fetal existence, moreover, this case allowed a cause of action for recovery of damages when the physician was not the cause of the damage to the child. This point is very frequently overlooked by commentators and courts in this area of law who analogize from the cases that allow recovery for prenatal damages resulting from automobile wrecks and other acts that in themselves are harmful. In the automobile accident case, the defendant is the agent who caused the child to be damaged, i.e., if the automobile accident had not occurred, the child would have been born healthy and the fact of the accident was the other driver's fault.

In *Jacobs* and similar cases, however, the German measles, not the negligent misdiagnosis, caused the child's problems. The court in *Jacobs* went into detail in pointing out that if the rubella had been diagnosed, neither Mrs. Jacobs nor the fetus could have been treated and that the only alternative to the birth of a defective child was abortion. In almost all other successful misdiagnosis cases, it is necessary for the plaintiff to prove that if the diagnosis had been correct, the condition would have been cured or at least substantially remediated by treatment. For example, if a physician negligently fails to realize that a patient has a terminal illness for which he could have offered no effective cure if he had recognized it, the patient cannot normally recover damages for diagnostic malpractice. He may do so only if proper treatment was denied, but if given would have made a substantial difference in the outcome of the illness. It is really most difficult to argue that abortion is either a 'cure' or a 'substantial remediation' of fetal disease.

Jacobs was the first case recognizing a cause of action for damages by the parents of a defective child against the physician, based on the claim that the physician had failed to tell the mother that the infant might be defective and, as a result, she failed to abort. If the damages awarded are to the parents for the expenses of child care in or out of an institution, then the cases such as *Jacobs* would seem to be in no way conceptually different from the usual malpractice awards; the only unusual aspect of these cases is the elements of damage the courts have allowed. Mrs. Jacobs, the patient, was denied adequate care with foreseeable damage to herself. On the other hand, in those other cases in which the child is the plaintiff and asks for "damages for being born", a very substantial departure from the basic concepts of tort law has occurred.

An unanswered but interesting question is to assume the fairly obvious situation in which a physician does, in fact, advise a woman that she should have amniocentesis for purposes of determining whether her baby would be born with severe problems but she refuses on the grounds that even if it is, she will not abort because she does not believe in abortion. The baby is born defective. Does it have the same right to sue its mother as it does to sue the physician who fails to advise of amniocentesis? If we wish to use the concept of negligence for not discovering prenatal damage and arranging an abortion, it is arguable that 'parenting malpractice' is as logical as medical malpractice in this situation, although there are, presumably, policy reasons for preserving parental immunity. One of them is, of course, that the parent is already legally obliged to provide support for the child. The conflict between the woman's right to control her own body and the child's right to be born, if at all, free of major defects, is a very interesting one.

Quite recently, two cases have allowed recovery of damages on behalf of children who were not even conceived at the time the damage occurred. In the very recent case of *Renslow v. Mennonite Hospital* [29], a woman sued a hospital and the physician on her own behalf and on behalf of her minor daughter, seeking damages for personal injury sustained by her and the child. These damages were a result of the fact that when the mother was thirteen, in 1965, she had been a patient in the defendant hospital and had been given two transfusions of Rh+ blood when she was Rh–. This was not discussed with her and she did not know about the problem until blood tests were performed while she was pregnant. The plaintiff infant was born on March 25th, 1974, suffering from erythroblastosis fetalis, for which she was treated by an exchange transfusion. It was alleged in the suit, however, that she had permanent damage to various organs, including her brain. The trial court dismissed her case because she was not in existence at the time she was allegedly injured; the Supreme Court of Illinois reversed and allowed recovery, on the grounds that the consequences to the plaintiff were foreseeable at the time of the negligent transfusion.

This case follows another, *Jorgensen v. Meade-Johnson Laboratories* [23], in which a woman had taken contraceptive pills, had stopped, had gotten pregnant and had twins, both of whom had Downs syndrome. It was alleged that the birth control pills had caused her chromosome damage. The parents brought an action on behalf of the mother and, as guardian of the twins, on their behalf, suing the manufacturer and asking for damages for breach of warranty and negligence. The trial court upheld the mother's right to sue for her own damages, but dismissed the action for the infants' pain and suffering and physical damage, on the grounds that they were non-existent at the time the cause of action accrued. On appeal, however, it was held that the twins did have the right to sue. While these cases are normally discussed as 'wrongful life' cases, they, of course, are not.

The Court of Appeals in New York had quite a busy year in 1977, hearing appeals in several 'wrongful life' cases.

Howard v. Lecher [20], decided in June, was a case brought by parents of an infant daughter who had died of Tay-Sachs disease. They sued the physician, arguing that he should have told the woman to have amniocentesis because of the risk of the diseases in their particular ethnic population. The trial judge denied the physician's motion to dismiss the action for damages for mental distress and the intermediate appellate court reversed and allowed the physician to prevail. At the Court of Appeals, the highest court in New York, it was held that the parents were not entitled to recover. As the court put it in that appeal,

> "The question before us is whether the doctor should be held liable for the trauma suffered by the parents allegedly caused by the birth, degeneration and death of the child". The court stated: "Since we are of the opinion that to afford the parents relief as against the doctor would require the extension of traditional tort concepts beyond manageable bounds, we are in agreement with the determination below that the complaint fails to state a cause of action".

Since the child, not the parent, was physically impaired, the court held that the parents could nor recover damages for their own metal anguish, in the absence of any physical or mental injury to themselves.

The court did not deal in *Howard* with whether the child herself, if she had survived, could have brought an action. Several months later, the intermediate New York court decided the case of *Park v. Chessin* ([8], [28]). That case involved the following facts: the parents had one child who died of a fatal, hereditary disease, known as polycystic kidney disease. They discussed with the obstetrician the possibility of having another child with the same disease and were told not to worry about it. The second child was born with the same disease and died at age 2½. The complaint alleged negligence on the part of the physician for failing to tell them that there was a high risk of having another child with the disease or to refer the woman for amniocentesis. The court held that the parents could recover medical malpractice damages for their medical expenses, except that the wife's mental anguish or emotional distress were not compensable. The important point was, however, that the court held that there existed a cause of action on behalf of the child.

The court pointed out that the facts of the present case were strikingly different from those in *Howard v. Lecher*. The plaintiff alleged in *Park v. Chessin* that they affirmatively sought a specific medical opinion of the defendant, with respect to the risk of having another child. Under the circumstances in which the defendant, who had delivered the first baby, knew that they had genuine cause to be concerned, the court found the physicians liable because the parents had specifically asked and the physicians had given them incorrect information about the genetic risk, not because the physicians had failed to initiate discussion of the subject.

One segment of this opinion is extremely interesting:

> ... No new duty is imposed on any physician in these circumstances; rather validating the parents' cause of action in the instant case merely extends to a physician a preexisting duty widely recognized in numerous fields of classic tort law, that one may not speak without prudence or due care, when one has a duty to speak, knows that the other party intends to rely on what is imparted and does, in fact, rely to his detriment.

In upholding the child's claim for 'wrongful life' the court pointed out that since abortion became legal, potential parents have the right not to have a child. This right extends to instances in which it can be determined with reasonable medical certainty that the child would be born deformed.

> The breach of this right may be said to be tortious to the fundamental right of a child to be born as a whole, functional human being. Under the circumstances presented, the portion of the complaint which sought recovery on behalf of the infant for injuries and conscious pain should be permitted to stand.

Another New York decision of 1977 on the intermediate level is *Karlsons v. Guerinot* [24]. That case involved a 37 year old pregnant woman whose physician failed to inform her of the existence of amniocentesis, as a result of which, it is alleged, she had a child with Downs syndrome. The court, in that case, held that the parents could recover for pain, suffering and mental anguish as a result of the birth of the deformed child, but that the child could not recover for wrongful life. It found that the physician's non-disclosure of the risk of giving birth to a deformed child was not covered by the standard informed consent doctrine applicable in New York, since pregnancy is not a medical situation involving active treatment.

The informed consent cases to date, in New York and elsewhere, all involve failure to disclose risks relating to treatment *procedures*. The court in *Karlsons* distinguished that situation from disclosure of risks peculiar to the condition of pregnancy itself, finding that allegations such as these had formed the basis of conventional malpractice actions but not informed consent cases. As to the child's cause of action, the court simply found that birth itself is not a suable wrong that is cognizable in court. Since damages are, in a tort action, compensatory in nature, the existence of such damages, according to the *Karlsons* opinion, is grounded on the premise that but for the negligence of the defendant, the plaintiff would be in a better position than he was as a result of it. In the instant case, the court held that recognition of the infant's cause of action would necessitate a finding that she was injured by the defendant's negligence in the sense that she was in a worse position than she would have been in had the defendant not been negligent. Thus, the threshold question was, according to the court, not whether life with deformities is less preferable than death, but whether it is less preferable than "the utter void of non-existence". This decision was, however, written two months prior to the *Howard* decision and thus its future effect on the jurisprudence is at present unclear.

An analysis of these cases indicates that provable negligence in disclosure to parents does, in fact, constitute malpractice in terms of the mother's right to recover ([6], [7]). This may, in fact, include as an element of her damage the expenses of raising the handicapped child. This conclusion, however, raised a collateral question: Is the father, who has the primary legal responsibility for support, an appropriate plaintiff, since he was not in a physician-patient relationship with the physician and thus was owed no duty of care? In the usual malpractice situation, where there is no physician-patient relationship there cannot be a breach of duty, and therefore there can be no suit.

There are, therefore, two questions which have yet to be discussed by the courts. The first is the right, if any, of the child to sue his parents for a decision not to abort if they knew or should have known that he would be born deformed. The second, and probably more realistic, question involves the right of the child if abortion is not available.

In many, probably most, cases which allowed parents to recover damages for the cost of child care, the courts have held that *Roe v. Wade* [32], *Doe v. Bolton* [15], and the other decisions giving a woman the right to decide to have an abortion confer on her the right, as a matter of constitutional law, as opposed to a matter of negligence law, to have a child born without defects. The right to be born without defects is explicitly discussed in *Park v. Chessin* as a 'fundamental right' of the child's, not the mother's as well and this idea is certainly implied in several other opinions. In view of the current restrictions on Medicaid payments for abortions, as upheld by the Supreme Court in *Beal v. Doe* [9] and *Mahrer v. Roe* [26], the question arises as to whether or not, if the mother knows that she will have a deformed child, she has a constitutional right to state payment for the abortion. Further, if Medicaid in the state of her residence will not pay for the abortion and the child is born deformed, does the *child* have a cause of action against, among others, the

United States government, the Department of Health and Human Services or the Secretary of Health and Human Services and the state Medicaid Director for wrongful life for failing to allow his mother to exercise her choice not to have him?

In view of the holdings in the cases to date, it can be argued that the government would, in fact, be liable in a suit brought by the child for failing to allow payment for such an abortion. If courts are going to hold either that the mother has a *fundamental* right to have a healthy baby or that the baby has a *fundamental* right to be born without defects (as opposed to either or both having an ordinary cause of action in negligence), it is logically inconsistent to make a physician liable in malpractice for failing to tell a woman that she may have a deformed child but not have the government liable if he does tell her but she cannot have an abortion because payment for such is beyond her means, and the government refuses to pay for it. If this is a right protected by the Constitution, the government must make it available.

The entire constitutional system of the United States is predicated on the assumption that fundamental constitutional rights are not just for those who can afford them. Voting is a constitutional right, thus poll taxes are unconstitutional, for one example. The abortion cases did not say that a woman has a *fundamental* constitutional right to an abortion. They said that she had a constitutional right to privacy with which the state may not interfere when she and her physician decide that she wishes to have an abortion. Performance of an abortion had been a criminal offense; the Supreme Court removed the penalties. The cases did not, for example, guarantee a woman that a doctor would be available who would be willing to perform it. Thus, from the perspective of the woman's constitutional rights, the Supreme Court's decisions on Medicaid payments are probably constitutionally proper, however much one may disagree with them or think they are socially unfair. The issue here, however, is that if courts are going to rule that a *child* has "a fundamental right . . . to be born as a whole, functional human being", (if he is born at all), as opposed to a non-Constitutionally-based, non-fundamental cause of action on behalf of the child against a physician who did not advise his mother about amniocentesis, then the denial of payment would appear to violate the child's rights, even if it does not violate the mother's.

The wrongful life cases will be one of the more interesting aspects of tort and perhaps constitutional law to watch in the next several years. I foresee that in cases of failure to perform amniocentesis and unsuccessful sterilization operations, where the parents are the plaintiffs and can prove enormous expenses as a result of the birth of a deformed child, courts in an increasing number of states will hold that the cost of care of that child is an element of compensable damage. Whether or not the courts should properly undertake to decide whether the child himself should have a compensable right not-to-have-been is another question to which I have no answer. I would foresee extreme reluctance by the courts in most jurisdictions to try to determine the damages in these cases, since the final question as a practical matter is "how much is it worth not to be"?

Yale University School of Medicine
New Haven, Connecticut

BIBLIOGRAPHY AND CASES

1. Capron, A. M.: 1976, 'The Law Relating to Experimentation with the Fetus' in *Appendix: Research on the Fetus*, The National Commission for the Protection of Human Subjects of Biomedical and Behavioral Research, DHEW Publication No. (OS) 76–128.
2. Fox, M. L.: 1974, 'Remedy for the Reluctant Parent: Physician's Liability for the Post-Sterilization Conception and Birth of Unplanned Children', *U. Fla. Law Rev.* 27, 158.
3. Holder, A.: 1970, 'Prenatal Injuries', *JAMA* 214 (11) 2105.
4. Kass, M. and Shaw, M.: 1976, 'The Risk of Birth Defects: Jacobs v. Theimer and Parents' Right to Know', *Am. J. Law and Med.* 2, 213.
5. Mark, D. J.: 1976, 'Liability for Failure of Birth Control Methods', *Columbia Law Rev.* 76, 1187.
6. Milunsky, A. and Annas, G. J. (eds.): 1977, *Genetics and the Law*, Plenum Press, New York.
7. Reilly, P.: 1977, *Genetics, Law and Social Policy*, Harvard University Press, Cambridge.
8. Wright, E. E.: 1978, 'Father and Mother Know Best: Defining the Liability of Physicians for Inadequate Genetic Counselling', *Yale Law J.* 87, 1488.
9. *Beal v. Doe*, 432 U.S. 438, 1977.
10. *Bonbrest v. Kotz*, 65 F. Supp. 138, DCDC 1946.
11. *Brooks v. Serrano*, 209 So. 2d 279, Fla., 1968.
12. *Coleman v. Garrison*, 281 A. 2d 616, Del., 1975.
13. *Custodio v. Bauer*, 59 Cal. Rptr. 463, Cal., 1967.
14. *Dietrich v. Northampton*, 138 Mass. 14, 1884.
15. *Doe v. Bolton*, 410 U.S. 179, 1973.
16. *Doerr v. Villate*, 220 N.E. 2d 767, Ill., 1966.
17. *Dinner v. Thorp*, 338 P. 2d 137, Wash., 1959.
18. *Gleitman v. Cosgrove*, 227 A. 2d 689, N.J., 1967.
19. *Griswold v. Connecticut*, 381 U.S. 479, 1965.
20. *Howard v. Lecher*, 366 N.E. 2d 64, at page 364, N.Y., 1977.
21. *Jackson v. Anderson*, 230 So. 2d 503, Fla., 1970.
22. *Jacobs v. Theimer*, 519 S.W. 2d 846, Tex., 1975.

23. *Jorgensen v. Meade-Johnson Laboratories*, 483 F. 2d 237, CCA 10, 1973.
24. *Karlsons v. Guerinot*, 394 N.Y.S. 2d 933, 1977.
25. *Libbee v. Permanente Clinic*, 518 P. 2d 636, Ore., 1974.
26. *Maher v. Roe*, 432 U.S. 464, 1977.
27. *Morgan v. United States*, 143 F. Supp. 570, D.C.N.J., 1956.
28. *Park v. Chessin*, 400 N.Y.S. 2d 110, at page 113, N.Y., 1977.
29. *Renslow v. Mennonite Hospital*, 367 N.E. 2d 1250, Ill., 1977.
30. *Rice v. Rizk*, 453 S.W. 2d 732, Ky., 1970.
31. *Rieck v. Medical Protective Co.*, 219 N.W. 2d 242, Wisc., 1974.
32. *Roe v. Wade*, 410 U.S. 113, 1973.
33. *Scott v. McPheeters*, 92 P. 2d 678, Cal., 1939.
34. *Sherlock v. Stillwater Clinic*, 260 N.W. 2d 169, Minn., 1977.
35. *Stewart v. Long Island College Hospital*, 296 N.Y.S. 2d 41, 1968; 283 N.E. 2d 616, 1972.
36. *Sylvia v. Gobeille*, 220 A. 2d 22, R.I., 1966.
37. *Terrell v. Garcia*, 496 S.W. 2d 124, Tex., 1973.
38. *Troppi v. Scarf*, 187 N.W. 2d 511, Mich., 1971.
39. *Verkennes v. Corniea*, 38 N.W. 2d 838, Minn., 1949.
40. *Williams v. New York*, 223 N.E. 2d 849, 1963.
41. *Zepeda v. Zepeda*, 41 Ill. App. 2d 240, 1963.
42. *Ziemba v. Sternberg*, 357 N.Y.S. 2d 265, 1974.

N.B. Since this article was written, with one exception, the courts which have considered the concept of wrongful life have rejected the concept that a child has a right to sue for damages in such cases. The New York Court of Appeals, the highest State Court in New York, upheld the parents' right to sue physicians for negligent failure to diagnose severe birth defects during the period in which the mother could have elected to abort the pregnancy, and allowed parents in two cases to recover as damages the cost of child care. The New York Court, however, rejected the two infants' claims to 'wrongful life' [1], [2]. In one of the two New York cases, *Park v. Chessin*, the jury ultimately returned a verdict in favor of the defendant physicians so no damages in fact were awarded [3]. A federal district court in Pennsylvania [4] and the Supreme Court of New Jersey [5] allowed parents to sue a physician for negligent failure to carefully interpret the results of amniocentesis which resulted in the birth of children with Tay-Sachs disease. The courts in each case, however, held that the children could not sue. The California Court of Appeals, however, has allowed a child to bring a wrongful action against a laboratory that negligently reported negative results of a Tay-Sachs screening test [6].

BIBLIOGRAPHY

1. *Becker v. Schwartz*, 413 N.Y.S. 2d 895, 386 N.E. 2d 809, 1978.
2. *Park v. Chessin*, 413 N.Y.S. 2d 895, 386 N.E. 2d 809, 1978.
3. *The Times, New York*, April 9, 1979, p. B2.
4. *Gildiner v. Thomas Jefferson Univ. Hospital*, 451 F. Supp. 692, D.C., PA., 1978.
5. *Berman v. Allan*, 80 N.J. 421, 1979.
6. *Curlender v. Bio-Science Laboratories*, 165 Cal. Rptr. 477, 1980.

PETER C. WILLIAMS

WRONGFUL LIFE: A REPLY TO ANGELA HOLDER

The law is a system of social control. Even more than most branches of the law, the law of torts is an obvious 'battleground' for social theories. The broad question which I shall pose is to what extent and how the legal system should regulate the relationship between health care providers and consumers. The question that Professor Holder addressed was significantly narrower: Is existence ever an injury? She began by 'translating' that question into an even more practical and focused one, namely, whether or not being alive is ever, in law, something for which one should receive monetary compensation from another. Before addressing directly Professor Holder's inquiry, I would like to consider the *kind* of question she has posed.

To ask whether existence is ever an injury could be either a factual or an evaluative inquiry. If the former, we are asked to begin an empirical study. We might turn to a public opinion pollster and find out if people ever wish they had never been born. We might turn to the anthropologist and inquire if societies ever compensate parents for having children. Or we might do what Professor Holder did: conduct legal research and determine whether or not courts in fact ever view being alive as something for which they will award compensatory damages.

The question might, on the other hand, be evaluative: to determine what *should* happen in courts, not what *does* happen. Here the question is normative and requires philosophic, legal, and political argument. I tend to view the second formulation of the question as more important, but it cannot be addressed successfully without attention to the factual one. Professor Holder seemed to ask the evaluative question in her initial comments, but focused her subsequent remarks almost exclusively on the factual one. Let me follow her lead, then, and address the question whether courts ever consider life itself an injury. I will also share her assumption – it is no more – that the answer to this question is the same as the answer to the question, do courts ever award compensatory damages for 'wrongful' existence itself?

How, in fact, do courts behave? To begin with, there are a number of ways in which one might classify wrongful life cases. The complication arises because there are so *many* different sorts of cases loosely collected under the rubric 'wrongful life'. One way to catalogue them is according to the *form of*

S. F. Spicker, J. M. Healey, and H. T. Engelhardt (eds.), The Law–Medicine Relation: A Philosophical Exploration, 241–252.

action, the type of wrong the plaintiff claims has been committed. This seemed to me to be the general approach taken by Professor Holder. There are a set of cases reflected in the common law which deal with prenatal injuries. There is also case law interpreting and applying wrongful death statutes. Some cases deal with breach of contract or warranty. Still others are based on various torts, e.g., negligence (regular or professional), misrepresentation, etc.

Another way to organize the 'wrongful life' cases is by asking who the plaintiff is. Some are parents; others, siblings; still others, the 'victim' – a defective or sometimes normal child.

Finally, one might organize the cases according to the type of damages being sought. A number of cases – particularly those brought by parents – ask for the costs of birthing: hospital costs, pain and suffering, loss of consortium. Other cases ask for the ongoing costs of care for the victim. Compensation might be asked for the special, additional costs of caring for a defective or deformed child and that child's pain and suffering. Occasionally courts have been asked to award compensatory damage for the usual costs of raising a normal child.

There is only one conclusion to be drawn from this typology: some courts allow some recovery for some types of actions by some plaintiffs claiming some types of damages. I agree with Professor Holder that there is no pattern to these awards, and trends are hard to discern. Further, I think we agree that many of these cases are improperly described as 'wrongful life' cases. The issue of whether or not life itself is an injury is most sharply drawn when the child is the plaintiff and asks to be compensated *because it is alive*. Though the issue of wrongful life is accessible when the infant has deformities, it is more cleanly focused on the issue of life itself when the child is normal. What we want to ask, then, is whether a court has ever awarded damages to a normal child because that child was alive rather than non-existent. There has been, to my knowledge, no case of a child being awarded damages in this type of case. This is a factual claim about how courts have decided cases. If not false already, it will probably soon become so. The real question we should address, however, is not the factual one but the evaluative one: *ought courts to award damages to children in these cases*?

How might we answer this evaluative question? First, one might have recourse to metaethical and metaphysical arguments for and against appraisals of existence. This kind of argument is neither unavailable nor unheard of. In general this abstract approach is anathema to courts which claim to settle the issue without "intrusion into the domain of moral philosophy" ([12],

p. 513), and to decide "pretermitting moral and theological considerations" ([10], p. 174). Even Holder began her account by translating the abstract philosophic question into a more practical, though nonetheless philosophic, one: Should the legal system allow compensatory damages to be awarded to someone whose claim for them is based on the view that he would 'have been better off' not existing? If, out of respect for the discomfort or myopia of courts and commentators alike, we are going to try to avoid philosophic discourse, how can we answer this question? One approach is to analyze critically the reasons offered by courts for a 'yes' or 'no' answer to this question. To what considerations do courts appeal when rationalizing their holdings? What will be discovered is that, though courts deny it, they are engaged in normative inquiry. Hence court decisions become amenable to philosophic critique. I am going to consider the cases Professor Holder presented, and try to systematize the reasons on which courts often rely.

There is, happily, some jurisprudential literature that can help us organize our efforts. In particular, one can rely on a rather loose version of a set of distinctions cast by Ronald Dworkin in his essay "The Model of Rules" ([1], pp. 22–28).

There are three sorts of norms upon which courts rely: rules, policies, and principles. Each is a standard for decision making but they operate in importantly different ways. A rule is the most narrow of these. It applies in an all or nothing fashion. A rule has rather discrete criteria for application, and if those criteria are met the decision of the court is dictated. An example is the rule in baseball that after four balls, a batter may proceed to first base. The decision of the umpire is settled after the fourth 'bad' pitch. Dworkin's legal example is the rule that a will is invalid unless signed by three witnesses

Policies and principles operate in an importantly different way. Unlike a rule which requires or necessitates a particular decision, policies and principles give weight to a decision. Policies or principles tend in a direction or count in favor of some outcome. They share the characteristic of being, if you will, looser than rules. The difference between them is nicely stated by Dworkin himself:

> I call a 'policy' that kind of standard that sets out a goal to be reached, generally an improvement in some economic, political, or social feature of the community (though some goals are negative, in that they stipulate that some present feature is to be protected from adverse change). I call a 'principle' a standard that is to be observed, not because it will advance or secure an economic, political, or social situation deemed desirable, but because it is a requirement of justice or fairness or some other dimension of morality ([1], p. 22).

Courts, in deciding what to do in a case in which someone asks to be compensated for being alive, will rely on rules, policies or principles. Only by relying exclusively on the first could courts arguably avoid philosophizing. We shall see that courts must rely on more than rules.

One normal rule in tort law states,

> Where a party's negligence is directly responsible for physical injury to another, ... the injured party may recover for the actual physical injury sustained and for the concomitant mental and emotional suffering which flow as a natural consequence of the wrongful act. ([6], pp. 111 and 364).

If it could be established that a health care provider has been negligent, and if it could be established that there are net costs to being alive, then these principles of tort law seem to apply. Some courts view the steps between a prenatal breach of duty, proximate cause, and foreseeable injury easy to establish.[1] Other courts facing comparable facts have decided that such a rule is not applicable. There is no cognizable harm, i.e., no legal wrong. The rationale for not applying the traditional tort rule to wrongful life cases has been that (1) there is no duty to the not yet conceived embryo, (2) there is no proximate cause, (3) the 'injury' is not foreseeable, or, finally, (4) there is no genuine injury.

Whether or not, in the application of the standard rules about tort liability, the courts find for plaintiffs or for defendents, the explanations seem *ad hoc*. To pursue the baseball analogy, the decision whether or not a fourth 'ball' has been thrown depends on a decision on the question 'was that a pitch?' That question is often one that is settled by appeal to policies and principles, not rules. What is actually happening in wrongful life cases is that the judges are using policies and principles in order to decide whether or not the rule applies. This is a typical phenomenon in unique situations or in cases of first impressions. As Dworkin remarks:

> ... When lawyers reason or dispute about legal rights and obligations, particularly in those hard cases when our problem with these concepts seems most acute, they make use of standards that do not function as rules, but operate differently, as principles, policies, and other sorts of standards ([1], p. 22).

What are some other standards that judges apply in these cases?

The first is what Dworkin called 'policies', standards that aim at some target or goal. Because tort law so self-consciously tries to work toward various social ideals, it has always been a battleground for social theory.

There appear to be four public policies to which courts frequently refer when dealing with wrongful life cases.

(1) There is a generally acknowledged *public policy in favor of a particular model of the family*.

(A) One aspect of this view of the family involves the belief that *having children is socially valuable*. As expressed by the court in *Shaheen v. Knight*:

> ... The great end of matrimony is not the comfort and convenience of the immediate parties, though these are necessarily a part in it; but the procreation of a progeny having a legal title to maintenance by the father ... ([9], p. 23 and 45).

This claim is often proffered to bar a parent's claims for recovery of the costs of raising a normal, or even a defective, child.[2] One standard and telling response to this view is that children are not a blessing, not even a blessing in disguise. What the Shaheen court called "a universal public sentiment of the people" in favor of having children and the benefit of parenting seems no longer to be the case in the United States. Public programs to limit procreation are common. Contraception and abortion are practiced by a growing proportion of the population. Rational couples are deciding either not to have any children or to limit family size. Certainly a child is not always a blessing to parents.

But this entire dispute is inappropriate to genuine wrongful life cases. Since we are focusing on the child suing for compensation to cover the cost of living out his 'wrongful life', what one needs to ask is not whether the child's existence is or is not a blessing for the parents but whether or not life is a blessing to that child. Whether a child is a benefit to its parents is irrelevant for this particular set of cases.

(B) Another way in which a social policy in favor of the family impacts on 'wrongful life' cases has to do with the *relation between parents and their children*. This was addressed by Professor Holder when she discussed 'parenting malpractice'. By and large there is a strong sentiment against allowing children to sue their parents. If we allow 'wrongful life' actions to be brought by children against third parties, there is no conceptual reason why they could not be brought against parents who themselves chose not to terminate pregnancy. Since parents are already legally obligated to care for their children, such a suit seems unlikely.

(C) A final consideration grows out of a public policy favoring the nuclear family. In *Rieck v. Medical Protection Company* the court maintained that allowing parents (or a child) to recover would turn the doctor into a 'surrogate parent' [8]. The defendant in such an action would have a financial obligation to raise or support the child, while the parents would have control over what that child would do. The separation of responsibility from authority within a family is something our society does not wish to extend beyond normal divorce cases.

(2) Public policies favoring the conception of the family are not the only kind of policies which operate in wrongful life cases. A strong *public policy against negligent conduct* is another. What will be the deterrent value of leaving ourselves open to suits for wrongful life? One of the strong arguments in favor of the fault system of tort liability is its deterrence value. If we allow suits for wrongful life, physicians will be more careful in performing sterilization operations; pharmacists more careful in filling prescriptions; and so on. This argument supports the view that we allow children to sue.

(3) Courts rely on *public policy designed to protect the integrity of the court system*. Courts are reluctant to become involved in complicated calculations of ambiguous damages. The claim is then made that the determination of damages for wrongful life is either theoretically or practically impossible.

(A) The argument that *damages are theoretically* incalculable turns on the comparison of existence, even with maladies, with "the utter void of non-existence" ([5], p. 692). Though initially one might place non-existence at a zero point on a cost-benefit scale, further reflection shows this is incoherent. What courts compare when they measure damages is the actual status of the plaintiff versus the status of the plaintiff had the wrong not been done. In wrongful life cases that latter status is actually a 'nonstatus'. Placing non-existence on a scale of benefits is somewhat like putting humor on a color wheel.

(B) Some courts have argued that, though it is not in principle impossible to calculate the damages attendant to life itself, to do so is beyond the practical scope of courts since such *damages are speculative*. The proper calculation of damages would involve calculating the cost of existence and then subtracting the benefits of existence. Most of the discussion of the speculative nature of these benefits has occurred in cases in which parents have sued for the costs of raising a normal or a deformed child.

... [The] satisfaction, joy and companionship which normal parents have in rearing a child make ... [the] economic loss [of rearing a child] worthwhile. These intangible benefits, while impossible to value in dollars and cents are undoubtedly the things that make life worthwhile. Who can place a price tag on a child's smile, or in the parental pride in the child's achievement? ([11], p. 128).

The difficulty of appraising the costs or benefits of being alive with respect to the person who is alive is even more difficult. Some courts have argued that it is too subjective a matter to be settled. If objectivity is in fact one of the values of our court system, the subjectivity of these damages would seem to suggest that we not allow recovery.

Proponents of damages for wrongful life have maintained that courts often make the kinds of speculative judgment that is being called for here. Calculating damages for pain and suffering, damages in wrongful death actions, or 'necessary support' in divorce cases indicates that, though difficult, courts can and do evaluate subjectivities. The analogies drawn, however useful in cases in which the *parents* are suing for the costs they will bear in raising a child, are not apt in suits in which the *child* is suing for damages.

Though courts may calculate the cost of pain and suffering, they normally do so only after a finding of some physical injury. Perhaps the crucial point in wrongful life actions is that one construe being alive as injurious. Even then, courts would be called upon not merely to evaluate the monetary cost of pain and suffering to the plaintiff, but also the benefits of his pleasure and joy. That would seem difficult indeed. Again, damages in wrongful death actions are not closely analogous to those in wrongful life actions. Unlike the former, the latter award damages to the victim, not the survivors. Finally, calculation of support payments is not analogous because they are not compensatory. No evaluation of benefits of being alive is even attempted.

A public policy in favor of a court system that applies predictable, discrete and objective measures of damages argues against allowing recovery in wrongful life cases.

(4) The final public policy point that has been raised by courts dealing with these suits is *a policy in favor of life over non-existence.* This particular conclusion sometimes appears as a ruling on damages. The court will say that, as a matter of law, the benefit of being alive outweighs the cost.[3]

Analysis of this policy claim is possible only if we maintain a distinction between death and never existing. While the law certainly seems to favor life over death (though this is presently under challenge in so-called 'euthanasia' cases), there does not seem to be a strong policy favoring life over never existing. The growth of public programs promoting family planning manifests the current perspective on non-existence. It would be difficult to argue adequately that there is a strong public policy in favor of people's having children. Nevertheless once a person is alive, the public policy in favor of life over death tends to override the contention of the wrongful life plaintiff that being alive somehow damaged him.

To recapitulate: courts have employed four general public policy considerations in wrongful life cases: A public policy in favor of a certain kind of family; a public policy against negligent conduct; a public policy to protect the integrity of the court system; a public policy in favor of life. These policies are all goal oriented. In addition to policies, however, courts also rely on what Dworkin calls 'principles' – normative standards that are not prospective. Two of those applied seem to be especially important.

(1) That *wrongs ought to be redressed* is a principle of compensatory justice. One court has stated: "Where the purpose of the physician's actions is to prevent conception or birth, elementary justice requires that he be held legally responsible for the consequences which have in fact occurred" ([10], p. 174). The claim is that the costs of being alive must be borne by someone. Fairness dictates that those costs be borne by a wrongdoer, rather than an innocent victim. Obviously this argument presupposes that being alive involves net costs. The earlier discussion of the benefits and burdens of being alive is again relevant.

This principle of compensatory justice seems to be most persuasive in cases in which the negligence of the defendant is particularly gross. To have serious wrongdoing without having some redress strikes proponents of this principle as unjust, though here the purpose seems punitive rather than compensatory.

(2) A second principle applied by courts emerges from the first, namely that *there must be a proportion between the wrong done and the burden borne by the wrongdoer.* The argument proffered is that to allow recovery in these sorts of cases places an unreasonable burden on the physician. The 'reasonableness' of the burden is normally evidenced in cases where physicians are asked to pay extremely high costs when children with defects have been born. In the kind of case we are considering – where the child is normal – it is doubtful that the 'cost argument' would be as persuasive. Additionally, the proportionality in *compensatory* justice schemes is a proportion *between the award and the injury, not between the award and some view of the severity of the wrong committed.*

To conclude, it should now be clear that the normal rules of tort law will not settle wrongful life cases. Rules will not apply themselves and courts must turn to policies and principles in order to make decisions whether or not to extend tort principles to new situations. Courts are, of necessity, engaged in principle and/or policy decisions. The threshold issue is whether *courts* are the proper forum for decisions in these cases. One view of the courts is that they should only apply rules. Creating law or designing public policy is the job of the legislature. If my analysis is correct – that applying rules requires reference to policies and principles – then such a narrow view of the function of courts is untenable. Few would maintain that courts could apply rules without reference to policies and principles. However, one might well try to show that courts are not particularly adept at making what becomes almost purely policy decisions. While courts and the adversary system are adept at settling questions that can be answered 'yes' or 'no', they are not particularly good at providing answers to complex social problems. As one dissenting judge stated:

> Ramifications stemming from claims for damages for 'wrongful life' would be many and multifaceted. Undoubtedly they would affect drastically not only the doctor-patient relationship, but also the relationship of parent to child and parent to parent. Such questions, I submit, are for sober reflection by a legislative body in the first instance, and not for the courts ([7], p. 117).

What legislatures should do when confronted with such issues is a question I cannot begin to address here; but I suggest that awarding damages to a normal child seems highly questionable given the soundness of the traditional concepts of compensatory justice.

I would like to conclude my comments with a reference to two difficulties that are suggested by Professor Holder's essay. The first difficulty emerges from her discussion of abortion. The easy availability of and changing attitudes toward abortion may make two tort doctrines relevant to wrongful life actions. Both would shift the responsibility away from the offending health care worker to the mother involved in the case.

The first relevant legal doctrine is *the rule of 'avoidable consequences'* which denies recovery for any damages which could have been avoided by reasonable conduct on the part of the plaintiff. The mother can often forestall some damages to herself and all those to the fetus by aborting the fetus.

The second legal doctrine is *the last clear chance rule*. This is a doctrine that affixes the responsibility for damages on the person who had the last clear reasonable opportunity to avoid the harm. In many wrongful life cases that person will be the mother. Again, the opportunity for her to abort the fetus may mean that she has the last clear chance to avoid the harm.

The question which arises in each of these possible circumstances is whether or not having an abortion is 'reasonable'. Plaintiffs in wrongful life cases, in order to rebut a defendant's argument that the policy in favor of life is determinative, contend that there is a growing acceptance of various modes of family planning, among them the right to abort. In other words, for better or worse, abortions are becoming a more socially accepted act.

One implication of this view is that having an abortion, in our modern social climate, is reasonable. If abortion is reasonable, the mother might be the only proper defendant in wrongful life cases.

The second difficulty with Professor Holder's view is rooted in her speculative discussion concerning the right of children to be born without defects, or the right of mothers to have a healthy baby. If such a right exists and if it is fundamental, she argues, then the government is obligated to pay for the abortion of defective fetuses. The problem with this view is that she appears to ignore an important distinction concerning the nature of rights.

At least since Hohfeld's classic treatise which addresses the different ways in which we employ the term 'right' [2], there has been a generally recognized distinction between *affirmative rights and forebearance rights*. Affirmative rights operate in much the way Professor Holder's 'fundamental rights' do. One person's right to something means that someone else is obligated to provide that thing. Forebearance rights, on the other hand, do not impose that kind of duty on anyone else. At best there is a duty of non-interference imposed. Once that distinction is appreciated, her claim that a constitutional right to be born without defects obligates the government to provide resources remains unsubstantiated. She offers no argument to show that such a right is an affirmative one.

Though it is true that "the entire American constitutional system is predicated on the assumption that fundamental constitutional rights are not just for those who can afford them", it is erroneous to conclude therefrom that all constitutional rights are affirmative rights. She cites as one example the right to vote. That right is an affirmative one since it creates a correlative duty on the government to hold elections. Professor Holder's discussion of poll taxes, however, casts the right to vote as a negative or forebearance right. The Government is not allowed to put hurdles (poll taxes) between people and their right to vote. Actually most of our constitutional rights are negative ones. The right to free speech is not a right to a particular forum; nor is the government required to provide us with a podium or an audience. The right to free speech, the right to privacy, the right to an abortion, and the right to bear arms are forebearance rights. The government may not prevent us from behaving in certain ways and doing certain things, but it is not obligated to pay for or provide anything. There are examples of affirmative, constitutional rights; commonly mentioned are the right to a jury trial and the right to legal counsel.

The claim that the right to abortion is an affirmative constitional right would be difficult to maintain; and if Professor Holder hopes to make such a case, it will require an argument other than the one she has provided thus far.

Finally, a right to be born healthy, even as a forebearance right, could impose upon mothers special obligations of some magnitude. One can imagine claims for damages against mothers for failure to maintain during pregnancy an adequate diet, for smoking or drinking to excess, for taking drugs that could lessen birth weight or the Apgar score of a newborn, etc.

A claim that children have a right to be born without defects is an intriguing one, but before we embrace it, we need a more careful analysis of both the nature of constitutional rights and the duties that would be incumbent on us were these rights to exist.

Professor Holder's exploration of the rulings of different courts in so-called 'wrongful life cases' is nonetheless a useful prelude to any analysis of the policies regarding people who exist in spite of their parents' or their own wishes.

State University of New York
Stony Brook, New York

NOTES

[1] Cf. *Park v. Chessin*, 400 N.Y.S. 2d 110 (Sup. Ct., App. Div., 1977). *Sherlock v. Stillwater Clinic*, 260 N.W. 2d 169 (Minn. Sup. Ct. 1977) ("Analytically such an action is indistinguishable from an ordinary medical negligence action . . .", at 174).

[2] See, *Christensen v. Thornby*, 255 N.W. 620, 622 (Minn., 1934). (". . . the plaintiff has been blessed with the fatherhood of another child".); *Gleitman v. Cosgrove*, 227 A. 2d 689, 693 (N.J. 1967) ("the intangible . . . complex human benefits of motherhood and fatherhood"); *Shaheen v. Knight*, 11 Pa. D. & C. 2d 41, 45–6 (1957) ("the fun, joy, and affection which the plaintiff . . . will have in the rearing and education of . . . [his] fifth child").

[3] See, *Gleitman v. Cosgrove*, 49 N.J. 22, 227 A. 2d 689, 22 A.L.R. 3d 1141 (1967); *Ball v. Mudge*, 64 Wash. 2d 247, 391 P. 2d 201 (1964).

BIBLIOGRAPHY

1. Dworkin, R.: 1977, *Taking Rights Seriously*, Harvard University Press, Cambridge, Mass.
2. Hohfeld, W. N.: 1964, *Fundamental Legal Conceptions*, Yale University Press, New Haven, Conn.

CASES

3. *Ball v. Mudge*, 64 Wash. 2d 247, 391 P. 2d 201 (1964).

4. *Christensen v. Thornby*, 255 N.W. 620 (Minn., 1934).
5. *Gleitman v. Cosgrove*, 227 A. 2d 689 (N. J., 1967).
6. *Howard v. Lecher*, 42 N.Y. 2d 109, 397 N.Y.S. 2d 363 (1977).
7. *Park v. Chessin*, 400 N.Y.S. 2d 110 (Sup. Ct., App. Div., 1977).
8. *Rieck v. Medical Protection Co.*, 219 N.W. 2d 242 (1974).
9. *Shaheen v. Knight*, 6 Lyc. 19, 11 Pa. D. & C. 2d 41 (1957).
10. *Sherlook v. Stillwater Clinic*, 260 N.W. 2d 169 (Minn. Sup. Ct., 1977).
11. *Terrell v. Garcia*, 496 S.W. 2d 124 (Tex. Civ. App., 1973).
12. *Troppi v. Scarf*, 187 N.W. 2d 511 (Mich. Ct. App., 1971).
13. *Zepeda v. Zepeda*, 411 Ill. App. 2d 240, 190 N.E. 2d 849 (1963).

SECTION V

ROUND TABLE DISCUSSION – LEGAL RIGHTS AND MORAL RESPONSIBILITIES IN THE HEALTH CARE PROCESS

DARREL W. AMUNDSEN

PHYSICIAN, PATIENT AND MALPRACTICE: AN HISTORICAL PERSPECTIVE

As long as there have been those in Western civilization who call themselves physicians or doctors or surgeons and undertake to cure, alleviate or correct physical abnormalities, or provide prophylaxis, certain standards of competence, etiquette and responsibility have been assumed, if not always precisely defined in legal terms. This has been true whether the practice of medicine was held to be a right or a privilege. In the West, until the late Middle Ages, anyone who wished could call himself a physician and practise medicine. There simply were no provisions for licensure. But even under such laissez-faire conditions, standards of competence and responsibility were popularly expected of those who would assume a healing role in society.

Philemon the Younger, writing in the third century B.C., states that "only physicians and lawyers can commit murder without being put to death for it".[1] And three centuries later Pliny the Elder complains that "there is no law that would punish capital ignorance .... Only a physician can commit homicide with complete impunity" ([10], 29, 8, 18). It is often assumed, on the basis of such statements as these, that there were, in classical antiquity, no legal means for seeking redress against the dolose, negligent, or incompetent physician, particularly in light of the absence of any system of medical licensure. I have, however, attempted elsewhere ([4], [2]) to demonstrate that, in both Athenian and Roman law, there were mechanisms whereby a physician could be brought to court in what we would call a malpractice suit. Both legal systems, in this regard, were deficient from the vantage point of modern practice, but both were founded upon an unwritten assumption of certain responsibilities and liabilities imposed upon any who chose to occupy a specialized role in society, a role in which the level of the incompetence of the supplier of a service was in converse ratio to the potential harm to the person to whom the service was provided. The cardinal evil of Platonic thought, that of supposing one knows what one in reality does not know, is illustrated time and again both in Plato's and Aristotle's writings by the example of the physician, particularly the incompetent physician. In Roman law, standards of the *bonus paterfamilias* (similar to those of the 'reasonable man' of English common law), tempered by an intricate set of definitions of fault owing to incompetence or negligence, were applied to the physician.

S. F. Spicker, J. M. Healey, and H. T. Engelhardt (eds.), The Law–Medicine Relation: A Philosophical Exploration, 255–258.

In the primitive legal codes of the early Middle Ages, while sophisticated definitions of culpable incompetence and negligence were lacking, physicians, although still unlicensed, were singled out for regulation owing to the potential for damage to the public. More often than not specific procedures that were thought to be harmful were controlled and irresponsible physicians severely punished.[2]

The earliest impositions of medical licensure requirements, beginning in the 12th century, were of two sources: (1) imposed by civil or ecclesiastical authority or (2) obtained by guilds of physicians or surgeons who sought thereby an enforceable monopoly on the practice of their trade in their city or region. In the case of the former, the rationale consistently advanced was that, owing to the damage the incompetent physician could inflict on citizens, the state or king or church felt bound to protect the people by limiting the practice of medicine to those duly licensed by competent authority ([5], p. 407, n. 11 and 12). Likewise when guilds petitioned for a monopoly it was on the grounds that the benefit to the community would be immense since the people would no longer be at the mercy of quacks, charlatans, and pseudo-physicians, and the guild would ensure a high level of competence and responsibility of its members ([5], pp. 406ff.). In communities where licensure had been imposed and in those where guilds had achieved a protected closed shop, malpractice litigation continued and, in the case of the latter, the guilds more often than not appear to have sided with the aggrieved patient against the incompetent or negligent guild member.

When one observes the history of the physician-patient relationship one is struck by the consistency of the recognition that there always are some practitioners who indeed are incompetent or negligent, regardless of the presence or absence of licensure requirements. What varies from time to time and place to place is the definition of what constitutes malpractice. In the Crusader Kingdom of Jerusalem in the 12th and 13th centuries, spectacular cases such as burning out the intestines of a patient while attempting to cauterize hemorrhoids were specified as earning the physician a death sentence [3]. In Catholic Europe in the late Middle Ages canon law held physicians as liable who undertook the treatment of certain cases without the patient first having made confession to a priest, for failure to advise a terminally ill patient of imminent death (when such notice would have provided him with incentive to set his spiritual and temporal affairs in order), failure to exercise reasonable diligence in the care of patients generally, and conducting dangerous experiments on patients, to name a few of the relevant offenses recognized by late medieval canon law ([6], esp. p. 942ff.). In Romanian law of the early 20th century, merely the failure of a physician's efforts to cure a patient made him responsible for pecuniary damages ([9], p. 574).

While it is true that as long as there have been medical practitioners there have been standards of competence and practice and that there have always been some practitioners who fail to meet or maintain those standards (although the standards vary at different times and in different places), it is also true that there have been diverse and disconsonant popular attitudes towards physicians. The unique relationship that exists between the physician and his patient resulting in part from the dependence of the often helpless patient on the usually enigmatic and shibboleth-guarding physician, has given rise to a tension that Will Durant recognized when he wrote that "in all civilized lands and times physicians have rivaled women for the distinction of being the most desirable and satirized of mankind" ([7], p. 531). Even a glance at the entries under 'physician' in Stith Thompson's *Motif-Index of Folk-Literature* [11] will demonstrate the pervasiveness of the diverse motifs that impinge upon the medical practitioner in various cultures. And the attitudes range from contempt to adoration for physicians, with a major emphasis on the foibles to which physicians are most susceptible.

In various genres of Western literature, from classical antiquity to the present, there is abundant evidence of conflicting attitudes towards medical practitioners. Here we see those who hold physicians in contempt, believing that all or most practitioners are unscrupulous men, avaricious and proud, beguiling the naïve, deceiving the innocent and cheating the unwary. Such men see physicians as evil if competent, but usually incompetent as well. On the other hand we also see those who excessively venerate the medical art, attaching an unrealistic aura to physicians, credulously attributing to them the power to cure nearly all of man's physical ills. When the physician fails, such people may attribute evil intent or negligence to him, for surely, if he had so wished, he could have been effective. Or they might view the physician who disappointed their expectations as being incompetent in comparison with the ideal they had posited. The attitude of the individual perhaps to the medical profession as a whole and definitely to the specific physician has always been a determining factor in resolving the question of whether or not to sue the physician, especially as the question involves the physician's competence or negligence. At some times the mechanisms for bringing malpractice suits are more conducive to litigiousness, and this certainly is the case in 20th-century America. But the differences between the present situation and those of the past are only in degree. The root problems and relationships have changed little.

Western Washington University
Bellingham, Washington

NOTES

[1] The Greek text is found in ([8], Vol. 3A, p. 253).
[2] E.g., among the Visigoths. See [1].

BIBLIOGRAPHY

1. Amundsen, D. W.: 1971, 'Visigothic Medical Legislation', *Bulletin of the History of Medicine* 45, 553–569.
2. Amundsen, D. W.: 1973, 'The Liability of the Physician in Roman Law', in H. Karplus (ed.), *International Symposium on Society, Medicine and Law*, Amsterdam, New York, and London, Elsevier, pp. 17–30.
3. Amundsen, D. W.: 1974, 'The Medical Legislation of the Assizes of Jerusalem', in *Proceedings of the XXIII International Congress of the History of Medicine*, London, Wellcome Institute of the History of Medicine, pp. 517–522.
4. Amundsen, D. W.: 1977, 'The Liability of the Physician in Classical Greek Legal Theory and Practice', *Journal of the History of Medicine and Allied Sciences* 32, 172–203.
5. Amundsen, D. W.: 1977, 'Medical Deontology and Pestilential Disease in the Late Middle Ages', *Journal of the History of Medicine and Allied Sciences* 32, 403–421.
6. Amundsen, D. W.: 1978, 'History of Medical Ethics: Medieval Europe, Fourth to Sixteenth Century', in *The Encyclopedia of Bioethics*, New York, the Free Press, and London, Collier MacMillian, Vol. 3, pp. 938–951.
7. Durant, W.: 1953, *The Story of Civilization*, Part 5: *The Renaissance*, New York, Simon & Schuster.
8. Edmonds, J. M.: 1961, *The Fragments of Attic Comedy*, Leiden, Brill.
9. Fowler, G. R.: 1906, 'Surgical Malpractice', in A. M. Hamilton and L. Godkin (eds.), *A System of Legal Medicine*, 2nd ed., New York, E. B. Treat & Co., vol. 2, pp. 570–579.
10. Pliny the Elder, (n. d.), *Historia Naturalis*.
11. Thompson, S.: 1955–1958, *Motif-Index of Folk-Literature*, 6 vols., Bloomington, Indiana University Press.

LISA H. NEWTON

THE CONCEPT OF A RIGHT ORDERING

There can be no doubt that the dramatic increase in malpractice litigation in our time constitutes a serious social problem. Solutions to that problem do not seem to be forthcoming from medicine, which cannot guarantee that patients will always fully recover from every illness, nor do they seem to be forthcoming from law, which cannot make logical room in the *corpus juris* for any *a priori* limitations on the right to sue for damages. Nor will solutions be found, I am presently convinced, through attempts to assimilate the modes of thought appropriate to one profession into those appropriate to the other: to make lawyers somehow partners in a healing process, or to describe, or circumscribe, each facet of the physician-patient relationship in terms of legal rights, duties and responsibilities. I agree with Darrel Amundsen that the tension between lawyers and physicians drawn by the malpractice issue has certain ancient roots. But a partial resolution of our otherwise unprecedented present condition will require a fundamental reordering of specifically modern social expectations, i.e., the expectations that an individual is taught to hold toward his society – and not only with regard to the workings of law and medicine.

I. THE CONCEPT OF A RIGHT ORDERING: ITS NATURE AND LOSS

The first task, then, on the plan I offer, is to extract from the disputed disciplines the central concepts that have most clearly become confounded; this requires the analysis of the ancient concept of a 'right ordering'. From its earliest manifestations the fundamental principle of Order in the universe was conceived as a dynamic balance among diverse principles, conflicting but complementary: such as Male and Female, Hot and Cold, Dry and Wet, etc., or the opposing of the four simple Elements (Fire, Air, Water and Earth); they must unite to be fruitful, they must combine to make up the things of our experience. In all such interaction there is the danger, and the recurrent fact, of violation of the allotted jurisdiction of one principle by another; retribution must be exacted for any such violation, the balance restored and justice reestablished.

This orientation toward a proportion, of substances and of powers,

S. F. Spicker, J. M. Healey, and H. T. Engelhardt (eds.), The Law–Medicine Relation: A Philosophical Exploration, 259–264.

pervades the work of the Ancients in all fields of inquiry, including law and medicine. In law, this notion of Order became the root notion of *justice*, requiring reward for services and punishment for offenses. In medicine, it became the root notion of *health*, that state in which all bodily humors and tendencies are in equilibrium. Within each body of thought, there were of course disagreements about the application of the concept: whether justice, for example, meant equality, no more and no less, of all citizens with respect to rights and rewards, or some other ratio, between the more meritorious and the less meritorious. Early physicians often disagreed about the structural details of the human body, but they were thoroughly in agreement on the general processes taking place within it and within the universe as a whole.

The organic world of the Greeks regulated by Order is no static condition of perfection, but a necessarily dynamic interplay of forces which are prone to disorder and disproportion by their very nature. The attitude toward justice appropriate to such a world-order is a moderate pessimism: you may expect that flagrant violations of the natural order, flaunted before the gods, will be punished somehow, but you are best advised to expect, and to expect to have to endure, a multitude of minor disruptions, accidental consequences of the natural processes. Further, since all compound substances, including our bodies, are made up of contrary principles, coexisting in one boundary only by virtue of very precarious ratios, you should expect that all such substances will eventually disintegrate into their component elements; it is this condition we call 'mortality'. Applied to law and medicine, this orientation yields very modest expectations of the available systems of judicial relief and health care. Given the normal operations of mischance and human malice, human life is to be expected to contain losses and disappointments, and the custom of law should be to let loss lie where it falls, unless there are overwhelmingly good reasons of social policy to remove it elsewhere. Similarly, given the nature of the human body, a condition of health, perfect proportion and harmony among its warring elements, is to be taken as accidental and necessarily temporary, not as a right deserving protection. The recurrent disruption of that harmony, and its ultimate loss at the decomposition of the body, are accepted as part of nature.

As the Romans were our teachers in law and the Greeks our predecessors in medicine, as well as in art and philosophy, they transmitted their basically sound attitudes toward these subjects very effectively. So we find the relatively modest expectations of human justice and medical care persisting into our own time, reinforced by certain religious doctrines that emphasized the corruption and imperfection of a frail body in a sinful world, and held out the hope of perfection in a world to come. Perhaps that last 'teaching' was the fatal mistake. The Ancients had no perfect heaven; the Medievals did; and the Moderns, ultimately, wanted its heavenly health and justice on earth. In our century we have seen all our theories confounded by rising popular expectations; it is this change of expectation that has rendered the working relationship between our two most influential professions so alarmingly problematic.

The fact that transformations of expectations in the two fields have occurred in a parallel fashion in the last two decades suggests that the root of the transformations is embedded somehow in our popular culture, not specific to either field. And this in fact turns out to be the case: while the image of medicine in that culture (via its media) has changed from a limited range of palliative skills to a model of 'miracle cures', the image of law (civil, as opposed to criminal) has changed from a limited mechanism for the rectification of some wrongs to an unlimited instrument to secure compensation for all loss suffered by any individual or group, now or in the indefinite past. The new images are not only clearly distorted with respect to the profession that is imaged, they are clearly mischievous in professional life, leading directly to the problem with which we began: when a contemporary patient expects a miracle cure of the medical profession (since medicine is now established on a 'scientific' foundation), and restoration to perfect health, he feels damaged when he does not get it. Since he expects the law to remedy all his damages, he takes his problem, and his physician, to the law forthwith. Contemporary malpractice litigation, then, is a perfect sign and symbol of the over-inflated expectations brought to the professions by their clients and patients: itself the direct result of these expectations, it represents a whole society further out of harmony, using up its best energies in self-destruction. Of course I am exaggerating, but exaggeration is appropriate when we are attempting to fix an image, and a level of expectation is preeminently a function of the imagination. The point is simply that a national, perhaps international, imagination seems to have been working steadily in one direction over the last few decades, presenting our professionals and, while we are at it, our elected officials, with a single querulous demand: that human existence be brought into, and protected in, a static ideal condition, free from *all* hazards of change and decay.

This, then, is the nub of the evil. It is a disease of the imagination, which takes to be real and universally obtainable those states which serve properly only as ideals or limiting cases. Such distortion of expectation was not unknown to the ancients; generally speaking, they treated it indifferently as injustice (arrogance, trespass, the *hybris* that flaws the tragic hero) or 'sickness' (as in Book II of Plato's *Republic*, the 'fever' that expects too much), as requiring retribution or requiring a purge. In our day we do not seem to be able to perceive this distortion as clearly as they. We have lost that insight into the uncertainty of all matters, the inevitable conflict-ridden imperfection of all conditions in the realm of physical matter. Given this insight, of course, we might prefer, with Plato, to spend as little time as possible thinking about such a disappointing state of existence. But at least we would be able to keep our vision of Forms (or mathematics, or Heaven) separate from our perceptions of this physical world, and would not import expectations appropriate to one realm into the other.

II. RETURN TO RIGHT ORDERING

Such is the diagnosis of the sickness afflicting our professions and our society. Or perhaps, it is better read as the indictment of our popular culture. The two metaphors, medical and legal, seem equally at home in this topic, and so they should; we have found at the root of our misunderstandings a fundamental loss of our sense of order or right proportion, a rejection of an obtainable and appropriate portion in life in favor of an impossible ideal, and such overreaching, disharmony, is the very source of our concepts of sickness and crime. But discernment of the cause is only the first step to a remedy. When it comes to cures or proper reparations, restoring the right proportion of the parts and restoring the whole to proper functioning, the Greeks inspire less confidence as teachers. Retribution for *hybris* in the tragedies tended to leave the stage awash with the blood of all the major characters; the purges for fevers, medical or social, tended to kill as often as they cured; and Plato's solution – of rebuilding all societal institutions from scratch, excluding almost all poetry, music and opinions other than his own – can hardly serve as a model. Yet our objective clearly has to be the restoration of a sense of harmony and moderation, the lowering of expectations to a level where their satisfaction for each person is compatible with their satisfaction for all.

Such restoration cannot, in the nature of things, take place in any area of social existence unless it begins to take place in all; the disease must be attacked all at once or it will simply migrate to another part of the body politic. Malpractice litigation, for example, has entangled within it a multitude of demands and counter demands. Patients demand perfect health (and no slip-ups) from their physicians, and when they do not receive it they demand perfect justice from the courts, and when they do not obtain that, they demand full health insurance from the government. Meanwhile, malpractice insurance premiums go sky-high, and physicians demand that the government provide the insurance for them, while the insurance companies begin to consider the merits of socialized medicine. All demands lead finally into the government, to emerge on the other side as incredibly detailed regulations, designed, again, to forestall any and all accidents, errors, conflicts, and unforeseen happenings in general, i.e., to ensure the uniformity of perfection, in whatever area has originally given rise to the demands. In a society, and a world, characterized by diversity and change, the regulations inevitably miss their mark, by a margin that increases with time and with the degree of specificity of the regulation; the error is compounded by renewed efforts to 'update' or improve them, making them even more specific in the process. It is theoretically possible that all the energy available for an enterprise might ultimately be consumed in the writing, refining, and implementing of the regulations designed to govern it. It is the entire demand, the impulse toward total satisfaction and the expectation that the institutions of our society can provide it, that must be done away with. Can we discern any markers along that course?

At present only negative ones appear: possibly, for example, the exorbitant cost of achieving and maintaining successively more perfect conditions may arouse citizens to adopt more realistic standards. The cost may be in dollars. I am thinking here not only of any current 'tax revolt', but also of the current attempt by some insurance companies to confront the public with the connection between successful litigation and higher insurance premiums. I am not convinced that the insurance companies are really significantly affected by the infrequent large awards; but it is a sign of health that attention is being paid to that connection. Along these lines, much more attention needs to be paid to the economic impact of federal and state regulations in all activities. The cost may also be in human time, energy and freedom. Perfection in any matter of the human condition is approached as a limit, such that each successive unit of effort yields less improvement than the unit preceding it. At some point the diminished return is simply not worth the continuing effort. Time spent in hospitals and waiting rooms is time not available for living; energy spent in pursuit of compensation or revenge for injuries suffered is not available for projects central to an individual's life. And ultimately, the necessarily imperfect protections afforded by collective regulation fail to justify the limitation of freedom imposed by such regulating. Each of these remedial processes has a necessary place, of course, and up to a point the relief that they can provide for human suffering more than justifies their costs. The imperative is to avoid the unjustified hope that we may move from that point on to perfection; the problem is to determine that point. It shifts in each generation, forwards or backwards. Perhaps the best we can do is simply keep it in mind, and in print, that such a point exists, and that each stage in the pursuit of health or justice or complete protection should meet the inquiries, 'To what end?' and 'At what cost in means?' These queries, bequeathed to us by Socrates, may be Philosophy's only contribution to the twentieth-century world; if so, they are sufficient to justify the discipline's presence in every council in human society.

Fairfield University
Fairfield, Connecticut

GEORGE J. ANNAS

THE FUNCTION OF LEGAL RIGHTS IN THE HEALTH CARE SETTING

It has become fashionable to talk about 'rights' for everyone, and patients and their providers are no exception. While there are many groups in society that desperately need to have their rights recognized and enforced, such as prisioners, suspects, aliens, tenants, debtors, employees, etc., perhaps none is as vulnerable as the desperately ill patient. This vulnerability and the potential abuses it permits have led many to suggest that the provider-patient relationship should be made more equitable, and that the status of the patient should be improved with this goal in mind [1].

As this may be impossible, others wishing to change the role of the patient in health care delivery have concentrated their efforts on wider questions, such as our economic and governmental system. Such critics believe that fundamental change in the provider-patient relationship is possible only after basic changes in our social structure. The argument is that the health system is primarily a mirror of the larger social, political, and economic system of which it is part, and changes in health care policy and practices will come only from changes in that larger system. Problems of equity and access are thus viewed not as problems of physician discrimination or hospital policy, but as problems of poverty, social class, race, and geographic location [4].

Many issues cannot be resolved entirely within the provider-patient relationship, however. Providers not only have formal relationships with their patients, but also have relationships with other providers, health care institutions, and numerous governmental agencies. A provider's relationship with these institutions and individuals is often a very complex one, and providers often find themselves confused and therefore submissive in cases where they do not understand their rights. As health care has become the major service industry in the United States, and the government – federal, state, and local – has become one of the major sources of funding for the industry, private and public regulatory agencies and their decisions have become increasingly significant. Whether an operation is covered by insurance may depend on an interpretation of the policy by a bureacrat, or the review of its 'necessity' by another health care professional or committee; whether medical research may be done may depend on a determination of the hospital's Institutional Review Board and the Food and Drug Administration; whether a medical

S. F. Spicker, J. M. Healey, and H. T. Engelhardt (eds.), The Law–Medicine Relation: A Philosophical Exploration, 265–269.

student or foreign medical graduate may practice in a certain setting may depend on state statutes and licensing regulations; whether husbands are permitted in the delivery room may depend on hospital policy; and whether or not life-sustaining treatment of a terminally ill patient may be terminated may depend both on state law and hospital policy.

In all of these cases, both the health care provider *and* the patient will be better off if the status of the law regarding both the patient's *and* provider's rights is understood, and the means of change or challenge well delineated. I would go even further. An understanding of the law can be as important to the proper care of patients as an understanding of emergency medical procedures or proper drug dosages.

For example, ignorance of their rights to treat minors in emergency situations led health care providers to ignore the needs of a 17-year-old rape victim, who was left alone in a major Boston hospital for four hours without any medical assistance. And ignorance of the law in 1978 led to the following instances in Massachusetts: a terminally ill patient being defibrillated seventy times within a twenty-four hour period; a baby whose brain had been completely destroyed being kept alive by artificial ventilation, surgery, and antibiotics even though all agreed the case was 'hopeless' and the parents had asked that 'heroic measures' be discontinued; continual resuscitation of a terminally ill heart attack victim with almost no brain activity for more than 30 days after the doctors and nurses agreed the case was hopeless and the relatives asked that 'extraordinary measures' be discontinued; and incurable babies with Tay-Sachs or Werning-Hoffman's disease being continually resuscitated against the wishes of their parents. In all of these cases the health care providers were 'forced' to inflict such inhumane torture on their patients because they believed that directions to do so from hospital administrators had the force of the law and that they were powerless to refuse [2]. Unfortunately, this list could be greatly expanded.

So the understanding of individual rights of both patients and providers can be extremely important in the health care context. But how are rights to be understood, and how does a person know that he or she has a 'right' to something seen as desirable?

There is, of course, a formidable literature on rights in the archives of philosophy and jurisprudence. Rather than review it, I would note briefly the thoughts of two recent entrants who have written with great insight. The first is John Rawls. In *A Theory of Justice* [5], Rawls asks us to imagine that a group of men and women come together to form a social contract. Unlike provious formulations, however, these individuals all have ordinary tastes, talents, ambitions and convictions – but each is temporarily unaware of his own fate and must agree to the terms of the contract before his awareness of his own status is restored. The theory postulates that under such circumstances all will agree to two principles. Loosely stated they are: (1) each person shall enjoy the largest political liberty compatible with a like liberty for all; and (2) inequalities in wealth and power should exist only where they work to the benefit of the worst-off members of society. Applying such an approach to the health care delivery system, one could conceivably develop an entire system of 'patient rights' and/or 'provider rights' that would rest on these two premises. Such a document would, I suggest, be strongly pro-patient since this group is currently the one that generally lacks 'rights' and is always the group that will be viewed as 'worse off' in the health care setting.

A second approach is suggested in Ronald Dworkin's *Taking Rights Seriously*. Dworkin notes the great confusion in 'rights' language generally created by attributing to it different meanings in different contexts. He notes, "In most cases when we say that someone has a 'right' to something, we imply that it would be wrong to interfere with his doing it, or at least that some special grounds are needed for justifying any interference" ([3], p. 188). An example is the right to spend one's money the way one pleases. This is, of course, different from saying that the way one spends one's money, e.g., gambling it away, is the *right* thing to do, or that there is nothing *wrong* with it. The first lesson is that when we speak of rights, this distinction may be critical to understanding what we are talking about. For example, a woman may have a legal right to have an abortion, but such a decision may still be considered morally wrong by her and/or her spouse.

Dworkin argues that there are such things as rights that can be said to be absolute in the sense that the government is bound to recognize and protect them. Such rights, which we often denote as 'legal rights', or somewhat more restrictively as 'constitutional rights', are generally spelled out in statutes and court decisions. By respecting such laws the government guarantees to the weakest members of the society that they will not be trampled on by the strongest. In Dworkin's words:

> The bulk of the law – that part which defines and implements social, economic, and foreign policy – cannot be neutral. It must state, in its greatest part, the majority's view of the common good. The institution of rights is therefore crucial, because it represents the majority's promise to the minorities that their dignity and equality will be respected. When the divisions among the groups are most violent, then this gesture, if law is to work, must be most sincere .... [Taking individual rights seriously is] the one feature that distinguishes law from ordered brutality ([3], p. 205).

Without going too far afield, one can apply Dworkin's notions directly to health care and note that the respecting and enforcing of rights can form a useful way of guaranteeing to defenseless patients that they will be treated with dignity and respect. While the health care provider often has the option to deny certain rights almost at will, he or she does this only at the peril of the integrity of the delivery system itself. In the absence of patients' rights, the health care setting can become a jungle.

I have argued elsewhere [1] that it is critical that the rights of patients be spelled out in a document and enforced in a reasonable manner. Although such a mechanism can do much to foster respect for basic human dignity and equality, it is not, of course, the answer to every problem. Insofar as legal rights are firmly based on moral reasoning and values, one need not fear their legal definition and enforcement. But, as Alexander Solzhenitsyn warned in his much-maligned address at Harvard, while a society without an objective legal scale is terrible, "a society with no other scale but the legal one is not quite worthy of man either":

A society that is based on the letter of the law and never reaches any higher is taking very small advantages of the high level of human possibilities. The letter of the law is too cold and formal to have a beneficial influence on society. Whenever the tissue of life is woven of legalistic relations, there is an atmosphere of mediocrity, paralysing man's noblest impulse ([7], p. 22).

Many have argued, of course, that such a paralysis already exists in medicine, citing examples of the rise in malpractice suits, with the physicians' reaction in practicing both negative and positive defensive medicine. Others would cite the dehumanizing effects of 'mass-production' abortions or decisions not to treat defective newborns.

Solzhenitsyn, in *Cancer Ward*, provides a fitting note on which to conclude. One which ties together, in its own way, with his own theory of humanity, the theories of Rawls and Dworkin on rights. The description concerns an oncologist, Dr. Lyudmila Afanasyevna, shortly after she has been diagnosed as having cancer herself, but while still able to practice medicine:

She walked the wards as though she had been deprived of her authority as a doctor, as if she had been disqualified for some unpardonable act, happily not yet announced to the patients. She examined, prescribed, ordered, and gazed at the patients with an assumed weighty air, but within herself she felt, with a chill that ran down her spine, that she could no longer dare to judge life or death for others, that in a few days she would be lying in a hospital bed herself, just as helpless, just as stupefied, caring little for her appearance, and waiting to hear the judgment older and more experienced persons would pronounce. And fearing the pain. Perhaps regretting that she had entered the wrong hospital. Perhaps doubting whether she was getting the right care. And dreaming, as if it were the highest possible happiness, of the ordinary right to be rid of the hospital pajamas and to go home at night ([6], p. 521).

Boston University Schools of Medicine and Public Health
Boston, Massachusetts

BIBLIOGRAPHY

1. Annas, G. J.: 1975, *The Rights of Hospital Patients*, Avon, New York.
2. Annas, G. J.: 1978, 'Editorial: Where are the Health Lawyers When we Need Them?' *Medicolegal News* 6 (2), 3.
3. Dworkin, R.: 1978, *Taking Rights Seriously*, Harvard Univ. Press, Cambridge, Mass.
4. Navarro, V.: 1976, *Medicine Under Capitalism*, Prodist, New York.
5. Rawls, J.: 1971, *A Theory of Justice*, Harvard Univ. Press, Cambridge, Mass.
6. Solzhenitsyn, A.: 1967, *The Cancer Ward*, Dell, New York.
7. Solzhenitsyn, A.: 1978, 'The Exhausted West', *Harvard Magazine* (July–August), p. 22.

WILLIAM G. BARTHOLOME

THE CHILD-PATIENT: DO PARENTS HAVE THE 'RIGHT TO DECIDE'?

Unfortunately, one of the most frequent and frustrating tasks of the medical ethicist in a clinical setting is that of having to sort out tangled webs of claims to an almost unbelievable variety of rights. In most situations those involved in these perplexing clinical dilemmas fail to examine the nature or basis of these rights claims. Rights, as a number of authors have pointed out, function as what might best be called trump cards in an ethical debate or dialogue [6]. Debates about obligations, responsibilities, rules, principles and values can be conducted almost indefinitely. By an appeal to a right, the participant in an ethical debate can essentially 'call' the other participants in the dialogue to play their hands. Rights claims have a demand quality ([5], p. 137). Others involved in the decision are put on the defensive.

Since a radical pluralism of values is the accepted order of the day, appeal to rights seems to many to be the only solid structure in a sea of ethical relativism.

I know no better example of the dangers of such claims than the claim frequently made in pediatric medicine that the child's parents have 'the right to decide' – in other words, the right to make all medical care decisions involving a minor child. Those who would defend such a parental right usually insinuate that this right has some clear social, ethical or, at least, legal basis. Often the claim is couched in the language of consent. Several of my fellow workers in medical ethics have carried on a debate of several years' duration on the meaning and basis of what has come to be called 'proxy consent'.[1] I have taken every opportunity available to me over the past several years to expose this concept for what I think it is: namely, a pernicious and tyrannical concept that has had significant negative impact on the lives and welfare of children ([1], [2]). I have argued that to use the word 'consent' in descriptions of parental involvement in medical care decisions involves an assumption that does serious violence to what I have called the moral standing of the child. I was recently heartened by the recommended guidelines for research involving children, proposed by the National Commission for the Protection of Human Subjects in Biomedical and Behavioral Research. The Commission members claimed that *no* parent had a right to consent to the involvement of a minor child in research. In fact, the Commission argued that the language of

S. F. Spicker, J. M. Healey, and H. T. Engelhardt (eds.), The Law–Medicine Relation: A Philosophical Exploration, 271–277.

consent should be replaced by the language of *permission* "in order to distinguish what a person may do autonomously (consent) from what one may do on behalf of another (grant permission)" [10].

I would argue that this alleged right to consent on behalf of a minor child is no more valid in the so-called therapeutic setting than in the research setting. Health care professionals and parents have adopted the notion of a parental right of proxy consent primarily because both have assumed that (1) parents almost always act with at least the intention of pursuing their children's best interests; and (2) parents are in the best position of knowing what those best interests might be in any given situation. I call these the 'identity of interests' and the 'special knowledge' assumptions.

Yet, any professional who provides services to children is well aware that the truth of both assumptions is highly questionable. One example should suffice. Over 80% of newborn males in this country are subjected to an operative ritual within hours of birth. For at least ten years, it has been known that there are no medical indications for routine neonatal circumcision. Since 1971, the American Academy of Pediatrics has urged that routine neonatal circumcision be abandoned. "Circumcision of the male neonate cannot be considered an essential component of adequate total health care" [11].

Whose interests are being served by this operation? How are parents in a better position to know what is in the best interests of an individual child who is less than twenty-four hours old? I could provide many more examples, but most children's professionals already agree that both premises are false.

Some have argued that parents should have the right to make medical decisions on behalf of their children since they must live with the consequences of the decision ([3], [4]). But it has also been pointed out that having to live with the consequences is also an excellent basis for arguing that parents should *not* have the right to decide; i.e., this is an obvious conflict of interest. Several authors have pointed out that such an argument confuses medical care decisions and custody decisions [7]. Others argue that parents have a legal and moral duty or obligation to insure that their children receive needed medical care. In fact, the failure to insure the provision of this care can be the basis for a claim of child neglect. Since parents have this clear legal and ethical responsibility, it only seems appropriate to grant them the necessary power and authority to fulfill this obligation. Somehow from this confusing claim emerges the claim that parents have a right to decide. Those who argue in this manner clearly confuse a *parental duty* with a *parental right*. This parental duty may provide the basis for an entitlement of the child against his parents to adequate medical care, but it cannot provide an adequate basis for a parental right vis-à-vis the health care professional.

It might be argued that the basis of such a right is the contract established between the parent and the health care professional. Indeed, this contract may form the basis on which claims could be made, such as the parental right to be informed of the nature of their child's problems or the right to be notified of interventions under consideration by the professional. But to argue that this contract entitles the parents to an unqualified right to dictate the course of medical treatment is to fail to be aware of the most elementary features of third-party contracts.

John A. Robertson has examined the nature of legal relationships involved in pediatric medical practice in the case of the 'defective' newborn ([12], also see [13]). He points out that parents have a clear legal duty to insure the provision of necessary medical care, one that is recognized by statute in every state. In most situations, parents contract with a professional in order to fulfill this duty to their child. The contract, however, involves the creation of the professional-child relationship. The professional assumes a duty to provide care for the child. This professional-child relationship takes on a life of its own. Robertson points out that the professional's withdrawal from the relationship requires formal notice and procedure, and provision for the assumption of the legal duty owed to the minor by another professional. The parents cannot terminate the relationship or waive the obligation to the minor child if there exists the likelihood that the child would be substantially harmed. The law does not permit a professional to avoid criminal liability by submitting to the wishes of the parents, particularly if this will lead to injury or death of the child.

Nevertheless, studies of how decisions are actually made in cases such as those involving handicapped newborn infants demonstrate that the critical and decisive factor in decisions made about provision of medical services to these infants is the desire of the parents.[2] Physicians seem more than willing to allow parents an almost unlimited degree of power over the lives of the handicapped newborn infant.

Ethically, I would argue, the problem is even more clear than it is when viewed from a legal perspective. From an ethical perspective, the concept of proxy consent is seriously wanting. Arguments have been advanced which maintain that this concept can be based on a construction of what the child *would* want if he were capable of making the decision; or what the child *ought* to want; or what the 'reasonable man' would want; or what is medically indicated; or on the child's need for treatment, etc. All are constructions.

Some are more problematic than others. All involve the assumption that the child's parents are capable of knowing what 'doing right' by the child might entail. All involve a third assumption: that children are morally transparent to their parents. I would claim that children, particularly small infants, are the most morally opaque members of the human community. This opacity is essentially ignored by any who would argue that proxy consent is ethically valid.

When parents bring a child to a health care provider, they often feel that they are losing something, some measure of control over the life of the child. At one time the child was entrusted to the professional. Such blind faith in the goodness and compassion of the professional may no longer be appropriate. But what was and continues to be at work in these encounters is that the child ought to be rendered visible as a separate individual. As parents we live with our children. We do not constantly remind ourselves that the decisions we make about them are based on assumptions about who they are and what they need. We do not constantly make ourselves aware of our very limited perspective, of our biases and prejudices. As parents, we see our children as radically independent persons only when something happens that disrupts the normal flow of shared living. Seeing a child off to the operating room is often a shocking and sobering experience for a parent. Perhaps for the first time the parents are ruthlessly aware that *their* child is *not theirs*. To claim an unconditional right to decide on behalf of one's child seems to me from an ethical perspective to radically distort what is involved in the professional-child-parent encounter.

The ethical question is not "*who* has the authority or power or right to decide?" The issue is "*what ought* to be done to respond to the child's peril?" To construe the ethical question as a 'who' question is to incorrectly take a procedural issue for a very difficult substantive question: "what *ought to* be done for this particular child?" Or, "what is demanded of parent and professional in order to do right by this child?"

What appears to be involved in the claim that parents have the unconditional right to make medical care decisions on behalf of their minor children, is our society's failure to answer a basic social, legal and ethical question: "to whom do children belong?" Parents do make health care decisions on behalf of their children. They exercise a considerable degree of power over their children's lives. Those who would defend an unconditional parental right of consent confuse power with right. From a pragmatic viewpoint, professionals are dependent upon parental involvement in order to provide health care services to children. The child, particularly the infant, depends on parental willingness to bring the child to the professional. Children are dependent on parental willingness to pay for health-related services. Parents are often the primary caretakers and the professional is dependent on their willingness to give medications to the child and to perform monitoring procedures such as measuring temperature, etc. Since he/she is so dependent on the cooperation of the parent in order to care for the child, the professional may feel that parents have or should have an unqualified right to consent. Society and professionals who attend children are only permitted to explicitly challenge this parental power if the health or welfare of the child is in peril. We tend to behave as if children belong to their parents. Is it any wonder then that parents actually believe that they have a right to decide? Those who would question this particular assumption are judged advocates of some form of communism. If children don't belong to their parents, the only option must be state ownership, power and authority.

I suggest that there is another option. In fact, it is an assumption at work in many areas of the world that children primarily belong to themselves.

If, most fundamentally, children belong to themselves, and if the capacity to know what doing right by them might entail is limited to those in possession of crystal balls, then parents do not have the right to decide. Parents do not have a right to grant or withhold consent (as proxys) for medical interventions into the lives of their minor children.

In my view the denial of this alleged right would have important and positive repercussions in terms of what might be called "the moral policy of pediatric medical care".

In closing I would like to list some of these repercussions:

(1) Any proposed medical intervention that could be delayed, without significant adverse consequences, until the child could provide his own consent would be *prima facie* wrong.

(2) Any medical intervention for which there is no demonstrable need would be *prima facie* wrong; e.g., circumcision.

(3) Any medical intervention that holds out the prospect of demonstrable benefit to a child whose life or well-being were in jeopardy would be *prima facie* obligatory; e.g., immunizations.

(4) The most important consequence of the denial of this alleged right would be the candid and explicit admission that decision-making on behalf of a child is extremely difficult. Perplexity is the order of the day. Any facile solution to that perplexity is suspect. In the serious game of deciding on behalf of the voiceless, there should be no trump cards. None for the professional. None for the parents.

The redistribution of power and rights in the *adult*-professional-patient relationship may well be warranted. But in our zealous quest to increase the freedom and autonomy of the adult patient in the health care context, we compound the problems faced by children in peril. Parental permission for interventions into children's lives must not be seen as the unconditional right to demand or refuse a particular intervention because it is a proper exercise of parental authority over the lives of children. That children are largely dependent, at least for a time, on their parents is to be affirmed, but that dependency does not warrant the second-class social standing implied by a parental right of 'consent' in decisions affecting the health care of their children.

The University of Texas Medical School at Houston
Houston, Texas

NOTES

[1] This debate was started by Richard A. McCormick 'Proxy Consent in the Experimental Situation', *Perspectives in Biology and Medicine* **18** (1974), pp. 2–20. Replies came from a number of people: Ramsey, P., 'The Enforcement of Morals: Nontherapeutic Research on Children', *Hastings Center Report* **6** (1976), 21; May, W. E., 'Experimenting on Human Subjects', *Linacre Quarterly* **41** (1974), 238; McCormick then replied, in McCormick, R. A., 'Experimentation in Children: Sharing in Sociality', *Hastings Center Report* **6** (1976), 41; which was replied to by Ramsey, P., 'Children as Research Subjects: A Reply', *Hastings Center Report* **7** (1977), 40.

[2] Three articles provide good insight into problems of decision making concerning the defective newborn ([8], [9], [14]).

BIBLIOGRAPHY

1. Bartholome, W. G.: 1977, 'The Ethics of Non-Therapeutic Clinical Research on Children', in *National Commission for the Protection of Human Subjects of Biomedical and Behavioral Research. Appendix to report and recommendations: research involving children.* Government Printing Office, Washington D.C., pp. 3–1 – 3–22.
2. Bartholome, W. G.: 1978, 'Central Themes in the Debate over Involvement of Infants and Children in Biomedical Research', in van Eys, Jan (ed.), *Research on Children*, University Park Press, Baltimore, pp. 69–76.
3. Burt, R. A.: 1975, 'Developing Constitutional Rights of, in and for Children', *Law and Contemporary Problems* **39** (3), 118.
4. Duff, R. S. and Campbell, A. G. M.: 1973, 'Moral and Ethical Dilemmas in the Special Care Nursery', *New England Journal of Medicine* **289**, 890.

5. Feinberg, J.: 1966, 'Duties, Rights and Claims', *American Philosophical Quarterly* 3, 137–145.
6. Feinberg, J.: 1977, 'The Nature and Value of Rights', in Joel Feinberg and Henry West (eds.), *Moral Philosophy: Classic Texts and Contemporary Problems*; Dickenson, Encino, pp. 328–337.
7. Fost, N.: 1977, 'Proxy Consent for Seriously Ill Newborns', in Smith, D. (Ed.), *No Rush to Judgment*, The Poynter Center, Ind.
8. Gustafson, J.: 1973, 'Mongolism, Parental Desires, and the Right to Life', *Perspectives in Biology and Medicine* **16**, 529.
9. Iodres, I. D., *et al.*: 1977, 'Pediatricians' Attitudes Affecting Decision-making in Defective Newborns', *Pediatrics* **60**, 197.
10. *National Commission for the Protection of Human Subjects of Biomedical and Behavioral Research. Report and Recommendations: Research Involving Children*: 1977, Government Printing Office, Washington, D.C.
11. Committee on the Fetus and Newborn: 1975, 'Report of the Task Force on Circumcision', *Pediatrics* **56**, 610.
12. Robertson, J. A.: 1975, 'Involuntary Euthanasia of Defective Newborns: a Legal Analysis', *Stanford Law Review* **27**, 213–269.
13. Robertson, J. A. and Fost, N.: 1976, 'Passive Euthanasia of Defective Newborn Infants: Legal Considerations', *Journal of Pediatrics* **88**, 883.
14. Shaw A.: 1977, 'Ethical Issues in Pediatric Surgery: a National Survey of Pediatricians and Pediatric Surgeons', *Pediatrics* **60**, 588.

DAN W. BROCK

LEGAL RIGHTS AND MORAL RESPONSIBILITIES IN THE HEALTH CARE PROCESS

The topic of our discussion is extremely broad while the space to address it is rather limited. Consequently, any developed philosophical argument on some aspect of the topic would have to be so narrow that I have decided instead to offer some rather general remarks. In doing so, I shall say little that does not seem to me to be obvious, but I hope that at least it also has the merit of being true.

What are some of the natural features of the health care process, and the circumstances in which physicians encounter patients in particular, that affect its moral and, in turn, legal character? Perhaps most prominent are various inequalities. Physicians generally command exceptional amounts of respect, authority, power and income. They possess vast amounts of information and knowledge concerning health matters that the average patient not only does not possess, but is often not even capable of understanding beyond a very basic level. Their knowledge in turn gives them great power to affect our lives in crucial ways by the services and care they can provide. Patients, on the other hand, are not merely in an inferior position in terms of knowledge, status and power. They generally come to the physician in a condition of anxiety, vulnerability, often even fear. Something is wrong with their body, something they in all likelihood do not understand and about which they are worried and anxious. The care that they need will often affect in dramatic, frequently life and death, ways what their future will be like. Medical care, while having great potential to benefit the patient is rarely without uncertainty and risks, potentialities for failure and serious harms. And, of course, the extraordinary medical advances of recent decades have not only multiplied the potential benefits but also the potential risks and harms we may receive. It is the various features of this natural inequality in the usual physician-patient encounter that gives special importance to some of the broad features of the principal legal rights and moral responsibilities present in that process. These rights and responsibilities both reflect and in some ways serve to correct for this natural inequality. This occurs in the asymmetry in moral position between physicians (or other health care professionals) and their patients – the physician principally is bound by various duties and responsibilities, while the patient principally is protected by

S. F. Spicker, J. M. Healey, and H. T. Engelhardt (eds.), The Law–Medicine Relation: A Philosophical Exploration, 279–283.

various rights. I believe this is true on most accounts of the physician-patient relationship, but it is especially evident on the contract or agreement model. The patient contracts to have specified care provided by his physician, in return for payment by the patient. In so doing, the patient exercises his rights by granting permission to the physician to perform actions the physician would otherwise have no duty (or right) to do. In contracting or agreeing to perform these duties, a physician incurs an obligation to the patient to do so, and an obligation to do so with due care, as well as a right to be paid for doing so. The point to be emphasized is that the right to determine what is done to and for the patient, and to control, within broad limits, the course of the patient's treatment and care, originates and generally remains with the patient. In his role as health care provider, the physician then ought to be significantly guided, constrained and circumscribed by the manner in which the patient uses his rights. Apart from theoretical soundness, the practical importance of emphasizing the duties and responsibilities of the physician, and the rights of the patient, arises from the natural inequality in the physician-patient encounter, that these duties, responsibilities and rights have the effect of partially correcting for. Now it might then seem that the task facing us would simply be (though it would, of course, be a complicated matter) to work out these moral rights, duties and responsibilities in more detail, and their relation in turn to legal rights, duties and responsibilities. But there is a feature of the law-medicine relationship that makes this task both especially difficult and controversial, and to which I shall devote the rest of my remarks.

Several years ago when I first began to develop a serious interest in biomedical ethics I attended a conference on mental illness and its treatment in which a high proportion of participants were either physicians or lawyers. Perhaps it was naiveté on my part, but I was astounded at the degree of distrust and outright hostility that seemed to characterize the 'law-medicine relationship' or should I say the 'lawyer-physician relationship'. No doubt there are many possible explanations of this situation, but I want to suggest one that has its roots in a philosophical, specifically moral, difference. Physicians and other health professionals are trained to provide health care for patients. They rightly view themselves as providing important benefits for their patients when they provide such care; they see themselves as acting in the best interests of their patients. Since treatment decisions are almost invariably complex and uncertain, however, they are continually making what in effect are cost/benefit judgments about the potential risks and benefits of various alternative treatments. With their training and knowledge, and the inequalities in the physician-patient situation noted earlier, it is natural for the physician not only to reason in these cost/benefit terms, but also to view himself as in the best position to make such decisions knowledgably and intelligently. While I shall not take time to argue it here, such cost/benefit reasoning in its normative form is, I believe, implicitly one or another form of consequentialist or utilitarian moral theory. And the pressures on physicians and other health care professionals towards utilitarian thinking are diverse and powerful.

In this context, how will the progressively increasing legal intrusions into and exercise of legal regulation and control over medical practice likely be viewed? The physician's response to this legal oversight and control often takes two forms. First, he may view such legal intrusions as a questioning, challenging, or criticism of his capacity best to make the multitude of cost/benefit judgments he does make in the day-to-day practice of medicine. When his rights and powers to make decisions within the health care process are in various ways constrained and curtailed, he often views this as an attack upon his competence. This quite naturally leads to suspicion and defensiveness towards the sources of these constraints on his practice. The second sort of response of physicians to increasing legal control is to see it as an unjustified limitation on their capacity to treat and care for their patients, to produce the benefits that health care can offer. Viewed from their utilitarian perspective such legal intrusions, to the extent that they make physicians less efficient in delivering health care, are misguided and wrong. The treatment of mental illness illustrates this well. As a result of both court decisions and new legislation, it has become increasingly difficult in most states for mentally ill persons to be hospitalized and treated against their will. Moreover, the course of such treatment is increasingly controlled and burdened with legal requirements and proceedings. Many psychiatrists seem not only personally to resent such shifts in the law, but also to consider them wrong – they believe that they are not in the interests of the patients they are putatively designed to serve, since their effect is to prevent many mentally ill persons from receiving the treatment they need, or from receiving treatment in its most effective form.

The legal tradition tends to place the matter in a quite different light. This is in part a matter of the different training and professional goals lawyers have, but also derives from a deeper source, namely a different underlying moral conception. This moral conception will lead to a different definition of both the moral and legal rights, duties and responsibilities of various parties in the health care process. The principal point of contrast with utilitarianism in this other moral conception is the independent status given to individual rights, and in particular some right(s) to autonomy, self-determination, privacy, or liberty. Here, the good for persons is seen not simply in such welfare items as health, but independently and importantly in our continuing status as rational agents, able and free to form and revise our own conceptions of the good, and entitled within limits to pursue our own good as we see it. This view of individuals and their good will be given more specific content in a range of particular rights that individuals have first moral rights and, often as well, legal rights. The important point of contrast with utilitarianism is that it is not sufficient justification for interfering with a person's rights, for invading the areas of choice and control such rights protect, that in the instance at hand, to put it generally, utility would be maximized by doing so or specifically, that health care would be more efficiently delivered by doing so. This issue has important implications for how we view the proper purposes the law is to serve. At least one important and very general purpose of legal systems and legal sanctions is to secure persons from various sorts of harms to which they would otherwise be subject; the criminal law illustrates this well, as does much federal regulation of private activities. This fits easily within the general utilitarian framework, as does the assurance to all of various minimal levels of benefits such as education, health care, and so forth, that they would otherwise làck. But if we view the law entirely in these utilitarian cost/benefit terms we will have missed the point of many rights prominent in our moral and legal traditions – the protection of individual choice or autonomy noted above. I believe, though I shall not argue it here, that some such right to autonomy occupies an important place within both liberal political philosophy and the American constitutional tradition. If I am right in this, then it should be no surprise that the law gives a certain priority to many individual rights, and that lawyers professionally trained in that constitutional tradition should be especially sensitive to these rights that physicians often find 'in their way'.

Now I am well aware that the contrast I have drawn between medicine and the law, and the moral traditions they each tend to draw on and support, has been overdrawn. Many physicians and lawyers do not at all fit the molds sketched for them here, and the medical and legal traditions are vastly more complex than the neat distinction between them drawn above might suggest. Nevertheless, if there is anything to the contrast I have drawn, I would end by stressing that which moral conception is sound is not to be settled by anything about the training or features of one or the other profession, but rather is a matter for moral and legal philosophy. If the many complex issues concerning rights, duties and responsibilities are to be adequately addressed, they must be addressed first as issues in moral and political philosophy, and in turn as part of the complex problem of the relation of morality to the law, legal claims and adjudications. Doing this may well require both physicians and lawyers to break out of, or at least to critically examine, some patterns of thought that their professions promote and reinforce.

Brown University
Providence, Rhode Island

JOSEPH M. HEALEY, JR.

CLOSING REMARKS

Physicians and other health care providers engage in the provision of health care services by virtue of, and in accordance with, a mandate from their society. This is, in my judgment, as it should be since the practice of medicine unavoidably involves a social dimension as well as an individual dimension. This mandate varies from society to society. It may be expressed through the mores and traditions of the society, through legal institutions which regulate the conduct of citizens generally and physicians and patients specifically, and through the philosophical and theological principles and processes which are the source of values for the society. In addition to the differences which exist among societies concerning the sources of the mandate, there are also major differences concerning what the substance of the mandate is, how it is determined, and how it is enforced. Though elements of the mandate do vary from society to society, it is possible to identify some common themes:

(1) the range of permissible activity in the pursuit of health;

(2) the rights and duties of the physician;

(3) the rights and duties of the patient;

(4) the reasonable expectations of both physician and patient about the process and outcome of health care interventions;

(5) the goals of the physician-patient relationship.

The presentations of our panelists remind us that we in the United States today are experiencing major difficulties in understanding this mandate, particularly those aspects dealing with the rights and duties of patients and providers. In part these difficulties have arisen because of an absence of consensus within our society and within the medical profession concerning the mandate itself. Our situation has historical parallels as Darrel Amundsen points out, yet there are unique aspects as Lisa Newton demonstrates. In any event, the distinctive characteristics of the contemporary health care process, as highlighted by Dan Brock, of the contemporary physician-patient relationship, as emphasized by George Annas, and of such recurring problems as the parent-child relationship, as shown by William Bartholome, create for us an enormous challenge: How can these issues surrounding the physician's mandate be clarified and resolved?

In large part, the answer can only be provided if lawyers, physicians,

S. F. Spicker, J. M. Healey, and H. T. Engelhardt (eds.), The Law–Medicine Relation: A Philosophical Exploration, 285–286.

philosophers and patients reject the antagonism which has accompanied past attempts at interdisciplinary endeavors. There must be a spirit of cooperation which acknowledges a positive role for each participant. For lawyers, the role will be to understand and to help physicians and patients to understand the legal components of the mandate. For philosophers, the role will be to understand and to help physicians and patients to understand the ethical component of their mandate. For physicians and patients, the role must be to understand the mandate and engage in the on-going societal process of shaping and reshaping it. The goal for all will be to assure that the meaning and value of the vocation of service which health care must be, will not be lost in the extremes of either paternalism or indifference but will remain deeply rooted in the longstanding tradition of compassion and competence.

The University of Connecticut, School of Medicine
Farmington, Connecticut

NOTES ON CONTRIBUTORS

Darrel W. Amundsen, Ph. D., is Professor of Classics, Western Washington University, Bellingham, Washington.

George J. Annas, J.D., M.P.H., is Associate Professor of Law and Medicine, Boston University, Boston, Massachusetts.

William G. Bartholome, M.D., is Assistant Professor of Pediatrics, University of Texas Medical School at Houston, Texas.

Dan W. Brock, Ph.D., is Associate Professor of Philosophy, Brown University, Providence, Rhode Island.

Charles M. Culver, Ph.D., M.D., is Associate Professor of Psychiatry, School of Medicine, Dartmouth College, Hanover, New Hampshire.

William J. Curran, J.D., L L.M., M.S.Hyg., is Frances Glessner Lee Professor of Legal Medicine at Harvard Medical School, Harvard University, Cambridge, Massachusetts.

H. Tristram Engelhardt, Jr., Ph.D., M.D., is Rosemary Kennedy Professor of Philosophy of Medicine, Kennedy Institute of Ethics, Georgetown University, Washington, D. C.

Bernard Gert, Ph.D., is Professor of Philosophy, Dartmouth College, Hanover, New Hampshire.

Ann Dudley Goldblatt, J.D., L L.M., is Instructor of Law and Medicine, University of Chicago, Illinois.

Thomas Halper, Ph.D., is Associate Professor of Political Science, Baruch College, City University of New York, New York.

Joseph M. Healey, Jr., J.D., is Assistant Professor of Community Medicine and Health Care (Law), School of Medicine, University of Connecticut Health Center, Farmington, Connecticut.

Angela R. Holder, L L.M., is Associate Clinical Professor of Pediatrics (Law), School of Medicine, Yale University, New Haven, Connecticut.

Patricia King, J.D., is Professor of Law, Georgetown University Law Center, Washington, D. C.

John Ladd, Ph.D., is Professor of Philosophy, Brown University, Providence, Rhode Island.

Robert U. Massey, M.D., is Dean and Professor of Medicine, School of Medicine, University of Connecticut Health Center, Farmington, Connecticut.

S. F. Spicker, J. M. Healey, and H. T. Engelhardt (eds.), The Law–Medicine Relation: A Philosophical Exploration, 287–288.

Lisa Newton, Ph.D., is Professor of Philosophy, Fairfield University, Fairfield, Connecticut.

Michael A. Peszke, M.D., is Associate Professor of Psychiatry, School of Medicine, University of Connecticut Health Center, Farmington, Connecticut.

John M. Raye, M.D., is Associate Professor of Pediatrics and Director of Newborn Services, School of Medicine, University of Connecticut Health Center, Farmington, Connecticut.

John A. Robertson, J.D., is Associate Professor of Law, Program in Medical Ethics, University of Wisconsin at Madison, Wisconsin.

Kenneth Schaffner, Ph.D., is Professor of History and Philosophy of Science, University of Pittsburgh, Pennsylvania.

Mark Siegler, M.D., is Assistant Professor of Medicine, School of Medicine, University of Chicago, Illinois.

Stuart F. Spicker, Ph.D., is Professor of Community Medicine and Health Care (Philosophy), School of Medicine, University of Connecticut Health Center, Farmington, Connecticut.

Robert M. Veatch, Ph.D., is Senior Research Scholar, Kennedy Institute of Ethics and Professor of Philosophy, Georgetown University, Washington, D. C.

Peter C. Williams, J.D., Ph.D., is Assistant Professor of Philosophy, State University of New York at Stony Brook, New York.

William J. Winslade, Ph.D., J.D., Lecturer in Law and Psychiatry, University of California at Los Angeles, California.

INDEX

The Philosophy and Medicine Book Series

Editors

H. Tristram Engelhardt, Jr. and Stuart F. Spicker

1. **Evaluation and Explanation in the Biomedical Sciences**
   1975, vi + 240 pp. ISBN 90–277–0553–4

2. **Philosophical Dimensions of the Neuro-Medical Sciences**
   1976, vi + 274 pp. ISBN 90–277–0672–7

3. **Philosophical Medical Ethics: Its Nature and Significance**
   1977, vi + 252 pp. ISBN 90–277–0772–3

4. **Mental Health: Philosophical Perspectives**
   1978, xxii + 302 pp. ISBN 90–277–0828–2

5. **Mental Illness: Law and Public Policy**
   1980, xvii + 254 pp. ISBN 90–277–1057–0

6. **Clinical Judgment: A Critical Appraisal**
   1979, xxvi + 278 pp. ISBN 90–277–0952–1

7. **Organism, Medicine, and Metaphysics**
   Essays in Honor of Hans Jonas on his 75th Birthday, May 10, 1978
   1978, xxvii + 330 pp. ISBN 90–277–0823–1

8. **Justice and Health Care**
   1981, xiv + 238 pp. ISBN 90–277–1207–7

GPSR Compliance
The European Union's (EU) General Product Safety Regulation (GPSR) is a set of rules that requires consumer products to be safe and our obligations to ensure this.

If you have any concerns about our products, you can contact us on

ProductSafety@springernature.com

In case Publisher is established outside the EU, the EU authorized representative is:

Springer Nature Customer Service Center GmbH
Europaplatz 3
69115 Heidelberg, Germany

www.ingramcontent.com/pod-product-compliance
Ingram Content Group UK Ltd.
Pitfield, Milton Keynes, MK11 3LW, UK
UKHW020134290926
15471UKWH00003B/478
9789400984080